A HEART FOR THE WORK

A HEART FOR THE WORK

Journeys through an
African Medical School

CLAIRE L. WENDLAND

THE UNIVERSITY OF CHICAGO PRESS

CHICAGO AND LONDON

CLAIRE L. WENDLAND is assistant professor of anthropology at the University of Wisconsin–Madison and honorary senior lecturer in the Department of Obstetrics and Gynaecology at the University of Malawi College of Medicine.

The University of Chicago Press, Chicago 60637
The University of Chicago Press, Ltd., London
© 2010 by The University of Chicago
All rights reserved. Published 2010
Printed in the United States of America

19 18 17 16 15 14 13   3 4 5

ISBN-13: 978-0-226-89325-9 (cloth)
ISBN-13: 978-0-226-89327-3 (paper)
ISBN-10: 0-226-89325-1   (cloth)
ISBN-10: 0-226-89327-8   (paper)

Library of Congress Cataloging-in-Publication Data

Wendland, Claire L.
    A heart for the work : journeys through an African medical school / Claire L. Wendland.
        p. cm.
    Includes bibliographical references and index.
    ISBN-13: 978-0-226-89325-9 (hardcover : alk. paper)
    ISBN-13: 978-0-226-89327-3 (pbk. : alk. paper)
    ISBN-10: 0-226-89325-1 (hardcover : alk. paper)
    ISBN-10: 0-226-89327-8 (pbk. : alk. paper)   1. Medical education—Social aspects—Africa.   2. Public health—Africa.   I. Title.
    R822.W454   2010
    610.71'16—dc22

                                            2009045732

FOR EVERYONE WHO LABORS ON THE GOGO
CHATINKHA MATERNITY WING:
PATIENTS, DOCTORS, MIDWIVES,
STUDENTS, GUARDIANS

CONTENTS

A few years into graduate school, I came to the horrifying realization that anthropology was one big group project after another. For years I had avoided group projects, finding both the lack of control and the interpersonal negotiations required to be deeply unappealing. It turns out, however, that although its collective nature is indeed sometimes frustrating, it is also one of the great joys of this kind of work. This book and I have benefited enormously from the insights, quarrels, kindnesses, objections, solicited and unsolicited help, friendly suggestions, guidance, and commentary of many people, only some of whom I can acknowledge here. None of these people will agree with all of it: responsibility for errors of fact or analysis remains mine.

Chiwoza Bandawe, Robin Broadhead, George Kafulafula, Bonus Makanani, and Joseph Mfutso-Bengo made me officially welcome at the University of Malawi's College of Medicine. I am indebted to them all, but in one case, sadly, I can no longer offer my thanks directly. Dr. George Kafulafula, one of the first graduates of the University of Malawi College of Medicine, died unexpectedly as this book was going to press. With his colleague and fellow COM graduate Dr. Bonus Makanani, he patiently led the Department of Obstetrics and Gynaecology out of a dark period to a time when its faculty and learners can rightly feel proud of their work. That was only one of his many accomplishments. He was a kind and generous man, beloved of his family, his students, and his patients; a clinician and researcher who worked to improve the lot of Malawian women and their babies; a thoughtful teacher; and a visionary leader in the college. He will be missed terribly.

Chiwoza Bandawe also deserves special recognition. My debt to him is spelled out in the technical appendix that details research methods; here I simply offer warmest thanks to him for guiding my initial forays into the College of Medicine, for pushing me to work clinically and to think about that work in light of the students' experiences, and for keeping me out of trouble in many ways (some of which I probably failed even to notice). Conversations with him in the course of fieldwork and afterward have strengthened my analysis of "heart" as Malawi's medical students construe it.

For practical help, hospitality, and lively conversation during the two longest stretches of time I spent in Malawi, I thank Hannah Banda, Cam and Claire Bowie, Karen Crabtree, George Kafulafula, Perry Killam, Hlalapi Kunkeyani, Bonus Makanani, Roselyn Makunganya, Martin Matalulu, Ireen Mbalule, Wezi Mkandawire, Naomi and John Msiki, Liyaka and Elizabeth Nchiramwera, Jaisingh Niemer, Mary O'Regan, Simoni and Bertha Paulo, Roseby Phalula-Nkalapa, Rhoda Phiri, and Terrie Taylor. Terrie Taylor first brought me to Malawi two decades ago when I was a medical student myself, and so changed my life.

In Madison, I have found a welcoming intellectual community, especially but by no means exclusively in the Department of Anthropology. Ken George, Linda Hogle, Sharon Hutchinson, Maria Lepowsky, Kirin Narayan, Virginia Sapiro (now, to Madison's loss and Boston's gain, at Boston University), and Sissel Schroeder all deserve particular thanks for their patient mentorship of a middle-aged newcomer to academia. Lucy Mkandawire-Valhmu greatly improved my Chichewa and my *nsima* making; I have learned much from our discussions about Malawi and about the potentials and perils of the research and teaching we both do there.

For reading and providing valuable comments on pieces of this manuscript in preparation, I am most grateful to Anne Enke, Nan Enstad, and Kirin Narayan. My senior undergraduate writing seminar in spring 2009 collectively tamed some of the wildest sentences in a draft version. (Remaining unruliness is not the students' fault.) Linda Hogle, Stephanie Koczela, Mary Moore, Traci Simms, and Kathy Wendland all read complete drafts of the entire manuscript, and each provided me with very helpful guidance for revisions. Two anonymous reviewers for the University of Chicago Press gave careful critical readings that prodded me to enlarge the theoretical agenda of this book and gave me the tools to do so. All of these readings were great gifts, and I thank the readers from my heart.

At the University of Chicago Press, David Brent pulled this manuscript from a large stack and saw potential in it. I thank him for that, and for the subsequent shepherding he and Laura Avey did as the manuscript became a book. I am grateful also for Sue Cohan's careful copyediting.

Lynnette Leidy Sievert and Ralph Faulkingham of the University of Massachusetts at Amherst deserve special thanks for mentoring me through the initial writing. I hope they will be proud of the substantial transformation this project has undergone. The "Ho-Court" provided moral support and distraction at crucial moments: thanks, Rafi Crockett, Kim Koester, Kaila Kuban, Nita Luci, and Lisa Modenos, and also thanks to Jennifer Foster and Flavia Stanley.

I was fortunate to receive financial support from several sources that allowed fieldwork and writing time: an International Dissertation Field Research Fellowship from the Social Science Research Council, two Graduate Fellowships from the University of Massachusetts at Amherst, and funding from the University of Wisconsin Graduate School's annual Fall Research Competition all helped speed this work.

In Malawi, I am above all grateful to two groups of people I may not name. The first consists of all the students, interns, graduates, faculty members, nurses, and others who took time to talk to me, some of them many times. The generosity with which they shared reflections on their own experiences made this book possible. I hope that they will recognize their stories here—despite the pseudonyms—and that they will feel I have represented their lives faithfully. The second group is that of my patients there, one little subset of the women of Malawi: their capacities for humor and patience (both necessary in their encounters with my Chichewa as well as their navigation of the hospital), joy when loss was all too often close at hand, and grace in the face of pain all humbled me—and continue to. I think of them often.

My greatest thanks go to Mary Moore, my partner. She ungrudgingly worked, without pay, under very difficult conditions as a full-time midwife at Queens Hospital while we were in Malawi together in 2002–3 and again in 2007. She delivered some seven or eight hundred babies during our time there, and sometimes we both believe she earned a gray hair for each one. (She also earned a few on many sojourns to various immigration offices, but about those, perhaps the less said, the better.) Over the years, our discussions of the experiences we had in Malawi, some recounted in this book and many not, have enriched my understanding of medicine there immeasurably, eased some of the sadness of that work, and kept alive the joy of it. She has commented with depth and thoughtfulness on many drafts of many chapters. She is my best reader, and the companion of my life, mind, and heart.

ABBREVIATIONS

A&E	accident and emergency
AIDS	acquired immune deficiency syndrome
BBC	British Broadcasting Corporation
CIDA	Canadian International Development Agency
CO	clinical officer
COF	Certificate of Fitness (for vehicle safety inspection)
COM	College of Medicine, University of Malawi
CT	computed tomography
DFID	Department for International Development (United Kingdom)
DHO	district health officer
DIC	disseminated intravascular coagulopathy
DNA	deoxyribonucleic acid
DO	Doctor of Osteopathy
GDP	gross domestic product
GNP	gross national product
HIPC	Highly Indebted Poor Countries Initiative
HIV	human immunodeficiency virus
HSA	health surveillance assistant
IMF	International Monetary Fund
IV	intravenous
JHPIEGO	(formerly) Johns Hopkins Program for International Education in Obstetrics and Gynecology; now used as a word, not an acronym
KA	Kamuzu Academy
KCH	Kamuzu Central Hospital
LP	lumbar puncture ("spinal tap")

MACRO	Malawi AIDS Counseling and Resource Organization
MBBS	Bachelor of Medicine, Bachelor of Surgery (basic Malawi physician credential)
MCP	Malawi Congress Party
MD	Doctor of Medicine
MK	Malawi kwacha (unit of currency)
MOH	Ministry of Health
MP	member of Parliament
MSCE	Malawi School Certificate of Education
MYP	Malawi Young Pioneers
NAC	Nyasaland African Congress
NGO	nongovernmental organization
OPD	outpatient department
PPP	purchasing power parity
SAP	structural adjustment program
TB	tuberculosis
UK	United Kingdom
UNAIDS	Joint United Nations Program on HIV and AIDS
UNDP	United Nations Development Program
UNESCO	United Nations Educational, Scientific and Cultural Organization
UNICEF	United Nations Children's Fund
US	United States
USAID	United States Agency for International Development
WHO	World Health Organization

Arrival Stories

"When you hear hoofbeats, think of horses, not zebras!" Faculty members in American medical colleges love to use this aphorism to exhort medical students—who tend to imagine obscure diagnoses everywhere—to think about common problems first and foremost when they encounter patients. I must have heard it a dozen times or more in my own medical-school years. Then in 1990, during the last few months before graduation, I worked in Africa for the first time, on the obstetrics and gynecology wards of a sprawling urban referral center in southern Malawi: Queen Elizabeth Central Hospital. At "Queens," as the locals called it, zebras were everywhere. Malaria, parasitic diseases, even witchcraft-related illnesses, were everyday problems. I was confused about diagnosis and clueless about therapy in such cases, but the Malawian nurses and clinical officers handled them easily. On the other hand, horses were rare. One day a well-traveled overweight businessman with high blood pressure presented with chest pain. In the urban Michigan emergency room where I had trained, cases like this were everyday events, routine enough that we distilled them into a four-letter acronym: *r/o MI*, for "rule out myocardial infarction," or heart attack. At Queens, though, the case was so unusual that the more junior doctors had to go to the textbooks, and the consultants organized an educational "grand rounds" for the entire staff.

It was not just diagnosis that was different. I struggled with what it meant to practice medicine in a part of the world where drugs ran out, equipment was scarce, one or two nurses might be responsible for a ward of sixty incredibly sick patients, and many important diagnostic and therapeutic measures were completely unavailable because of the price tags they carried. No CT scanners. No ultrasound machine. No chemotherapy drugs except methotrexate, and then only if you could get your patient signed up for a special study happening in Lilongwe, four hours away by bus (in the unlikely event that the patient could afford a bus ticket and that the bus did not break down). No radiation therapy at all. No newborn ventilators, so babies born before thirty-two weeks gestational age rarely survived.[1]

The doctors and midwives who taught me were well aware that things were different elsewhere. Some were angry, others philosophical about their work: "Even with the little we have, we can do a good job for people." I was less sure.

When I left Malawi for the first time, plans were already well under way to start a medical school there. I wondered how Malawian students— not born, raised, and trained in the land of CT scanners and hypertensive executives with chest pain—would cope with the experiences I had found so troubling. Would they take deprivation in stride? Would they even recognize it as deprivation? When they learned to be doctors, would they be destined for frustration? Would they, like me, at one moment want to stay forever and at the next count the days until they could leave, while feeling guilty for counting? Or would something different somehow happen? Who would they learn to be?

Years later, I returned as an anthropologist to explore these questions just at the moment when Malawi's new medical school was graduating its first fully domestically trained doctors.

⸎

I am back in Malawi, walking to Queens Hospital in the cool early-morning shade of the blue gum trees, down the same dirt path that I walked every day years ago. Now, though, a Malawian medical student walks by my side. She is slim and tidy in appearance, braids pulled into a neat knot at her nape, white coat covering her simple dress. She is in her third year of school, and she is telling me about her studies. This year is a real challenge, she says (pronouncing the word in the Malawian way: "chah-*lenj*"). You have to move back and forth from the microscopes and textbooks to the hospital, learning pathology in the classroom block and then seeing it in real life—and death—among the patients at Queens. But it is fascinating, too. When yet another thin man with a high fever and a cough walks into the outpatient department, she can "zoom into his body" with her mind. She can actually picture what the inside of his lungs would look like under magnification and how the processes she could see there would cause his symptoms. She doesn't yet know how to treat the problem, but at least she knows what's causing it. I ask if she feels like a doctor yet. She laughs. "Maybe almost."

At the junction with Chipatala Road, streetside vendors hawk hard candies and Fanta, fruit and groundnuts, dried fish dusted with orange pepper, and giant yellow bread rolls that taste a little like sawdust (and are rumored to contain it). A young woman under an umbrella has a telephone at the ready propped on a cardboard box: at "phone bureaus" like these, new innovations in the last year or two, you can pay to make a call anywhere in the country. An herbalist used to work this corner, too, between the shoe repair fellow and the pharmacy, a tall, worried-looking man who sold remedies from a wooden table edged with colorful decoctions in used gin bottles and piled high with a tangle of roots and bark. His private consultation booth was a frame of branches wrapped with tattered black plastic. Did he leave because of the crackdown on street vendors, or is he gone for another reason? He was beginning to look very thin before he disappeared, and you don't have to be a doctor, or a medical student, to know that is never a good sign.

My student companion stops for a moment to make a purchase. She's good at bargaining, and the vendor gives her two tangerines for her five kwacha, about a third of what I would pay. She begins peeling a tangerine, telling me that she's missed breakfast to study. Back at the medical-school complex behind us, students get breakfast free in the noisy and chaotic cafeteria—"the caf"—but then you sacrifice what she's found is the best time to hit the library. Over fifty students are sharing two textbooks and half a dozen microscopes. There is no way to avoid the line at the microscope, which stays locked in the lab, but during mealtime there is much less competition for the books.

Her small book stipend for the year wouldn't buy even the one text she was reading this morning, the fat fifteen hundred–page guide to the pathologic basis of disease. All the Malawians she knows have very good memories, she tells me, but even among them her memory is exceptional, praise God, and she can make do without photocopies. I wonder whether, like many of her fellow students, she is trying to save the book stipend to help out with school fees for her siblings or other family obligations, but I don't feel I know her well enough yet to ask.

We've just turned to enter the hospital grounds when a small boy calls out: *"Thandizani, mai!"* Please help, madam! He's run after us, surprisingly fast given the homemade crutch and the leg missing below the knee. (Traumatic amputation? Congenital defect? Postsurgical complication?) The boy is one of a few regular beggars at this corner. They run into traffic to knock on the windows of the shiny four-by-fours with "Save the Children" or "UNICEF" or "Johns Hopkins" painted on the side and white people behind the wheel. Most of the *azungu* just stare straight ahead and pretend there's no one there at all, but once in a while someone rolls down a window and hands out a couple of coins or a small bill. The boy looks at us steadily, eyebrows up in an appeal. He is wearing a tattered shirt that announces "Michigan State Spartan Pride," probably a last-minute gift from a departing medical-student visitor. I shrug and say "*Ndilibe*," I have nothing; I've brought no money along. The student next to me hesitates a moment, then tosses him one of her tangerines. (*Muthu umodzi susenza denga*, the saying goes: One head cannot carry the roof. We all have to help each other.) The boy flashes her a grin and hobbles rapidly away, finding himself a quiet corner of the brick-walled hospital compound to enjoy his prize in peace before moving into the traffic again.

I'm walking on to the obstetrics and gynecology ward, but my student companion is headed for the main hospital block, and we say our good-byes as she turns off toward the big double doors. She quickly peels her remaining tangerine and pops the cool, juicy pieces in her mouth before she reaches the entrance. It's always tough to leave behind the smoky, faintly eucalyptus-scented air of Chipatala Road for the bloody, bleachy, sweaty smell of the hospital; the residual fragrance of tangerine helps, I know. My watch says it's a couple of minutes before half seven. It will be time for her to find the other students and the consultant for morning rounds. Time to stand quietly at the edge of the group and try to soak up the knowledge she will need soon when she's sent out to run a district hospital, time to figure out how to make a diagnosis without most of the laboratory tests in the pathology textbook and to treat an illness without most of the drugs in the pharmacology book. Time to learn to be a doctor. I watch her square her shoulders inside her white coat, pull open the door, and walk in to begin the day.

⟨∽⟩

Every day, African students learn to be African doctors in medical schools and hospitals all across the continent. They cope creatively with limited resources. They experience fatigue and frustration, joy and commitment, doubt and fear and anger. They bring their own histories and cultures to the places in which they are supposed to learn a transnational medicine, and sometimes they craft something new out of that encounter. Yet their stories are nowhere articulated in the social science literature on medicine and medical education, an extensive and rich body of scholarship limited by its geographical confinement within the wealthy North.

My argument in this book is that paying close attention to the experiences of a cohort of African medical students, and to the ways the students themselves make sense of those experiences, forces us to reexamine what we think we already know: about the effects of biomedicine in poor places, about medical science and African healing, and about what happens as students become doctors.

CHAPTER I

Introduction:
Moral Order and Medical Science

Medicine is full of stories. Medical tales circulate in the dramas and comedies of popular culture, in public and private conversations, and within the workplaces of biomedicine. Sick people recount the stories of their afflictions to their clinicians, who then translate them into the specialized narrative form of "medical histories." Doctors in training and in practice exchange other stories, less formal and more dramatic: someone makes a challenging diagnosis just in time; one unexpected complication after another produces a cascade of catastrophic results; a last-ditch intervention saves the patient—or doesn't. (We call these "war stories." Like Aesop's fables, they transmit morals from one generation to the next: "Always check the X-ray results yourself," for instance, or "Never believe the teenager who says she didn't have sex—get a pregnancy test.") Narratives of biomedicine employ plenty of stock characters. Doctor archetypes alone include the anachronistic small-town general practitioner (with or without a heart of gold); the obstetrician in a hurry to get a baby delivered before tee off; the prima donna surgeon, technically gifted and interpersonally impossible; the courageous medic who wields the tools of the trade in refugee camps and epidemic zones. There are certain common plot lines, too. There is a plot in which the naïve medical student becomes the accomplished doctor, for instance, and another in which heroic emissaries bring modern medicine to the parts of the world in direst need.

Thinking of medicine's many stories *as stories*, for me, helps in getting past the issue of whether they are true or false (although that is also an important question) to ask other questions of interest: how they circulate, to whom and by whom they are told, how complete they are, what endings to each story are possible—or not. Some narratives are created and exchanged primarily by those who practice medicine, others—often very different—by those social scientists or historians who study it, still others by politicians or advertisers or television screenwriters. These various stories do significant work, as anyone who has seen some mobilized and others suppressed in arguments over health care infrastructure reforms will be aware. Primarily reflecting the lived experiences and scholarship of people in the global North, they are also important, I will argue here, for the ways we think about biomedicine in the global South.[1]

Doctors, like other practitioners of science, most often tell a story of biomedicine in which its science is neutral, transcending culture. Scientific knowledge might be translated into different languages to be learned, but the translation is understood to be transparent, the knowledge communicated to be universal. Similarly, scientific practices are seen as transferable technologies. While cultural "barriers" in some places may require altering the packaging of a given technique—say, a vaccine or a contraceptive—to improve acceptance, the technologies are in themselves *neutral*: their implementation, indications, and effects the same in all locations of practice. Medical knowledge and practice, because they are scientific and beyond culture, are thus eminently portable; as a faculty physician in Malawi's College of Medicine put it, "If anything lends itself to globalization, medicine does."

Neutrality is hard work, and it is work that must be learned. The very definition of medical competence is the ability to see past the individual patient's subjectivity, specificity, cultural and social embeddedness, to get at the underlying pure organic pathology that will define diagnosis and dictate therapy. Such competence also requires the clinician to move beyond her own culture and social location. New doctors must learn to take the "view from nowhere," the objective perspective of medical science, uncolored by particularities of social class, ethnicity, gender, or sexuality—their own or their patients' (Beagan 2000; J. Taylor 2003).[2]

The story of science that depicts it as neutral and culture-free—whether the scientific project in general or the sciences in their particularity—stands up poorly to scrutiny, and few if any social scientists or historians would now accept it.[3] Most now understand science to be *deeply* cultural: scientific facts and social or cultural values are impossible to separate. How does a scientific fact get to be a fact at all? What issues will be understood as legitimate scientific problems? What questions can and will be asked about those issues? Who can ask them? What investigations can get funded? What constitutes evidence in those investigations? Which possible answers are within the realm of consideration? Which metaphors and models are used in the analysis? Which results are then disseminated widely, and which

disappear? All of these are essentially *social* and *cultural* questions, laden
with value, and the answers to these value-laden questions determine what
constitutes scientific knowledge.[4]

Applied sciences like medicine are even more evidently cultural. How
knowledge is put into practice, by whom, for whose ends, and with what
constraints can readily be shown to reflect—and to perpetuate—values and
relations of power in the wider society. Because medical science is so thoroughly embodied, learned and practiced on the real bodies of real people, it
has been more difficult to maintain the illusion that biomedical knowledge
is culture-free and "disembodied." In clinical medicine, then, the mutual
construction of medical fact and cultural value is perhaps even more obvious than in other applied sciences.

Very often, as the story of medicine as a cultural product goes, those
medical values have worked to legitimate domination. Work in anthropology, sociology, and history shows medicine to have entrenched the second-
class status of women by depicting them as unruly bodies in need of male
regulation, made social oppression based on racial categories appear only
"natural," and furthered the control of colonial powers over their subjects.
These effects were not simply the products of bad science or bad medicine,
corrupt research or sexist scholarship (although there was plenty of that,
too). Even good-quality, widely accepted medical science could extend the
power of the already dominant, reaffirming oppressive cultural values and
propping up social hierarchies. It could do so all the more effectively because it was so commonly accepted as value-free, merely *technical* (and
therefore inherently apolitical) knowledge and practice.[5]

Medicine in Export

Whether one understands medicine as cultural product or as culture-neutral
technology will, of course, have serious implications for how one thinks
about its effects when it moves from Europe and North America to the poorest parts of the world. That move has been substantial. The geographical
expansion of medicine over the past century and a half compares in scope to
the spread of the monotheisms or of economic regimes, although in recent
years it has encountered little of the resistance met by (for instance) mission Christianity or "free-trade" alliances.[6] Instead, the techniques, structures, and purveyors of biomedicine have very often been welcomed by
those in the global South to whom they are exported, and medical schools
and hospital buildings have become measures of a donor's generosity or of a
nation's modernity and commitment to health.[7] Since the turn of the mil-

lennium, "global health" interventions have accelerated greatly, pressed both by commercial interests in the name of market share and by activists, academics, and politicians in the name of human rights and development.[8]

Constructing biomedicine as a culture-neutral body of knowledge and technical practices allows it to be more readily bought, sold, traded, and exported. Such commodification and exchange has occurred in the service of a variety of ends and under a variety of motivating rubrics. One motivation is purely mercenary: biomedical technologies are profitable products; their export expands the market and serves the interests of transnational capital. Medical aid as a commodity, however, can also be exchanged for other desirable ends. Among medical missionaries, for instance, pills, vaccines, and surgeries may be quite openly understood as a means to bring people closer to Christ, or to Allah.[9] In secular versions of this particular global health narrative, it is not religious conversion but political influence that is sought. At least one prominent conservative American think tank has argued explicitly for health promotion as a crucial component of US foreign policy in the post-9/11 era. The pragmatic potential of global health promotion could be much more than "a matter of 'doing good' or of advancing moral purposes about the future of humanity," the authors of a RAND Corporation policy paper contended.

> Rather, promoting health abroad is also a critical aspect of foreign policy
> and, indeed, of national security—both for now and for the future. . . .
> No other area today offers the United States a greater chance to pursue
> a purposeful vision of the future, to exercise leadership, and to promote
> our core values and interests. (Hunter, Anthony, and Lurie 2002)[10]

In justifications like these for promoting biomedicine abroad, it is often very difficult to disentangle the desire to address tremendous suffering; the desire to open new markets for pharmaceutical products, tests, and devices; and the desire to use health care as an effective arm of foreign policy that can promote a consumerist form of democracy while mitigating anti-Northern (or specifically anti-American) sentiment.

Other narratives also construe biomedicine as a commodity, but instead of understanding medical care as something to be exchanged for other things of value, see it as itself a "good" that good people should provide to those who lack access. In one iteration of this narrative, drugs and doctors and surgical procedures are humanitarian interventions, the charitable duty of the rich toward the poor. In a stronger rhetorical move, they are basic human rights, and their provision is the moral obligation of the "haves"

to the "have-nots." A social justice analysis that calls for the export of biomedicine to the Third World makes a graver argument yet by diagnosing
poverty and endemic disease there as direct consequences of the exploitation of these regions by colonial powers, neocolonial superpowers, and
transnational commerce (see, for example, Farmer 1999; Kim et al. 2000).
Biomedicine in this view is not simply the moral duty of the fortunate to
the unfortunate. It is, rather, one part of the restitution due from those culpable to those exploited.

Whatever the featured motivation and desired outcomes in each of
these variations on the story of biomedicine in export, it is notable that
in all of them, the central character remains the same: that is, biomedicine, its knowledge, its practices (and arguably its practitioners) are depicted as culturally neutral, universally beneficial, unqualified goods. As
Paul Farmer has it, "Nothing is wrong with high-tech medicine, except
that there isn't enough of it to go around" (Farmer 1999:14). Such interventions as vaccination campaigns and iron tablets, mosquito nets and hernia
repairs, antiretroviral medications and tuberculin tests, are technologies to
be appropriately distributed, not culture to be imposed or contested. In the
popular depictions of global health efforts, when "culture" appears at all,
it is the culture of the intended recipients, and it is usually depicted as a
problem to be solved in order to enable effective delivery of medical care.

Whether it is traded for cash, political legitimacy, or religious alle-
giance, given as a charitable humanitarian duty, or demanded as recom-
pense in the name of social justice, this medicine is in all cases seen as a
set of knowledges and practices that is, in itself, culture-free. A radically
different story of biomedicine is told by analysts who argue that its ties
to Western culture are in fact inherent and inextricable: that it is not simply a commodity that can be used to sell or sweeten Western culture (as
the RAND analysis would suggest) but that it is itself a cultural product
and its export an instance of cultural imperialism. Introducing a volume
that strongly critiques biomedicine as a form of domination, two historians
of medicine argue that "the values of Western scientific medicine were exported to the rest of the world along with the theory, practice, institutions
and social relations of that medicine" (Cunningham and Andrews 1997:10)
and that because only "true believers" can practice medicine, "where the
medicine goes, so does Westernization" (11).

An extensive multidisciplinary critical scholarship on health and disease, in fact, mostly takes a perspective closer to the one that sees biomedicine as culturally embedded, inherently Western, and part of an imperial
project. Political economic medical anthropologists, critical geographers of

health, and social epidemiologists are among many researchers who have turned attention to the multifarious routes by which global inequities create suffering among the poor. This scholarship emphasizes the dependence of health, illness, and healing systems upon material conditions: relations of power and production.[11] Labor, capital, and the social structures they create are understood to be consequential for health. From the perspective of this critical scholarship, the heroic narrative of biomedical care and cure as morally urgent humanitarian export looks very different. Hospitals, doctors, and medical schools at best slap superficial and inadequate bandages over the deep wounds of inequality, interfering with oppressed peoples' capacity to perceive and address the injustices of global exploitation. At worst, high-technology medicine becomes an active agent of oppression, promoting the interests of elites at the expense of the poor. Doctors dismiss chronic hunger as "nerves" and treat it with tranquilizers for which poor patients must pay (Scheper-Hughes 1992); health campaigns attribute cholera outbreaks in the shantytowns of South America not to the breakdown of public water and sewer systems but to inadequate personal hygiene among the poor (Paley 2001). Biomedicine constructs HIV infection, alcoholism, and a hundred other problems as failures of individual will and matters of individual pathology (see, for example, Singer et al. 1998). It thus neatly conceals structural violence, the systematic inequalities and injustices that further enrich the powerful while they exact a disproportionately heavy toll on the bodies of the most oppressed. In the scholarship that takes this perspective, medicine functions, in essence, as a Trojan horse, concealing within its outward "gift" the deadly force of its embedded cultural, political, and economic interests.

The debt of this literature to Marxist social theory will be clear to many readers.[12] In one version of orthodox Marxism, biomedicine (like philosophy, religion, law, and other systems of thought) can appear to function as a mystification of the real causes of human suffering: labor and exploitation. Those who seek medical help, in this view, are victims of "false consciousness." In the early days of political-economic approaches to medicine, some theorists interpreted it in precisely this way (see, for example, Stark 1982). Most critical medical anthropologists, however, prefer the subtler concept of hegemony to explain biomedicine's dominance and spread.

Antonio Gramsci (1971) used the term *hegemony* to extend and refine Marx's linkage between the ideological superstructure and material base of human society. Gramsci recognized that ruling classes come to dominate not only by exerting power through the state, or by deliberately mystifying the working classes with ideology, but also by perpetuating their worldview through the structures of civil society (the schools, the churches, the clinics, etcetera) in ways not always fully recognized by either rulers or workers. The ways of thinking and acting espoused by the dominant, according to Gramsci, are not imposed upon the subordinate. Instead, not visibly linked with their origin at the site of social power, they are internalized widely in a society as popular opinions and "commonsense" values, norms, modes of speech, and behavior. Hegemonic values, because they appear not to be values at all, are exceptionally powerful. Hegemony, then, is an entire symbolic order in which coercion and consent are both at work, in which the origin of power is elusive, unrecognized—and is for this very reason more difficult to contest. But it is also never complete. Other ideas and assumptions, often also sedimented into common sense or popular opinion, compete with hegemonic ones and provide bases for potentially counterhegemonic ideologies and actions.[13]

The concept of hegemony helps critical medical anthropologists to analyze the ways in which healing systems are linked with dominant power structures. Anthropologists working from this theoretical position understand biomedicine to be a form of social control and cultural authority, perpetuating dominant-class interests by detaching human suffering (in the eyes of both patients and health care workers) from the socioeconomic systems that produce it (see, for example, Taussig 1980). Seen through a Gramscian lens, biomedicine could be understood as a set of norms, values, tools, and technologies with which the powerful think about, measure, inspect, discipline, and work upon the bodies of the disempowered, with nearly everyone involved accepting such interventions as appropriate—or even as moral goods.

Critical scholars of health raise several concerns about the hegemony of biomedicine in export. Some perceive the spread of medical science as delegitimating (or co-opting) indigenous healing knowledge (among others, see Maier 1988; Shiva 1988). Some argue that medicine's focus on technology will inevitably produce demands for unsustainable and inappropriate biomedical interventions (Lewis 2007). In the most widespread argument, many contend that medicine's near-exclusive focus on curative therapy for the individual (as opposed to preventive measures to promote public health or structural changes to the social relations that underlie illness) means that practitioners and policymakers steeped in biomedical ways of knowing are unable to see influences on health beyond the level of individual biological predisposition and individual behavioral choices. Biomedicine in the global South, as elsewhere, will therefore inevitably act to obscure the roles of social, political, and economic factors—in short, structural violence—in the production of disease and death.

Some historical and contemporary research supports this concern. In Nigeria, for instance, because physicians dominated the public health sector, good health came to be measured by numbers of doctors and hospitals, and the source of good health seen as good health *care*, not healthy environments. Effective disease prevention and examination of the socioeconomic roots of illness were ruled out of the bounds of consideration (Alubo 1994; Gusau 1994).[14] Julia Paley has described a similar process in Chile (2001: see chapter 5). Faced with a cholera scare, the Chilean Ministry of Health conducted an educational campaign urging individuals to wash their hands, cover their trash, and peel their vegetables. A disintegrating system of public sanitation, irrigation of crops with human sewage, inadequate access to treatment for those suffering from diarrheal disease, and the widespread lack of potable water were not up for discussion. The state's biomedical officials construed their responsibility as the education of individuals who were then to be responsible for their own health, not as the provision of an infrastructure that made health possible.

Medicine's sociopolitical effects are so significant that historians writing on postcolonial medicine often depict biomedicine as an inherently colonizing—or neocolonial—enterprise (W. Anderson 2000; Keller 2006). Medical competence, like scientific competence more generally, is "a *social authority* which legitimates itself by presenting itself as pure technical reason" (Bourdieu 1999:32; his emphasis). Because medical knowledge is marked as neutral and scientific, doctors and other medical workers can assume a high degree of social control even while disavowing any such intent.[15] In the postcolonial world, the authority of medicine replicates colonial authority structures that privilege the exogenous over the indigenous, scientific reductionist rationality over other forms of rationality, male over female, European over African or Asian, white over black. Doctors' bodies are perceived as white (W. Anderson 2003) and medicine as a construction of global whiteness that surpasses national identity. In the words of political scientist Alfred Fortin:

> Medicine is not the simple administration of culturally or morally neutral procedures and technologies. Western medicine reproduces a cultural order, and in its dealing with the needs of the non-white, the non-male, and the non-Western, medicine is beset with problems generated by its own hubris and perceived universalism. (Fortin 1991:18)

None of this critical literature suggests that biomedicine is the only healing system to reproduce a cultural order (in Fortin's terms). Jean Comaroff, in a now-classic paper, has argued that *all* forms of healing represent "human intervention in disorder—culturally specific self-conscious attempts to mend the physical, emotional and social breaches caused by illness" (Comaroff 1982:51) and that *all* forms of healing incorporate social interests into visions of corporeal reality. The crucial theoretical turn that began around 1980 was to note that biomedicine was not exempt from this cultural specificity, and therefore could not be used as a neutral truth against which other systems of therapy or experiences of suffering could be measured. By putting biomedicine on an equal epistemological footing with other healing practices, as cultural product rather than neutral science, historians and anthropologists could better understand its effects in the colonial and postcolonial world. Western concepts of individualism, for instance, turned out to be at the heart of colonial-era healing missions in southern Africa. Missions among the Tswana, as Comaroff (1993) showed, focused on the black body—presumed to be greasy and dirty—and the need for hygiene and sanitary control. In its individual and corporeal focus, as practitioners and their technologies acted upon the physical body and ignored social relations, medical science in Africa symbolically reaffirmed the ontological primacy of the physical world and the individual body (cf. Vaughan 1991).

In the two stories of biomedicine abroad, whether it functions as salvation or oppression, humanitarian obligation or tool of domination, biomedicine itself is credited with relatively durable core characteristics. It is high-technology. It inevitably focuses much more upon cure of the individual than on prevention for the public, although the latter is sometimes an important collateral benefit of the former. It is essentially secular, essentially scientific, essentially reductionistic: the distractions of patients' social, cultural, spiritual, and psychological worlds must be ignored to perceive with accuracy the pathological processes of that ontologically primary universal individual body.

In all of these respects, it is also essentially Western. Reading the literature referred to above, one comes away with the strong sense that both those who embrace it and those who see it as cultural imperialism tend to understand biomedicine in the poorest countries of the world, and perhaps especially on the African continent, as an export—whether a crucial one or a destructive one—from wealthier places. Its practitioners, at least by imitative aspiration if not by origin, are for all intents and purposes Northern elites: an indigenous biomedicine would be an oxymoron. Whether gift or curse, medicine remakes people and the world but is not itself remade to any great extent in its encounter with other ways of being, of working, of thinking.

Biomedicine and Its Moral Order

What is this remarkably durable set of ideas and values attached to biomedicine? What is often written and spoken of colloquially as medical culture (even if that is a "culture of no culture," as Janelle Taylor [2003] has it) may be usefully narrowed to something we can think of as medicine's *moral order*. The terms are not identical. *Culture* is a famously slippery concept, but in most attempted definitions, the word ends up indicating something like a body of beliefs and behaviors learned and taught within a given social group.[16] In this sense, "medical culture" will include—for instance—the ways medical professionals dress, socialize, and interact among themselves and with other people. Those are useful and interesting things to examine, and some will make appearances in the pages that follow. For those most interested in the deep values that undergird medical work, the term *moral order* can be more precise. Livingston (2005:20) defines a moral order as "a shared set of values held by society that guides its members in expected conduct and provides a way to judge or interpret the actions of others." It is *moral* because it is about assigning value, about deciding what is good or bad, and it is an *order* because it is an organizing schema with which we understand our own and others' actions.

How could we think about a moral order of contemporary biomedicine? Almost no one argues that medicine is monolithic. Most scholars who take late twentieth- or early twenty-first-century biomedicine as their object of study, however, understand this set of knowledges and practices to be rooted in certain core values that are shared with science as a whole, even if these values are not usually consciously articulated by medical practitioners or educators. I find it useful to organize these values into four major components: reductionist rationality, authority over nature and the body, individualism, and technological orientation.[17]

Reductionist Rationality

Practitioners perceive the empirical knowledge cumulatively produced by science through examination of ever-smaller components of the body as evolving toward truth. For medical professionals, this reductionist knowledge becomes the only objective and rational way to understand the human body, its illnesses, and its healing processes. (In human health and disease, there are no ultimate mysteries of the sort that would require theological explanation. Laypeople might see certain mysterious forms of suffering or processes of healing as evidence of divine action; for medicine, these are simply realms in which scientific discovery lies in the future, not the past.) Human suffering can best be understood by a deep knowledge of the body as an intricate and complex piece of machinery, one profoundly influenced by (yet somehow separate from) the mind.[18] A malfunction of the smallest part—a gene, a protein, a cell membrane receptor—may have devastating effects. Clinicians analyze illness by disaggregating the individual into a collection of organs or molecules (Luhrmann 2001), and health by breaking down people or societies into assemblages of risk factors (Castel 1991; Petersen and Lupton 1996). In other words, medical knowledge is secular, mechanistic, materialist, reductionist, and Cartesian (Lock and Scheper-Hughes 1996).[19]

Authority over Nature and the Body

Science claims authoritative knowledge about nature. The phenomenal growth of specialized knowledge and technology increases this authority by distancing people from other ways of knowing nature or the body. Scientific medical knowledge requires more and more specialized apparatus in the age of molecular biology. As we move from the stethoscope to the microscope to the thermal cycler that analyzes DNA samples by polymerase chain reaction, the evidence of one's own eyes or subjective states becomes less trustworthy and the deference to professional-technical authority greater (Foucault 1975; Starr 1982).[20]

In the applied sciences, authoritative knowledge is often converted to a more instrumental authority: in medicine, it legitimates interventions into the human body and those afflictions that plague it.[21] Medicine's social hierarchy makes the locus of authority clear, as the metaphors used to describe physicians' roles in hospitals and clinics and operating theaters reveal. A decade or so ago, the doctor was often "captain of the ship," while now the superficially more collegial "team leader" is more common. Still, it is clear in whom medicine's instrumental authority is embodied. Metaphors used for nonphysician clinicians make it even clearer: in the bureaucratic logic of health care systems, they are often called "physician extenders," as if they were prostheses of the doctor-captain-leader.

Individualism

The individual is the locus of both responsibility and pathology, and the site for curative work. There is a curious paradox to this individualism, however. As many critics have pointed out, in medical diagnosis and therapy—and perhaps especially in medical research—the vagaries of real individuals (whether patients or research subjects) are steadily stripped away (see, for example, Fox and Swazey 1984; Good and Good 1993; Gordon 1988). The social connections, community commitments, cultural constraints, and resources that make a person who she is are irrelevant to the work of medicine, which treats her as an autonomous—yet universalized—individual. Doctors see pathology as the result of individual genetic predisposition coupled with individual behavioral choices. Medicine is therefore poorly equipped to examine, or even to see, effects of wider societal forces such as racism or poverty (Krieger and Smith 2004).[22]

Technological Orientation

Those who work in medicine commonly perceive technology as central to their work, and value highly any opportunity to intervene technologically in the course of an illness. Byron Good (1994) has argued that technology actually becomes central to a secular redemption drama for doctors: health, not salvation, is the ultimate moral good—and it is to be achieved by technological means. The orientation to technology in a setting in which medicine has authority over the body means that doctors feel compelled to intervene where technological intervention is possible in the course of any illness. In fact, in a converse working of this process, the mere availability of technology that can rework the body means that potential sites of such work can be reconstituted as illness: normal birth becomes a site for medical intervention, as does normal death, or cosmetic or psychological variations from some normative ideal, such as an "overly large" nose, "underdeveloped" breasts, or shyness pathologized as "social anxiety disorder."[23]

⌒

The four central values of this moral order are not unique to medicine but are shared with science as a whole. In medicine, they converge upon the body. The individual body is the site from which medical knowledge is generated, whether in the clinical encounter or in the research setting. What constitutes evidence for doctors, what prompts them to action, is visible or measurable dysfunction within the confines of the individual body. The site of their work is that same body. For many physicians, these unspoken values provide criteria by which possible courses of action can be evaluated, by which other clinicians' behavior can be judged as good or bad medicine, by which knowledge is deemed useful or irrelevant. Reductionist rationality, authority over the body, individualism, and technological orientation are values common to both stories of medicine discussed above: necessary to produce "neutral" knowledge and practice, they also cognitively structure a medicine seen as neocolonial domination. They are underwritten by medical ethics. They are also thoroughly encoded by medical training.

Hegemonic Moral Orders and Medical Enculturation

Previous scholarly work on medical training has made the transformation from novice to physician seem ineluctable: students come into medicine as one sort of person (or many sorts of persons) and are molded, often quite violently, into someone else. The very language used to describe this process—"socialization"—reveals how little agency is ascribed to students. The narrative arc usually goes like this: The idealistic premedical student begins her medical training just wanting to help people. Seven to ten (or more) years of rote memorization, sleep deprivation, fear, and ritual humiliation later, she emerges on the other end of training a fully credentialed doctor. She has become technically skilled, medically knowledgeable, emotionally detached, cynical, convinced of her own status and authority; she is less the idealist who wants to help her fellow humans and more the technocrat who wants to do procedures on compliant bodies and be handsomely paid for it. She sees individual biology and behavior as the root causes of disease and is blind to larger social and political concerns—or if not completely blind, she at least sees attention to such concerns as well outside her job description. The transformation is so profound that Frederic Hafferty (1991) has compared it to a doctrinal conversion in which old values are repudiated and new identities assumed.

Much evidence supports this familiar story, evidence that has remained quite consistent over five decades of research on medical training and despite major changes in both the content of medical curricula and the diversity of entering students. It is a narrative reaffirmed in the many memoirs and fictional depictions of medical education turned out since the late 1970s. In these tales of training, the narrator himself typically escapes (albeit narrowly) the dehumanized fate to which his classmates succumb, but the normative arc remains—and is in fact reinforced by the example of the exception that proves the rule. Medical students eagerly consume and reproduce such tales, seeing reflected in them the doctors they wish, or fear, to become.

Research on medical training has mapped an extraordinarily consistent moral trajectory among students since the foundational studies conducted in the 1950s, through the neo-Marxist and feminist analyses of the 1980s, to the Foucault-influenced works of more recent scholarship. When the now-classic studies *Boys in White* (Becker et al. 1961) and *The Student-Physician* (Merton, Reader, and Kendall 1957) first reported on what happened to students as they became doctors, the medical students studied were nearly all white, upper-middle-class males. Most were Protestants; many were the sons of doctors.[24] In North America, student demographics have changed markedly since those early studies. Women make up over half of many entering medical-school classes; ethnic, sexual, and (to a lesser extent) socioeconomic minorities have a visible presence in many. School selection criteria and curricula have also changed, in part as deans and faculties of medicine responded to the critics of medical socialization by trying to produce a more humane and more "diverse" generation of doctors.[25] Despite these shifts, the process and outcome of medical socialization in the twenty-first century look strikingly similar to those of five decades past.[26] Individuals' experiences of medical training, of course, do vary to some extent. This research shows that *as a collective*, however, doctors-to-be predictably experience several interrelated changes during their training.

Medical students quickly take on a mechanistic and depersonalized view of humans. Students themselves notice this depersonalization and usually describe it as beginning during the early part of their training, starting with anatomical dissections in the cadaver lab. One of the most important mechanisms by which it comes to seem normal and appropriate is through the learning of a new medical jargon, a formal scientific language that embeds a profound reductionism and rejection of subjectivity.[27] Hand in hand with a mechanistic perception of the body comes a greater valuation of technology and of opportunities for technological intervention; technical skill becomes a crucial marker of good medical work.[28]

Doctors-in-training exchange their early idealism for a profound cynicism. Other people now become either means or obstacles to some desired end, such as learning, demonstration of competence, or sleep. These others may include their friends and teachers, but cynical attitudes about patients are particularly common and are reflected in the disparaging slang terms medical trainees use to discuss patients (who may be called "gomers," "crocks," or "toads," for instance).[29] Loss of idealism is related to the dou-

ble standards that students find are accepted as normal in the profession—
for instance, a formal commitment to doing no harm, coupled with "back-
stage" encouragement to practice procedures on poor, terminally ill, or
otherwise marginalized patients. Such double standards have been usefully
analyzed as medicine's "hidden curriculum": never formally stated but evident in the institutional policies and evaluation practices of the medical
school. Students who see their role models saying one thing and doing another become disillusioned and cynical. These feelings are exacerbated by
students' own choices not to speak up about things they find unacceptable,
a silence most view as both necessary (given medicine's rigid social hierarchies) and despicable (given their own ideals of ethical practice).[30]

Student doctors identify strongly with their new profession. Many note
growing difficulty relating to nonmedical family and friends, a change that
people who study medical socialization often understand as another mani-
festation of detachment and depersonalization. However, medical students
themselves often explain their relationship difficulties as in part stemming
from a sense of alienation from those who do not share the "lived experience" of medicine and simultaneously tend to develop intense bonds with
other medical personnel (particularly their fellow trainees).[31] This progressive alliance with their future profession is one factor contributing to a
deep internal reluctance to criticize medicine or their fellow physicians.
(Another factor is the strictly enforced institutional hierarchy of the training program, which effectively prohibits criticism of higher-ranking professionals by lower-ranking ones.) It can contribute to a feeling of—or a desire
for—authority.[32] Medical students typically see themselves as holding ambiguous status: on the bottom of a complex hierarchy of medical personnel,
yet identifying with the exalted professionals at the top. The ambiguity
of their role often results in a defensive authoritarianism and an increased
need for power.

*Students don a "cloak of competence" even when they do not feel
competent,* to mask uncertainty, consolidate status, and demonstrate authority.[33] They routinely pretend to greater knowledge, experience, and certitude than they actually possess. This cloaking increases in the clinical
years, as they negotiate between their own inexperience and their need to
demonstrate the technical ability (and the eagerness to intervene) that will
mark them as real medical professionals.

They come to desire "anonymity," as some researchers have called it:
not to stand out as different or to make waves. A more accurate term is
probably *conformity.* Students in fact compete to stand out from the crowd
and be noticed by faculty, but *not* for uniqueness, rather as exemplars of a

type: the ideal doctor. They modulate the ways they dress and speak. Aspiring to ideological or political "neutrality," they come to embrace the status quo in ways that in fact mark a shift to political conservatism.[34] Empirical research describes students as both fearing and welcoming some of this homogenization, as a sign that they are becoming real doctors. First-person accounts often depict it as a destructive process of personal dissolution: an oft-quoted lament from one memoir calls medical training "that hamburger machine that chops up nice kids and turns them into the doctors I know" (LeBaron 1981:58).

A substantial and high-quality body of research on the process of medical socialization, then, seems to argue strongly for the existence—and persistence—of a durable moral order in medicine. As students become technically competent physicians, they demonstrate increasing emotional detachment (the "affective neutrality" of the professional, as it is sometimes called) and reductionism. They also come to value technology and authority highly. That these findings hold across time, and despite changing demographics among medical-school entrants, supports a view of biomedicine as a powerful hegemonic.[35]

A serious weakness of such research as done so far, however, is that it generally fails to address extra-institutional factors that might plausibly be expected to shape professional identity: regional history and culture, access to capital and resources—the wider material and cultural contexts of medical training. Part of the problem is one of location. How generalizable can these findings be, when virtually all the research has been conducted in the global North? Of the more than seventeen hundred medical schools worldwide, fewer than 10 percent are located in North America (see table 1.1), yet the great bulk of literature on physicians' professional socialization is based on and reflects the experience of North American medical schools and residency training programs.[36]

What Is an African Biomedicine?

To what extent are the values attributed to the process of professional education in fact historically, geographically, culturally, and economically contingent? Where access to the machinery of technoscience is extremely limited, do medical students still create a moral drama in which technoscience is the savior of the afflicted? Do doctors-to-be still identify as elite white males in a world where the elite white male was historically the colonial agent or the missionary? We simply do not know the answers to these questions. We do know that colonial medicine and at least some

TABLE 1.1. World medical schools

Region	1955	1970	1985	1996	2007	Change 1955–2007 (%)
Africa	15	44	75	113	135	+773
Asia	260	422	592	755	816	+214
Australia and Pacific	6	12	14	15	18	+200
Europe	188	233	268	310	321	+71
United States and Canada	97	132	158	157	157	+62
Central and South America	80	161	235	290	322	+303
World	*646*	*1,004*	*1,342*	*1,640*	*1,769*	*+174*

Source: Data compiled and calculated from the second (1957), fourth (1973), sixth (1988), and seventh (2000) editions of the *World Directory of Medical Schools*, published by the World Health Organization (Geneva: WHO), and the updates through December 2007 found at http://www.who.int/hrh/wdms/en/.

Note: Qualifying medical schools are all those leading to credentialing as a physician within the countries reporting; curricular content and nomenclature of terminal degrees (e.g., MD, MBBS, DO) vary.

postcolonial medicine has reinforced concepts of disease that look much like the individualistic, mechanistic, decontextualized, and depoliticized explanations Northern medical students learn. At the same time, however, the historical record also shows that doctors in Africa, Latin America, and Asia have been heavily involved in radical political movements, including movements directed at revolutionary and anticolonial change.[37] This kind of collective activism, quite often in the name of medicine, does not look like the apolitical "neutrality" of the North. What does it look like?

Biomedical practices in the global South, and perhaps especially in Africa, are often constructed as deeply *philosophically* divided from indigenous healing practices that stress the social nature of illness and healing (Comaroff 1982). Perhaps for that reason, there has been very little anthropological analysis of African biomedicine as a form of cultural meaning-making, and no anthropological study of African practitioners of biomedicine.

Discussions of the ways people use various therapeutic options can and do list biomedical remedies alongside nonbiomedical therapies such as the use of herbal remedies or incorporation into cults of affliction or various other healing measures. The therapeutic itineraries of Africans seeking amelioration of suffering often include stops at all of these types of practices (see, for example, Hutchinson 1996; Janzen 1978). The anthropological literature on the *provision* of healing practice, rather than its consumption, is not so inclusive. In this literature, African practitioners are indigenous healers who use "traditional," neotraditional, or spiritual modalities, sometimes while also drawing on the symbolic power of biomedicine: spiritists, herbalists, prophets, witchfinders, *asing'anga*. These figures stand in stark contrast to biomedically trained physicians who, when they appear, are almost always European whites. Anthropological scholarship on the learning and practice of biomedicine and that on the learning and practice of African healing traditions have, in essence, comprised mutually exclusive discourses, intersecting only in discussions of the tension and conflict between the local and the global. This binary persists despite the fact that biomedicine has been in Africa for well over a century, and its practice *by Africans* has long been widespread. Across the continent, biomedically trained African physicians, nurses, and others examine and diagnose patients, give injections, perform surgeries, and dispense medications—yet they remain functionally invisible in the anthropological literature: African healers are not biomedical; biomedical practitioners are not African.[38]

Megan Vaughan (1994) noted over a decade ago that this distortion leads to several false dichotomies: between the scientific knowledge of biomedicine (her term is *scientific medicine*) and the social knowledge of indigenous healers; between bodily curing of pathogens and symbolic healing of social ruptures. If African biomedicine is not an oxymoron, what is it? Without empirical examination of how contemporary African biomedicine is learned, lived, and practiced, we will describe medicine only in relation to its own theory of itself (as found, for instance, in textbooks) rather than in all the richly contextualized historical and cultural complexity of its actual local instantiations. That omission allows biomedicine (either the culture-neutral medicine of the doctors or the culture-laden medicine of the social scientists) to serve as a straw man in our analyses of healing in Africa: presumed to be both technically effective and inherently individualizing, seen as a set of readily mobilized technologies—whether technologies of curing or of dominion.

The Purpose of This Book

I do not dispute that medicine is a cultural system and that, as such, it has powerful political and social effects. The evidence that connects medical facts to values is too good. In the remainder of this book, I will argue, however, that the values that underlie medical science are far more culturally specific than previously understood, and therefore not consistently and inevitably reproduced across locations where medicine is taught and practiced. My evidence is an ethnographic exploration of medical training in the southeast African country of Malawi. This research, like all research to date on medical training, shows that students take on powerful values as they learn to become doctors. Those values, however, are in significant respects different from the ones previously assumed to be inherent in medical science. In addition, while some seem to be acquired fairly passively during the process of training, others are actively forged, hammered together from the cultural materials at hand in the heat of clinical encounters in which overwhelming need meets inadequate resources. The experiences these students have as they become doctors, and the ways in which they come to reconfigure what being a doctor means in this poor country of the South, upset ideas about science that are common in the wealthier countries of the North. Serious attention to this African story reaffirms and expands the literature that discredits naïve depictions of medical science as culture-free, but this story also complicates understandings of biomedicine as neocolonialism.

In this book, I ask what happens to the moral order of medicine when much of the material technology required to manifest biomedical practice is unavailable, when scientific medicine is entwined with spiritual or political mission, when clinicians' working lives are in every respect shaped by the same structural violence that produces patients' suffering. If, for example, sub-Saharan Africa is materially and technologically impoverished, and biomedicine is definitionally an expensive high-tech practice, then what does an African biomedicine look like? And if in fact the practice *is* altered by its incarnation in the specific setting, as I will argue it is, how does this in turn alter medicine's relationship to structures of inequality? What are the implications of an African biomedicine for the stories doctors, medical students, and academics have been telling ourselves and one another about what medicine is and how it works (or fails to)?

Malawi is a small, landlocked country at the southern tip of Africa's Rift Valley, wedged between Mozambique, Tanzania, and Zambia and bordered to the northeast by a vast lake. It is known for the beauty of its tropical fish, the friendliness of its people (some travelers know Malawi affectionately as "Africa for beginners"), its poverty, and its wide array of deadly diseases. I have been there on several extended journeys since 1990. Since 2001, I have been engaged in ethnographic work among students and doctors at the country's new College of Medicine.

Malawi's medical students become doctors in one of the poorest countries on a poor continent, where maternal and child mortality are high and life expectancy is low, where the dual scourges of HIV/AIDS and international economic policies ravage the hospitals and threaten both biomedical workers and their patients. In this country, the presence of biomedicine is both long-standing and rapidly increasing. Locally trained doctors are desperately sought by the public health sector, even while training programs are derided by some donors as an unjustifiably intensive use of scarce resources—in essence, an inappropriate technology for the region. It is my contention that the African student who takes on the identity of African doctor here is a figure whose very existence confronts and destabilizes the theoretical oppositions mapped above. These students are not "us," elsewhere. To this very challenging clinical milieu they bring experiences and histories that matter for the doctors they ultimately become. Attention to the lived experience of these trainees, then, provides a unique lens on the natures of biomedicine and the biomedical healer.

This study engages with many different bodies of literature: the history of medicine (in Africa and elsewhere); ethnographic work on African healing; postcolonial theory; scholarship on medical socialization; work on global health. It is impossible to do them all justice, and I have not. Any reader will be aware of more work with which I could have fruitfully engaged. I have elected to frame this project primarily in light of previous scholarship on how trainees are inducted into the medical profession: how one becomes a scientifically trained doctor. This Malawian ethnography corroborates some of the findings of this large body of research, extends other findings, and challenges the overall explanation quite significantly in several respects.

Readers in a hurry should be able to evaluate my major argument by reading chapters 1, 5, 6, and 7. Those who want richer detail should read it all, including the stories that separate the chapters, and the footnotes in which most of the academic references lurk.[39]

A more detailed description of methods is available in a technical appendix; here I will simply sketch major sources briefly. This book is based primarily on a year's fieldwork I conducted in 2002–3 and on follow-up conversations and observations during five months of additional fieldwork (while I was again in Malawi working on a different research project) in 2007. I refer occasionally to material from shorter visits in 1990 and 2001. I collected, transcribed, and analyzed all the data myself, but the research design was improved tremendously by the collaboration of a Malawian colleague, Dr. Chiwoza Bandawe, and his insights have also strengthened my analysis. Materials include data gathered primarily at the University of Malawi College of Medicine: four focus groups, 61 formal interviews (of

which 42 were with students, interns, and recent graduates), 121 questionnaires, and field notes based on thousands of hours of informal interviews,
conversations, observations, and interactions. Because the medical school
was new, I also had access to some of the key personnel involved in its development, and thus to their understandings of their project. For two days
each week during fieldwork, I examined, spoke with, treated, and operated
upon obstetrical patients at the adjacent teaching hospital. Working where
the students work in the labor wards and operating theaters of this large
and decrepit urban public hospital, I gained additional valuable insight into
their lived experiences. Because I most wanted to understand how students
constructed meaning out of their experiences, however, among all this data
I pay the most attention to their own stories.

As I will show in the course of this book, Malawi's poverty affects
physicians' working lives and thus their self-understandings. The strategies Malawian doctors use to reconfigure the work of medicine do not arise
de novo, however; they reference older regional concepts of the healer as
indigenous intellectual and political leader, responsible for explaining and
treating illness by attending to disorder in the wider community. They also
reflect the profound influence of African Christianity and the long-standing
association of medicine and mission in this part of the world. Chapter 2
situates the research historically. I provide an overview of healing traditions from the precolonial era to the present, in Malawi specifically and
southeast Africa more generally, and explain why healers of all sorts may
reasonably see themselves both as elite and as endangered. To give readers
insight into the current state of Malawi's patients, clinicians, and health
sector, I also briefly explore factors contributing to the country's terrible
health indicators.

Chapter 3 lays out the routes to becoming a doctor in Malawi, including the intersections of gender, class, and religion on the paths to medicine.
I also address the explanations students give for choosing medicine, and the
costs of that choice for themselves and others. This chapter draws heavily on fieldwork sources and begins the primarily ethnographic center of
the book.

Chapters 4, 5, and 6 look at the experiences of Malawi's doctors-to-be
during their training and early practice years. Chapter 4 follows them into
the laboratories and lecture rooms of basic science training and examines
their early experiences of learning medicine. Trainees learn to "see" the
universal body through processes of dissection and microscopy. They also
take on a medical habitus that has some homogenizing effects, even as they
never fully escape the effects of their class and gender identities. In parts of

this process, we can see hegemony at work; like all hegemonies, it has fissures and gaps.

The fissures deepen in chapter 5, which accompanies trainees into the hospital. With the move from the microscope to the bedside, these students' experience begins to diverge more radically from the one described in the classic studies of medical socialization. At this juncture, Northern students face the challenge of translating intellectual theory to embodied practice, as they pick up and begin to develop competence in the deployment of the tools of their trade. Malawian students enter the hospital with the same expectation of developing mastery, only to find the tools of the trade in very short supply. Instead, they face a painful reality of risky communicable diseases, overwhelming workload, and patient and health-sector poverty. This chapter charts the ensuing crisis.

Conditions of practice extend beyond the walls of the hospital. Chapter 6 attends to the wider social, political, and economic factors that engender both opportunities and constraints for the new doctors. Financial concerns are particularly salient, as junior public-sector doctors in Malawi—although without question a local elite—still live in poverty by Northern standards. Responsibilities to their extended families and communities raise the stakes on the difficult choices they make. This chapter highlights newly trained doctors' articulations of the complex practical and moral dilemmas they face, and of the solutions they seek to construct. I explore how they improvise responses, both in the course of their day-to-day labor and in the meaning they give to their work, by drawing on available resources of many kinds.

The concluding chapter steps back to consider the theoretical consequences of this work. Malawian medical students' struggles to understand, embody, and—in many cases—break down and rebuild the identity of doctor illuminate more than their individual trajectories, interesting as those are. They challenge current understandings of both medical enculturation and biomedical hegemony in Africa. I argue that technologies can be potent actors even when they are materially absent; that medicine's moral order can better be understood as one of many possible moral economies; and that the experiential knowledge students of medicine learn can lead just as effectively—if to ambiguous ends—to a politicized identification with "the people" as it can to a depoliticized detachment.

Throughout the book, I have kept the focus tightly on the narrative voices of those with whom I worked and spoke. Cheryl Mattingly has suggested that the narratives we construct, which we commonly understand as simply *representing* our experience, actually *structure* it, giving our lives meaning and purpose, "provisional answers to the question 'Who Am I?' among a limited range of historical possibilities" (Mattingly 1998:128). Or, as Clifford Geertz put it, "We assemble the selves we live in out of materials lying about in the society around us . . . from birth on we are all active, impassioned 'meaning makers' in search of plausible stories" (Geertz 2000:196).[40] Narratives are subjective constructions, then, and they are also social. Social processes determine what stories *can* be told, what stories *must* be told, what stories *cannot* be told. Those who narrate select from a vast store of events and memories, putting the selections into temporal and causal orders: this happened and then that happened; this happened *because* that happened. In narratives, what may have seemed random is made coherent. Narratives join affect and cognition, what we think about and how we feel—not only for tellers (or writers) of tales but for the ones who listen (or read). Narrator and audience can relive experiences and reflect upon them simultaneously.

Within the chapters themselves, I have used medical trainees' comments and my own observations as snippets of data, arranged them according to an analytical framework, and thus imposed on them a narrative coherence. I have tried to be responsible in this process but am well aware that there are other ways of selecting and arranging and interpreting this material, and therefore other stories that could be told with it. In part for that reason, and in part to ground the theoretical material in the lived experiences of those incarnating biomedical practice in Malawi, I have also included between chapters the narratives of several specific students, doctors, and patients. In the accounts that the trainees themselves related—about their paths to medicine, about their expectations for their future—we can see them taking up various locations in other stories: of their nation, of their families, of medicine.

Paths and Locations: My Journey to the Field

Why Malawi, why this project? If one were looking for an economically impoverished, culturally non-Western site in which to investigate what happens to medical students as they become doctors, it would be difficult to come up with a place better than Malawi's new medical school. I also chose Malawi because (as the prologue recounts) I had been there before, during my own transition from student to doctor, and because that experience was distressing, fascinating, and unsettling to my early assumptions about what biomedicine was and could be. There is more to the story, of course. A couple of months on the wards in an African hospital, compelling and troubling as they were, did not in isolation make this project one for which I would return to school, struggle to learn another language at which I demonstrated no natural talent, repeatedly hazard Malawi's hospitals (and what is probably worse, its public transit), and ultimately change careers.

It has become a convention of ethnographic writing to spend some time exploring the social and cultural positioning of the anthropologist, in part as one way of allowing readers to interrogate the value of the work. Feminist scholars (for example, Haraway 1988; D. Smith 1990) have long argued that all researchers work from social locations not easily extricable from our theoretical locations. Our positions influence (or even determine) what questions we choose to explore, what our investigations illuminate and what they obscure, and whose ends our research serves.[41] Specifics of the ethnographer's experience and social location are not to be somehow magically subtracted from our work to create an illusion of objectivity, most anthropologists now argue, but rather should be acknowledged, explored, and negotiated in the field and in our writing.

Social location unquestionably influenced this research. Even on a modest research fellowship, I was wealthy compared to nearly everyone I interviewed and worked with. I was a social scientist working in a medical school that valued "hard" science, a physician slowly transitioning from clinical medicine to anthropology. I was American, white, a woman. In most cases, I tried to mitigate the distancing effects of my own identity where possible, through designing research carefully and collaboratively, living and dressing modestly, using Chichewa when it was appropriate and I could manage it, avoiding entrenchment within the expatriate community. At other times, I capitalized freely on social position. I doubt, for instance, that I could have walked into mission and public hospitals and talked with the staff as readily were I not a white doctor. Some aspects of who I am made for ready alliances, some created social distance. Most did both at one point or another, depending on the specific circumstances. After the first few weeks of (predictable) alienation, I never felt either completely marginalized or readily assimilated—nor have I ever since.

The social location that influences this research most significantly, I suspect, is that of physician. I am an obstetrician-gynecologist. It was therefore possible for me to work in the same field as my informants, to follow their medical language and stories, and—after we came to understand each other at least partially—to share some of the risks, triumphs, joys, and griefs of the work. Sharing a profession meant I had greater access to many parts of my informants' worlds, yet it also no doubt blinded me to aspects of medical socialization that others might have noticed and I took for granted. I probably felt more sympathy for the students and interns than many other researchers would have, and suspect that to be both a liability and a strength of this work.

As a doctor, of course, I have also undergone my own process of professional socialization, and that, too, influences this work, likely both for good and for ill, and likely in ways I do not fully understand.

I have been thinking about medicine's moral order (although I would not then have used that term for it) for well over twenty years, since before I started medical school myself in 1986. Like my fellow would-be doctors, early in training I had eagerly consumed the med-school memoirs and fictional accounts that were a hot new genre at that time (Pollock 1996). Even as first-year students, most of us had read the classic *House of God*, hoping we would never be that cynical or that exhausted, but also picking up the world-weary toughness and the medical slang of the very cool. It would be several years before television's *ER* became an instant medical-student hit, but we watched its predecessor, *St. Elsewhere*, identifying with the interns and feeling incredibly proud when we knew enough to pick up the occasional medical errors. The medical school I attended tried to encourage reflexive thinking, discussion, and mutual engagement on the subject of socialization: Why were physicians so often autocratic, detached, and insensitive, even hostile to patients? How might we avoid such a fate? Subsequent years of specialty training elsewhere were humbling. In a setting of abuse and overwork, I saw some of these unwanted characteristics blossom rapidly in my friends and in myself as, embittered and exhausted, we found our efforts to resist them waning. The face of the first patient I hated, not five months into internship, is still burned into my mind. So is that of the first patient—a miserable and angry young woman whose cancer had metastasized and would not be cured—I wished would die so I could go to sleep. All that time and all that effort: I would not consider quitting. In many ways, I genuinely loved the work, and still do, but for a long time, I felt as if the price for learning it was my soul. I came to appreciate how powerful a system of socialization really can be, and how it both requires and manufactures the consent of those being socialized.[42]

When it was time for me to teach medical students and residents myself, the question of socialization grew even more complicated. In the mid- to late 1990s, I was clinical faculty for several Navajo medical students on elective attachments in the Indian Health Service hospital where I worked. Many of these students described feeling torn between the values of their home communities, which they described as highly collective and kin-oriented, and their new medical culture, which they perceived as motivated by individual achievement and competition. They questioned whether they could make these two worlds mesh. This issue hadn't come up for me or my mostly European-American colleagues, and (like anyone who has spent many years in school) I looked to the library for help. But when I tried to find books or journal articles on this sort of culture clash, I came up empty-handed. In the medical literature of the time, those who wrote on "cross-cultural medicine" tended to assume that Otherness was located in the patient, and that the doctor was unmarked by culture, ethnicity, or gender. Put in other terms: patients had culture, doctors had knowledge. This curious omission made me eager to learn more about medical culture and how it fit or conflicted with the other cultural reference points of its practitioners. When I pursued graduate training in anthropology, I developed the tools that would allow me to do so.

This personal engagement with the research topic makes a book more interesting to write (and, I hope, to read). It will also raise red flags for some readers. The evolutionary biologist Stephen Jay Gould, writing about just such engagement, once claimed:

We have a much better chance of accomplishing something significant when we follow our passionate interests and work in areas of deepest personal meaning. Of course such a strategy increases dangers of prejudice, but the gain in dedication can overbalance any such worry, especially if we remain equally committed to the overarching goal of fairness, and fiercely committed to constant vigilance and scrutiny of our personal biases. (Gould 1996:37)

I hope that both the passionate interest and the fierce vigilance of which Gould writes are evident in the material that follows.

⌒

This book depicts a constellation of people, events, and structural forces that occupied a particular moment in a particular place. It has already changed, as all constellations do; their light continues to reach us long after the stars themselves have moved or flamed out.[43] A few of the people of whom I write are dead. Some have left medicine or Malawi, not always by choice. At the time I write now, much of Malawi seems a little better off than it was when I began this research, although some parts of the hospital, the school, and the city in which I worked seem a little worse. One of the arguments I will make in the pages that follow, however, is that very little ever really goes away completely. Just as the histories of mission medicine, of a doctor's dictatorship, of the confrontations between witchcraft and science, have left their traces on Malawian medicine, I hope that this evanescent narrative of ordinary human beings, struggling to make difficult decisions where there is no morally clear option, will leave its own trace on the story of what biomedicine is and might be.

⚜

All Part of the Same Big Mess
Mkume Lifa

Mkume Lifa was one of the youngest students in his class, only eighteen when he began medical school. I first met him in his premedical course, when he hung out with a much older group of experienced clinicians who were "upgrading" to become doctors. He seemed then naïve and idealistic, more than a little awestruck by the breadth of real-life experience his classmates had. His seriousness (and his habit of wearing a suit and tie to class) made him the occasional butt of classmates' joking. Five years later, as he neared graduation, he had become a student respected for his hard work and scholarship. He retained a quiet, wide-eyed, and serious demeanor, and he still wore a tie under his white coat.

Mkume had grown up in one of Malawi's largest cities and spent much of his childhood in the staff housing compound of a big central hospital. His parents were both part-time missionaries who also held down other jobs. His mother ran a small business and farmed the family's land. His father had worked his way steadily up through the medical ranks from a relatively humble beginning as a health surveillance assistant to a high administrative position.[44] Mkume told me that in secondary school, one of his major goals had been to do better than his father.

> I had my own ambitions. And most of those ambitions were defined by how much [money] we were going to have as we were working, how much we would be getting, because I wanted to get out and be somewhere above what my father was doing. So like most other Malawian children, who like me were finishing their secondary education, I wanted to do either business administration, economics, or law. But later on I turned and decided I should do medicine because my priori-

ties now changed. I started looking at things differently. . . . Not only looking at my own life but at the lives of the people around me. And I started seeing that in life you don't only have to be yourself; you live with other people around you. And I saw that I wouldn't do much for them if I chose to enrich myself and not find ways of helping. I could get a million kwacha per month. But I wouldn't be able to help them, because *my* needs would also increase with that amount of money. But if I became a doctor, I could help a lot of people. And that thought is what drove me to change my priorities. I came to find that life isn't in order—basically, we're all part of the same big mess, really—and that I should do something for everybody.

This realization was "definitely a part of growing older," Mkume added, but it was not only that. It connected with other people's ideas of what it meant to be a good person. "You hear what certain people say. Not directed at me, but what they would—what they think an ideal person ought to be like. It just grasps the soul listening to them, when you're making your decisions." It also connected with experiences visiting poor relatives.

My father used to take me to his home in the village. And when I got there, I could see very poor people struggling for basic necessities. And there was a way in which I could reach out to them and help them, if I had the knowledge. And I just had that burning—that burning *will* within me to acquire that knowledge that I should be able to help, that knowledge with which I could reach out to those very needy people. Because for example, we would go—my father, my uncle, and I—and these two guys would carry with them groceries to give to the numerous old people. Because we have very extended families in Malawi! So you give to numerous people. But you discover that the things they give them will only last two weeks, a week at most. But I thought: I could give them something which would last them longer than two weeks.

The knowledge Mkume believed he would accrue as a doctor might enable him to give more lasting gifts. The satisfaction of using this knowledge would be one of the few rewards of his profession.

The most rewarding thing about being a doctor in Malawi—and, of course, anywhere else—is the satisfaction that you get, the personal satisfaction as you do your work. Apart from that, there is a lot of respect in Malawi. The other thing is that you have the potential of contributing a lot to your community. And basically that is *all* that is rewarding about being a physician. You can't talk of the financial situation, because here, you see, doctors do not receive a lot of money. They keep telling us it is very expensive to train a doctor. But it is not just money; it takes hard work, commitment. The course is difficult. And then you finish and earn four thousand Malawi kwacha [about forty-two dollars per month at that time]. It isn't much, so doctors here, they are not wealthy.

At the end of the interview, I asked Mkume to imagine his working life after internship was done. He laid out a grand vision of medicine's potential (and status), and an ambitious set of goals. He finished by urging other Malawians to join him in pursuing those goals. As he spoke, I thought that I could hear the cadences of his missionary parents.

After finishing my internship, I would want to work at a small hospital, preferably a rural hospital. And mostly what I see is a lot of responsibility: somebody who people would be able to look up to, to help them not only medically but psychologically, spiritually. That's what I aspire to. And the kind of establishment that I would like to have is that of somebody who can mix well with the community. That they can feel comfortable with.

Clinical practice alone would not be enough, given Malawi's current straits.

Mostly what I want to do is preventative health. I would like to see an initiative that is free of the political ties that it has now, to prevent HIV, and eventually TB and the rest of it, too. So I would start initially with HIV. And I'd be one of the persons who has contributed to fighting, not as somebody who has found a cure for HIV/AIDS but as somebody who in a way has helped a lot of lives and who has contributed enough to stop the spread of this nationally. . . . Malawi as a nation needs us, to make decisions in our lives that are good decisions. And when you're making those decisions, you've got to look at: What are the priorities? What does our country need ultimately? I do not believe that our country needs more modern industry, more motor vehicle mechanics. It needs more doctors. So, as you make your decisions in life, do not only think about yourself. Think about others in the community. Everybody needs money to survive, but many need a doctor to survive more than they need money to survive. So we do need doctors, and it's a cry out to our nation: many people should come forward and do medicine. And to those doctors who graduate—let us stay in our country. If we don't develop our country, nobody will develop it for us. We have taken the contribution of our country for our education, and we owe that to our nation. Life is not only to make it financially. We should not only think about what we shall get but what we shall give unto others: that's how we will make a better Malawi.

CHAPTER TWO

Medicine and Healing in
a Postcolonial State

When Malawi's new doctors began studies at Malawi's new medical school, they brought with them concepts of medicine and healing, some shared with medical students in the global North and some not. When they left at the end of their internships more than six years later for postings around the country, they faced regionally distinctive challenges as well as challenges common to physicians elsewhere in the world. Both their ideas and their challenges emerged within a Malawian history in which transnational movements of people, beliefs, diseases, healing practices, goods, and money have had profound effects.

This chapter explores briefly the contradictory legacies of vernacular healing, colonial medicine, and mission medicine that shape what being a doctor means, in a place that has long been a crossroads of Africa, a place where globalization has been both an immiserating and an enriching force for hundreds of years. Malawi's history is notable for the blurring of spiritual, medical, and political power. Healing power and the healer's status were often used for political advancement or rebellion; healing movements and medical activities were often seen as moral cleansings of society. The healer has long been an ambiguous figure of high status, but also at high risk—endangered bodily, politically, morally. The story and its contradictions are embodied in individuals: Hastings Banda, a doctor who was also a dictator; Chikanga, a healer whose pan-Africanist philosophy made him charismatic and dangerous; John Chiphangwi, a physician-educator who put himself at risk to help his patients; David Livingstone, the missionary explorer whose medicine for Malawi was—at least in part—capitalism.

In Malawi, *all* forms of healing have complex legacies. They represent at the same time state power and antistate struggle, nationalism and transnationalism, innovation and tradition. And they do so in a place in which dire poverty and entrenched health problems create both enormous needs and enormous obstacles to meeting those needs. These legacies affected the ways that students there came to interpret the meaning of their work as doctors and delimited the paths these new doctors could take.

Healing in Southeast Africa: Dualistic Power Working on Social Bodies

Southeast Africa encompasses the Anglophone and Lusophone countries from Tanzania through the former British Central Africa region to South Africa. As Steven Feierman (2006) has pointed out, there are good reasons to consider this area a coherent region when examining healing traditions: a close linguistic kinship stemming from the Eastern Bantu expansion in the first millennium CE (see also Janzen 1992); an especially violent shared history of colonial conquest; and long-standing intraregional exchange of healers and medicines (West and Luedke 2006).[1]

Healing practices in southeast Africa are also famously innovative and open to outside influences. The integration of exogenous and endogenous is part of what gives them power, and part of what makes it difficult to disentangle healing from religion or politics. Healers have crossed regional and conceptual boundaries for at least as long as the historical record exists, incorporating ideas and practices from Islamic medicine, Pentecostalism, colonial bureaucracy, biomedicine, and elsewhere (Flint 2001a; Probst 1999; van Binsbergen 1991; West and Luedke 2006). They are so pluralistic that nearly any generalization about African healing risks being an overgeneralization. From the cults of affliction that arrived in southeast Africa centuries before the colonial powers did, to the Pentecostal prophet healers of today's Malawi, many healers have been religious practitioners (and vice versa). They have also often been figures of considerable political influence, acting to bolster or destabilize the authority of the state (Janzen 1982; Luedke 2006).

Healing in southeast Africa is typically public, collective, imbued with moral purpose, and sometimes violent. In the region's oldest known traditions, "health" and "illness" are seen as broader-than-bodily concepts for harmony and disruption; healing has been strongly oriented to the social body for at least four centuries, and probably much longer. An individual's physical health is inseparable from community well-being or even from the fertility of the land.[2] Fractured social relations are expressed in sickness or in other forms of suffering that most Northerners would consider nonmedical: misfortune in business, for instance, or crop-imperiling drought.

In addition to empirical therapies, therefore, the appropriate treatment for such misfortunes consists of attempts to heal ruptures in the social milieu. Healers' tasks are to diagnose the sites of those ruptures and advocate treatment. A child's illness, for example, might result from the failure of her parents to adhere to customs of postpartum sexual abstinence, or the jealousy of a neighbor, or the intervention of an ancestor angered by inadequate funeral practices—for the relevant social realm does not consist solely of the living. In each case, specific remedies apply. This focus on the repair of social ills does *not* mean, however, that African healing must be seen as an essentially homeostatic mechanism, restoring the status quo by punishing transgressions of accepted norms. Healing practices can also be seen as forms of resistance to modernity or ways to push for change by shifting existing balances of power. Whether employed on behalf of continuity or change, healing ritual continues to represent an inherently social process that cannot be understood as directed solely toward the individual suffering body.[3]

In southeast Africa, many people attribute certain misfortunes and illnesses to witches (who may or may not be conscious of their supernatural powers), and healing of witchcraft-related injury has attracted considerable attention from ethnographers and historians.[4] Witchcraft is usually rooted in envy, and those at either end of the economic spectrum are therefore particularly vulnerable to witchcraft accusations. In Malawi, the economically successful often face suspicions that their gains have been gotten with supernatural aid. The extremely poor, on the other hand, are suspected of causing harm through their envy of the wealthy. Material goods are not the only relevant form of wealth. Childlessness, for instance, may be inflicted by witchcraft but may also lead a woman jealous of the fertility of kin or rivals to work witchcraft against them. As in other regions and other times, barren women are at high risk of being targets during periodic witch-cleansing movements.

Healing of witchcraft-related injury requires entry into the same supernatural world in which witches work their harm, and therefore in southeast Africa (as in much of the rest of the continent), the nature of healing power is seen as fundamentally dual: the power to heal *is* the power to harm, something—like sex or like fire—that is essential to life but that must be controlled to mitigate damage (Davis-Roberts 1992; West 2005).[5] Healing and harm can both be accomplished using substances that in Malawi are called *muti*—a word translatable as either "medicine" or "poison." *Muti* can be used to heal, to promote good fortune, to aid one person at the expense of another (as in the *muti* of human body parts, used to ensure business success and typically procured by violence against some hapless stranger), or to injure. The ambiguity of *muti* tends to attach also to the person who wields it. Those who diagnose spiritually caused misfortune and advise appropriate treatment are able to do so precisely because they have access to the realm of the invisible in which witches work. This access to the occult can be easily used to work harm, intentional or not.

Perhaps paradoxically, the personal experience of spiritual injury—whether caused by witchcraft or by other forces—often becomes a vital qualification to heal, and one that may protect the healer to some extent from accusations of evil intent. Initiates, recruited into healing "cults" or "drums" from the ranks of sufferers as part of their own healing process, must transcend human and epistemological boundaries to gain healing power. They must then learn to wield this power with caution (Friedson 1996; Willis 1999).

"African healing" can be rather frustrating to contain analytically, given the pluralism of practices, the way the capacities to heal and to harm are not readily separated, the mingling of influences and of traditions, and the wide conception of what constitutes illness. In practice, African healing is often defined primarily by what it is not: biomedicine. But biomedicine, too, has a long history in this region—and specifically in Malawi—and it, too, is not always easily separable from other types of healing, religious, or political practice.

The Arrival of Mission and Colonial Medicine

Historians often depict biomedicine, in its mission and its governmental incarnations, as a handmaid of colonialism in Africa. In southeast Africa, the lines between the missionary and colonial projects were blurry; medicine played an ambiguous role—or rather, several potentially contradictory roles—in both. Certainly, colonial medicine could be oppressive. At the same time, in this region it tended to be thin on the ground, only intermittently effective, and usually not very relevant to people's lives. Although (or partly because) medicine was associated with whiteness, many Africans used it as a route to power. African medical assistants, doctors, and nurses who were able to procure training often threatened existing class, professional, and racial divisions.[6] Some worked for the state; some became anticolonialist leaders. Like the "traditional" and prophet healers who were also active in anticolonial and postcolonial politics, these ambiguous figures sometimes reinforced the legitimacy of political leadership. In other cases, they undermined it.

Even before formal colonization, biomedicine was entwined with religious and political power. The most famous explorer to reach the area now known as Malawi was also its first Western-trained physician and missionary: David Livingstone.[7] When Livingstone first arrived in the mid-nineteenth century, the area was already populated by ethnic groups that had arrived in serial waves of migration over a thousand years, intermarrying and trading but also retaining some group-specific languages and cultural practices. Most of these peoples were loosely clustered into a state known as the Maravi, a state whose major function was to regulate trade in ivory and slaves.[8] This earliest known integration of the region into the global economy, as Harvey Sindima (2002) has pointed out, prefigured effects of colonial and postcolonial economic integration by displacing thousands of people, by weakening rural agricultural economies, and by producing entrepreneurial agents of foreign powers who undermined other types of authority. Abolitionist missionaries like Livingstone hoped that the slave trade could be reduced and eventually eliminated by the introduction of other profitable commercial ventures. In his famous Cambridge speech of 1857, Dr. Livingstone had claimed, "My desire is to open a path to this district, that civilization, commerce, and Christianity might find their way there" (Chambliss 1881:257). The first and last of these aims, at least, were soon to take the shape of medical missions.

By 1861, a mission stood at Magomero in the south of what was by then sometimes called Nyasaland ("land of lakes") district. Within a few years, the first African medical dresser had trained in surgery and microscopy and was working with missionary doctors farther north (King and King 1992).[9] Through the late nineteenth century, medical missions gained in number and strength, despite the shocking mortality rates of early mission personnel. Hospitals and training programs were to heal the sick and bring to Africans the advances of civilization. In fact, the nineteenth-century concept of mission medicine may have had more commonalities with African beliefs than either the white doctors or the black healers recognized: missionaries tended to see sin as the ultimate cause of sickness and suborned the cure of individuals to a moral cleansing of society.[10] In Nyasaland, missions thrived especially in the Shire River highlands town the missionaries called Blantyre (after Livingstone's birthplace in Scotland) and in the northern Livingstonia Mission, run by Dr. Robert Laws with an emphasis on higher education and hospital building. As discussed below, training of medical assistants, nurses, and midwives—but not doctors—soon grew to be a major mission function.

Where the missions led, European farmers, traders, and corporate investment soon followed, although the small and economically marginal territory never attracted the numbers of white settlers drawn to some of its neighbors. By 1878, the African Lakes Company was trading in Blantyre, and soon afterward Cecil Rhodes's British South Africa Company procured a charter to develop the area. By 1891, the British Foreign Office, anxious both to protect British interests and to fend off rival claims by the Germans and Portuguese in the infamous "scramble for Africa" (Pakenham 1991),[11] had claimed most of present-day Malawi as a protectorate.[12]

Medical science was elsewhere used to justify oppressive and exploitative European rule, most egregiously when Leopold II of Belgium disguised his brutal regime in the Congo as a humanitarian effort bringing medical care to the disease-afflicted natives (Hochschild 1998). Colonial medicine also participated in controlling African subjects; public health rationales could be used to keep Africans from congregating freely, or to limit movement over government-imposed but culturally meaningless borders (often, as in the trypanosomiasis "control" measures Maryinez Lyons [1992] describes, without sound epidemiologic premises). In Nyasaland, however, colonial government medicine initially had little to do with Africans at all. It was mainly targeted toward treating sick or injured Europeans[13]— although mission medicine after its first few years did have a wider purview.[14] In Nyasaland, as elsewhere in southern Africa, colonial medicine later expanded to treatment of Africans only when plantation owners and others sought to maximize the productivity of their labor forces.

Medicine and Healing: Routes to Power, Mobility, and Danger

Colonizers were not the only actors of the colonial period, nor the only medics: Africans sought training in the esoteric techniques of medicine from the beginnings of European contact (Ranger 1981; Vaughan 1991), not only as a desirable form of knowledge but also as a route to social and intellectual advancement. Nyasalanders were likely to find that paths to education and advancement led north. Paradoxically, even while they opened the way for capital investment and abusive labor extraction by their fellow Europeans, many of the northern missions openly espoused a then-radical "Africa for Africans" philosophy and promoted higher education as a means of African liberation (Jeal 1973; Ross 1997).[15]

Both mission medicine and the medical training of Africans expanded rapidly in Nyasaland at the turn of the twentieth century. Blantyre Mission Hospital opened in 1896. Within three years, the mission's doctors had added a ward for malaria research, sponsored and often staffed by the London School of Tropical Medicine. They had also begun a hospital assistant program for Africans that was much more extensive and formalized than earlier ad hoc training programs. Candidates had to pass a standard exam developed by the mission physicians and upon graduation were licensed to perform surgery and dispense medications (King and King 1992). By the 1920s, medical dressers and hospital assistants were being exported from Nyasaland to Dar es Salaam and beyond, as East Africa then had no training programs for Africans (Beck 1970).

Mission-educated Africans may have extended the colony's power and reach, but they were also at the forefront of anticolonial unrest, which came to a new peak in Nyasaland with the Chilembwe rebellion of 1915. The first African who graduated from the Blantyre medical assistantship program, John Gray Kufa, was also a Presbyterian deacon who worked at the Blantyre Mission for several years before going on to staff a dispensary for workers on a large tea plantation in the highlands. There he fell in with John Chilembwe, an African Baptist preacher who had studied with radical missionaries in Nyasaland and later in the United States, then returned to open the Providence Industrial Mission. Many of Chilembwe's parishioners worked on the surrounding tea plantations, as did Kufa's patients. Chilembwe became increasingly aware of—and vocal about—the devastating effects of forced labor on the people of Nyasaland.[16] With Kufa as his second-in-command, he led an armed uprising in 1915. It was one of the earliest anticolonial rebellions in British-colonized Africa, and it was crushed vigorously. Kufa and Chilembwe were executed; Providence Industrial Mission was razed by the British government.

Chilembwe's mission was not rebuilt until 1928, when the executed preacher's former student Daniel Malekebu returned to Nyasaland to reopen the church as a medical mission. Dr. Malekebu, who had been sponsored by African-American missionaries to attend Meharry Medical College in the United States, was Nyasaland's first African physician. When he tried to return to his home country, he was initially turned away by a colonial government grown extremely wary of educated African radicals. After spending some years in Liberia, he was able to return to Nyasaland after convincing the government that he did not intend to involve himself in politics. He worked at Providence Industrial Mission preaching for many years.[17]

Colonial surveillance of Nyasaland's educational structures increased after the Chilembwe rebellion. Like all other branches of education, training of Africans in biomedicine came under government control, even if the actual teaching was still mostly done by the missions (Shepperson and

Price 1987). In the 1920s, a National Medical Council was established to register hospital staff who qualified by passing a National Approved Course run at the Livingstonia Mission, and the colony's first midwifery school opened at Mlanda Mission (King and King 1992). By the mid-1930s, the first government-run medical training school opened at Zomba to train medical dressers, nurses and midwives, laboratory assistants, and sanitary inspectors. The government also set up district hospitals at the urging of settlers who wanted medical services available for themselves and their workers (Ngalande Banda and Simukonda 1994). Although Nyasaland now trained all manner of subordinate medical personnel, those at the head of the hierarchy continued to arrive from overseas: all physicians were still Europeans or the rare African sponsored by missionaries to attend medical school abroad.[18] Training programs may have increased in this era, but actual clinics and hospitals remained sparse and for the most part confined to the towns. Whether for this or other reasons, most Nyasalanders continued to seek guidance and care from diviners, herbalists, prophetic healers, and *asing'anga* (Lwanda 2005).

In the 1930s, a particular focus of healing work was an apparent rise in the incidence of witchcraft. The surge in witchcraft accusations reveals some of the social tensions brought by colonialism, and the syncretic rituals with which southern Africans responded illustrate their integration of biomedical and colonial practices into innovative healing forms. After forty years of colonialism, some entrepreneurial or well-placed Africans had become substantially more prosperous, while most suffered, and the proliferation of antiwitchcraft or *mchape* movements in the 1930s is generally thought to be a response to growing inequality (see, for instance, Marwick 1952). Nyasaland escaped neither the increased inequality nor the witchcraft purges that followed. (In fact, Audrey Richards's informants from Northern Rhodesia believed that *mchape* had originated in Nyasaland [Richards 1935].) The *mchape* movement of the 1930s swept from village to village, as suspected witches—or sometimes entire villages—faced trial by poison ordeal. The concept was not new. Historically, such ordeals had involved the administration of an infusion of ground bark to suspected witches at the request of a chief. Any witch who had not renounced all evil practices and turned in all *muti* and magical accoutrements would be killed by the poisonous drink. Every innocent who drank it would be protected against witchcraft—for, like other healing substances, this one had both the power to cure and the power to kill. The 1930s movement had several distinctive features, however. Not initiated by the chiefs, it was brought to the villages by groups of young men, often migrant laborers laid off when

the global economic depression hit the mining industry in Northern Rhodesia and South Africa.[19] The actual drinking of *mchape* was surrounded
by imagery and practices reflective of colonial bureaucracy, of medicine,
and of Christianity. Richards (1935) noted that these young men lined up
villagers for inspection in a manner reminiscent of a census, used mirrors
to identify witches, opened their ceremonies with sermons in which the
"washing of sins" was a major theme, and stored the poison itself in stop-
pered chemists' bottles rather than the traditional horn containers. This
syncretic social healing project reflected and helped to accomplish a shift
in authority from a rural chiefly gerontocracy to a cadre of mobile young
men, and signs of medical and bureaucratic modernity added to the movement's symbolic power.

In the years during which Nyasaland was under colonial control, then,
healing movements and healers themselves sometimes reinforced authority, sometimes changed it, and often challenged it outright. Institutions of
healing (whether biomedical or not) stood in tension with other structures
of power, a tension that was to continue into postcolonial times.

The End of Empire

The conscription of Africans into two European wars, blatantly racist laws
and policies,[20] the wide-ranging effects of taxation and migrant labor, perceptions of social decline, and the brutal treatment many Africans experienced at the hands of white settlers had created fertile ground for nationalist movements in much of Central Africa by the 1940s. In Nyasaland, the
last straw was the unwanted Federation of Northern and Southern Rhodesia and Nyasaland in 1953. The British government, hoping to minimize
colonial bureaucracy while maximizing the movement of capital and labor
across regional borders, imposed federation despite vocal and organized opposition by the new Nyasaland African Congress (NAC) and by traditional
chiefs. Nyasalanders rightly feared the racially discriminatory politics of
settler-governed Southern Rhodesia (Rafael 1980) and were outraged that
the colonial government ignored their protests. But the British were concerned about the draining of labor to the South African gold mines and
wanted to redirect it to the copper mines and settler-owned plantations of
the two Rhodesias. Federation went ahead.[21]

The colonial government attempted to sweeten the unpalatable arrangement with medical and other inducements. Nyasaland would be allowed to send promising secondary students to Salisbury in Southern Rho-

desia or Lusaka in Northern Rhodesia; some might be eligible for grants to train as physicians. Federal funds were supplied to improve the country's infrastructure: roads, railways, and especially hospitals. The old Blantyre Mission Hospital closed, and the gleaming new four hundred–bed Queen Elizabeth Central Hospital opened (with separate wards for whites and blacks). These measures could not buy off an angry and disenfranchised populace. The NAC, now headed by charismatic nationalist Dr. Hastings Kamuzu Banda, gained strength. Banning the party and jailing its leaders only fanned the flame. After several years of civil unrest and bloody suppression of agitators, the colonial government agreed to hold elections. Banda and the NAC (renamed the Malawi Congress Party) were victorious. The federation collapsed, and colonial Nyasaland became independent Malawi in 1964.

Malawi under the Doctor's Rule

Hastings Kamuzu Banda embodied much of Malawi's tangled colonial, religious, and medical history.[22] Born in an obscure village in central Malawi, he was educated at a Scottish mission and became a devout member of the Church of Scotland. He worked as a migrant laborer in Southern Rhodesia, from there traveling on foot to South Africa. At the Witwatersrand Deep Mine on the Transvaal Reef, he met African-American missionaries who sponsored him to further his education in the United States. There he eventually earned a degree in history at the University of Chicago[23] and an MD at Meharry. When called back to Nyasaland by the NAC, he had been in private medical practice for over twenty years, in Scotland, in Britain, and in newly independent Ghana.

The nationalist NAC leaders who hoped Dr. Banda would be a respectable elder spokesman for their movement were in for a surprise. They were confident but young, and knowing the nation would prefer an older leader, they had toured the country promoting Banda as the *ngwazi* (hero or lion-killer—essentially, messiah) Nyasaland needed to shake off colonial rule. The *ngwazi* was thought to be in his late fifties, qualifying as "old" in a place where life expectancy at the time was thirty-eight years.[24] But he had an unsuspected taste for power and few scruples about maintaining it, and he was to live and rule much longer than his promoters had expected. Within months of his election, he had driven potential rivals into exile—or worse—after the "cabinet crisis" demonstrated his unwillingness to brook even minor opposition. Malawian physicians in senior administrative posts were among those who fled the country. By 1969, he had amended laws and political structures to amass great personal control over Malawi's land, press, judiciary, and economy.

Banda's early political success stemmed both from his canny exploitation of potentially conflicting ideologies and from external factors that encouraged international interests to turn a blind eye to his regime's human rights abuses for far too long. As a highly educated doctor from a small Malawian town, he was able to draw explicitly if selectively on what he depicted as both European and traditional African mores (Chanock 1975), as well as on the Christian beliefs held by most Malawians.[25] Many of the "traditional African" ways he promoted were more pseudotraditional inventions, incorporating elements of older ceremonies into new forms designed specifically to enhance his own authority. In what he called a celebration of Malawi's matriarchal tradition, for instance, he organized women's movements—*mbumba*—whose chief function was dancing for him wherever he appeared. He valorized the Chewa people as the most Malawian of Malawians, while repeatedly marginalizing northerners by accusing them of tribalism. (Northerners were greatly overrepresented among Malawians with tertiary education, and thus a threatening source of potential rivals. For Banda, controlling them was essential, no matter the cost. In 1989, for instance, he dealt a great blow to the public health sector by expelling northern nurses from the central and southern regions with the specious justification that tribal fidelities would lead them to mistreat patients not from their own region. The simultaneous expulsion of northern teachers had a similarly significant impact on public education.) He made much of his own selection as an elder in the Church of Scotland, adding religious to political and traditional authority. He established an elite secondary school staffed solely by European teachers and teaching the classics, where the students played cricket and spoke only English. Yet he also denounced the University of Malawi for "destroying the character of our boys and girls" by promoting Western permissiveness, not to mention political ideas (Forster 1994).

The paradox here was that African tradition, higher education, and religion, while essential to the construction of Banda's legitimacy, also had the potential to be rival power centers. Banda's ambivalence about these important nonstate forces was evident. As long as adherents (students, healers, patients, congregants) gave uncritical support to the regime, they were relatively free, even encouraged, to flourish in Malawi. As sources of alternative allegiances, however, they were also vigilantly monitored (Forster 1997), and vigorously hounded if they gave evidence of threat. When Jehovah's Witnesses refused to buy Malawi Congress Party membership cards on religious grounds, for instance, "Young Pioneers" acting on orders from the government harassed, expelled, or even murdered them. The Jehovah's Witness Church was prohibited by law in Malawi for nearly three decades. *Nyau*, a Chewa secret society into which nearly all postpubertal males were initiated, was initially encouraged; its great costumed *gule wamkulu* dance was even adopted as a cultural icon for the MCP in the first years after independence. The masked participants of the *gule wamkulu* characterized themselves as wild beasts who could not be bound by human laws, so perhaps it is not surprising that the period of open approbation was short. Within a decade, the MCP leadership repressed or "domesticated" the society it had once promoted, and certain prominent and defiant dancers went to prison, ostensibly to ensure the security of civil society (Kaspin 1993).[26] Banda boasted of his own degrees but carefully restricted opportunities for tertiary education in favor of "locally appropriate" vocational training and put barriers in the way of other Africans seeking to become physicians (Lwanda 2005).

The leadership of traditional healers, especially when it crossed borders, was also suspect. Alison Redmayne provides an interesting case study on this topic by tracing the career of the healer Chikanga, who flourished in Nyasaland in the 1950s and early 1960s (Redmayne 1970). Born Lighton Chunda, after an illness Chikanga renamed himself and set up as a diviner, drawing seekers from four countries and cleansing professed witches— unlike other witch-cleansers, without killing them. His refusal to charge for his work convinced many of his authenticity and may have been part of the explanation for his far-reaching popularity, although for the Tanganyikan clients with whom Redmayne spoke, the long journey to him and back could eat up a year's wages. Another factor may have been his unusual power to summon sorcerers and witches to him, perhaps in part because he encouraged only cure and not revenge. Chikanga used a language of appeal to all Africans, regardless of creed or ethnicity, reflecting the pan-African ideals of the day. This language, coupled with his amazing popularity, also made him a serious threat. His career was cut short when Banda ordered him to stop his healing activities and move into internal exile near Blantyre to be watched.[27]

Banda's selective exploitation of tradition and his vigilance about rival powers might have been enough to sustain his regime, but the interests of powerful countries in the North also played a role. In the 1960s, armed and violent struggle against white rule began in Angola, South West Africa, Mozambique, Rhodesia, and South Africa. In each case, rebel movements had at least nominally socialist leanings. As the Cold War grew hotter, the superpowers found southern Africa very interesting indeed. A stable, pro-Western, business-friendly state like Malawi was a good investment, and Banda's government found it easy to get loans and donations. Malawi also maintained diplomatic and trade relations with both the white-minority government of Rhodesia and the apartheid government of South Africa, eventually becoming the only state in southern Africa to do so. It was therefore an attractive target for investment not only to South Africa but to allies like the United States.

By 1971, Kamuzu Banda had himself declared "president for life," and while he did not in fact hold the position for life, he came close. Twenty-three more years of increasingly repressive rule followed. Dissidents fled or were jailed without trial; journalists could publish only news flattering to the president. The abuses grew more extreme in the 1980s, when Banda's sense of impunity seems to have escalated. Many of his political opponents died in suspicious car crashes or unsolved murders. His henchmen tortured others in custody, assassinated some in exile with letter bombs or firebombing, or abducted them from their homes in other countries and brought them back to Malawi to rot in the prison at Zomba. Dr. Banda boasted openly on the national radio that the Shire River crocodiles had grown fat on the bodies of his enemies (Chimombo and Chimombo 1996). During this time, simply being an educated Malawian was extremely dangerous: surgeons, teachers, and lawyers languished in jail. Many who had gone abroad for higher education were afraid to return.

But opposition to these abuses also increased, and the economic distress of ordinary Malawians fueled the opposition. The country's economy had grown robustly during the 1970s, mostly due to a strong plantation sector, but in the 1980s, matters deteriorated drastically. A rapidly growing population and increases in estate holdings put greater pressure on the remaining available land. Rural households entered a period of shrinking landholdings and diminishing crop yields, exacerbated by drought and soil depletion. Rebels in Mozambique blew up the Nacala railway line that had transported Malawian goods to the coast, and export income dropped. AIDS, first confirmed in Malawi in 1985 but probably present since the late 1970s, began to take a toll on labor productivity and household income, while overloading and disrupting the social and kin networks used to cope with distress. Even migrant labor opportunities, long a standby for Malawians, began to dry up. The Employment Bureau of Africa stopped recruiting Malawians to work in South African mines in 1988, citing high HIV-positivity rates (Chirwa 1997), while the collapse of the copper-mining industry in Zambia and the deteriorating economy of Zimbabwe effectively closed off two other longtime opportunities for migrating Malawians.

Structural Adjustment: Wounding the Social Body

The state's acceptance of structural adjustment policies meant government could not cushion these blows. Most of sub-Saharan Africa had faced economic crisis by 1980, caused by a combination of dropping commodity prices in the mid-1970s, drought, worldwide increases in oil prices, and currency overvaluation. Governments throughout the region sought more loans to offset the crisis. Major lenders, firmly committed to neoliberal policies that advocated downsizing the state and allowing the "free market" to drive development, took the opportunity to set new conditions for loans. The World Bank's Berg Report (World Bank 1982) proposed solving Africa's economic woes in part by eliminating labor market "distortions" such as minimum wage laws, pension programs, and other labor protections; other recommended austerity measures included user fees for health and education services, privatization of state services, removal of subsidies and price controls, civil service reduction, and currency devaluation. Such measures were built into the structural adjustment programs (SAPs) upon which loans were to be conditional. No new loans were granted—and promised funds were withheld—until borrower countries signed the agreements (Schoepf, Schoepf, and Millen 2000).[28] In southern Africa, Malawi was the first country to sign on to structural adjustment.

The principles behind the SAPs were those of laissez-faire liberal economics.[29] What looked logical in economic terms, however, was brutal when translated into the language of human experience. For economists, imposition of user fees and abolition of price controls were to directly reduce government expenditure while bringing the efficiency of the market into (presumably) inefficient government bureaucracies such as education, health care, and the provision of food to the poor. In Malawi and elsewhere, the translation was that feeding, educating, and providing health care for its people were now by definition outside the responsibilities of a state; safety nets were luxuries poor nations were told they could not afford. In economic logic, removal of wage, labor, and environment protections would result in expanded production, as foreign capital would flow to where the costs of doing business were low. In human terms, when labor protections and occupational safety and health regulations were gutted, and collective bargaining was hamstrung, poor people worked harder in more dangerous jobs to make anything resembling a living wage. For laissez-faire economists, currency devaluation and the resulting inflation would reduce in-country demand, particularly when coupled with removal of price controls, making more available for export. Increased production and decreased domestic consumption would then favorably affect the balance of trade. For the laborers who experienced it, stagnant or dropping pay and inflated prices meant their wages would purchase less and less. When a nation's people must produce more in order to buy less, the proportion of resources that can be extracted from the country and sent abroad increases.

There has never been evidence that SAPs in any degree improve the health, nutrition, or well-being of poor people in poor countries. Even lending institutions ultimately acknowledged that austerity programs worsened health indicators, rationalizing that short-term pain was necessary to secure long-term gain (Kolko 1999). A quarter century after the first SAP agreement was signed, this long-term gain had yet to materialize, except in the profits of transnational pharmaceutical, agricultural, and manufacturing industries (Turshen 1999).[30] In Malawi, structural adjustment ended most government subsidies, including the fertilizer and seeds on which farmers counted. Health and nutritional status deteriorated as agricultural production moved ever more toward export crops, price controls were removed, and costs of basic foodstuffs soared.[31]

The changes required by SAPs hit Malawi's health sector particularly hard, and at a time when it was also staggering from the consequences of the AIDS epidemic. The rapid expansion of privatized medical care pushed by lenders was to be accomplished in part by starving the public sector. Patients were required to pay to access care; although the formal sums involved were minimal, the informal ones could mount quickly as they had to pay for drugs and supplies no longer available at their clinics (Turshen 1999). Salaries for civil service nurses, medical assistants, clinical officers, and others were frozen, and staff levels dropped. All the while the numbers of the sick, and the severity of their illnesses, rose rapidly. Hospital wards and outpatient clinics overflowed with patients who would never get better; many medical staff fled to places they could make a living wage, left clinical work in despair, or died.

Trouble and Transition

The deterioration of public health, education, and agriculture, exacerbated by externally imposed austerity regimens, fueled the already-smoldering fires of opposition to the Banda government. Ordinary people wearied of the contrast between the difficult realities of their own lives and the costly and elaborate pageantry intended to show the glory of the regime, and wearied also of the climate of intimidation and surveillance.[32] In the early 1990s, other sources of foreign aid began to dry up. Donors had become increasingly squeamish about reports of the regime's human rights abuses and about Banda's close ties with the apartheid government of South Africa. The end of the Cold War also meant that African countries no longer needed to be wooed away from the Eastern bloc with generous bilateral aid or with development projects that enriched government officials and their cronies. As conditions continued to worsen, unrest within the country could no longer be contained. Even some of the forces that had maintained the power of the dictatorship began to turn against the dictator. In March 1992, Malawi's Catholic bishops prepared a letter that was read aloud in every Catholic church in the country, calling for Banda to step down and condemning the excesses of his government. It is generally agreed that this pastoral letter was pivotal in Malawi's transition to democracy, particularly when Banda's own Church of Scotland disowned him as an elder and joined in the protest.

Banda's initial reaction was to crack down hard. Police acting on his orders imprisoned many office workers on suspicion that their fax machines and photocopiers were spreading seditious materials, and shot into a crowd of striking workers and bystanders, killing dozens. A prominent opponent of the regime suddenly died, almost certainly murdered, in prison. These actions only escalated the activist pressure from within the country and diplomatic pressure from without. Seven months after the bishops' letter, a group of major donors agreed to withhold all aid except drought and refugee relief.

By the end of 1992, it was clear to most observers that Dr. Banda had not much longer to stay in power. His Malawi Young Pioneers, ostensibly a youth group devoted to promoting agricultural development but actually paramilitary thugs who did much of the administration's dirty work, were crushed by the Malawi Army after a brawl in which MYP youth shot and killed two soldiers. Malawian exiles, university students, trade unionists, and church groups were involved in demonstrations and strikes against the regime. High inflation—averaging 30 percent a year—and droughts in 1992 and 1993 made for many hungry and angry Malawians. Tensions ran high. In 1993, Dr. Banda called a referendum on his rule, a referendum he apparently expected to win but in fact lost by a two-to-one margin. A multiparty election took place in 1994, and a new president, Bakili Muluzi, took office.[33]

Things did not go well for the new government, however, despite the initial public euphoria. Muluzi and his Parliament promised free primary education and improved health care for all, but the health sector continued on its downward spiral—and the education sector joined it. School enrollments increased by 50 percent, pupil-to-teacher ratios hit sixty-to-one, textbooks and supplies were lost or stolen and never replenished, and national exam failure rates skyrocketed. AIDS affected nearly every family and overburdened nearly every health care worker and unit in Malawi. Many homes disintegrated; orphans roamed the city streets.[34] A prophet healer named Billy Goodson Chisupe, a member of that same Providence Industrial Mission church founded by John Chilembwe and run for years by Dr. Daniel Malekebu, promoted a virus-eradicating remedy that had been revealed to him in a dream. One in twenty Malawians, including many health workers, flocked to his small town to drink Chisupe's medicine—called *mchape* after the poison ordeals of the 1930s (Doran 2007; Probst 1999). The state seemed passive and confused about how to respond, even while government officials using government transport to get there lined up to drink *mchape*, and its handling of the situation drew much criticism. Constitutional reforms provided for a free press, but Muluzi and his backers continued to monopolize public radio and the newly established public television station. The new constitution also set limits on presidential powers and duration in office, but the president's party soon sought to amend the constitution to allow for additional terms of office. In the massive protests that ensued, the Young Democrats of the president's party, imitating their precursors the Young Pioneers, beat and harassed opponents of constitutional change, including more than twenty members of Parliament. As Malawi's economic situation continued to deteriorate and government corruption scandals blossomed, many of the promises of multiparty democracy came to seem hollow. Political unrest was on the rise again by the time this research began in earnest in 2002, and some Malawians already looked back to the days of Banda's rule with nostalgia.

Poverty and Health in Twenty-first-Century Malawi

Malawian newspapers reported on the front page in 2002 that the country had been designated (by the United Nations Development Program) the poorest peaceful nation in the world, its per capita GNP that year at US$166. For decades, it had ranked among the poorest dozen countries, with a rapidly growing population of nearly twelve million people, a vulnerable economy based heavily on a few agricultural export commodities, and an external debt half again as large as the gross national product.[35] Like most other countries in sub-Saharan Africa, Malawi was heavily and perilously donor-dependent—about three of every four dollars spent on health and social welfare measures derived from donor aid (World Bank 1994).[36]

At the beginning of the twenty-first century, most Malawians eked out a living with subsistence agriculture, although the burgeoning population and deteriorating soil made this living insecure. Urbanization, held in check for longer than it was in neighboring countries, had begun to increase rapidly. Malawi's few real cities were surrounded by large slums in which recent arrivals from the countryside struggled to survive. Health was precarious, and life shorter than it ought to have been. Malaria, AIDS, respiratory and diarrheal illnesses, and malnutrition still killed many children. Malawi's hard-won improvements in child mortality were responsible for increasing life expectancy from about thirty-six years in 1955 to forty-nine years by 1995, but the impact of HIV erased much of this gain. By 2002, some estimates put life expectancy back in the late thirties. Other health indicators also lagged, although some have since improved (see table 2.1).

Health services of all kinds were uneven in distribution and quality, and various healing epistemologies coexisted and borrowed from one another. When Malawians needed health care for themselves or their children, most used herbal or over-the-counter remedies first. In rural areas especially, traditional practitioners like herbalists, *asing'anga*, or village birth attendants were often the next resort. Choices about which therapeutic resources to seek did not follow any simple pattern, however; decisions depended on many factors, including geographic and financial accessibility of those resources, influence of social networks, family funds available, and the severity and etiology of the diagnosis suspected (Chokani 1998; Mwanza 1982).[37]

Medical pluralism was tolerated and sporadically encouraged by the Malawian government (although, since the *mchape '95* incident, it was no longer legal to proclaim that one had a cure for AIDS). Most traditional healers registered with the Traditional Healers' Association of Malawi, but as a group, they did not seem to be as professionalized (or their remedies as commodified) as elsewhere in the region. Prophetic healing, including the casting out of demonic influences and the lifting of curses, had grown rapidly and rivaled traditional healing in prominence and legitimacy, especially in urban settings. Biomedical services consisted of small primary health clinics, district hospitals, and four central referral hospitals in the public sector; a number of mission hospitals that worked cooperatively with the Ministry of Health (and provided 30–40 percent of facility-based care in the country); and a small private for-profit sector mostly run by paramedical

TABLE 2.1. Selected economic and health indicators

Indicator	Malawi	Africa	World	United States
GNP per capita (PPP-adjusted US$), 2007[a]	750	2,141	9,872	45,850
Annual per capita health care expenditure (PPP-adjusted US$), 2006[a]	62	111	790	6,719
Physicians per 100,000 population, 2000–2007	2	19	126	239
Estimated % adults over 14 HIV-positive, 2007	11.4	4.7	0.6	0.5
Life expectancy at birth (years), 2007	50	52	68	78
Under-5 mortality rate (deaths per 1,000 live births), 2007	110	145	67	8
Maternal mortality ratio (deaths per 100,000 live births), 2005	1,100	900	400	11

Source: All figures except physicians per 100,000 population are taken directly from the World Health Organization's World Health Statistics 2009, available online at http://www.who.int/whosis/whostat/2009/en/index.html. Physicians per 100,000 population were calculated from health resource and population figures in the same source.

Notes: All figures are the most recent available. Life expectancy estimates have improved markedly in Malawi since the time of my fieldwork, in large part due to a dramatic reduction in under-5 mortality. Figures for HIV-seropositivity, maternal and under-5 mortality statistics, and physician-population ratios are all considered unreliable, as variability among countries in calculation and reporting is significant.

[a]Purchasing power parity (PPP) is a way of adjusting for the fact that a dollar could go further in Malawi for many basic necessities, such as food staples or child care (although imported consumer items such as cars or batteries tended to be more expensive).

personnel. Indicators of biomedical services and staffing remained bleak: in 2000, even as the medical school was already producing graduates, Malawi had both the highest population per physician and the lowest annual per capita health care expenditures in southern Africa.

Instituting a Medical School

Historically, Malawians who wanted to train as doctors—rather than the midlevel clinicians called clinical officers—faced nearly insurmountable logistical and financial hurdles.[38] In the 1960s, the medical school in Harare (then Salisbury) had agreed to take qualified Malawian students at in-country tuition rates, but this arrangement ended with the demise of the Federation of Rhodesia and Nyasaland in 1963. South Africa's medical universities were closed to black Africans from out of state. Training in other relatively inexpensive developing-world settings, such as Cuba or Mozambique, usually required students to master another language before completing the difficult medical curriculum. Historical and social linkages meant that most of those few Malawians who attended medical school abroad did so in the United Kingdom, sponsored by missions or, in a handful of cases in the 1980s, by the government (Ngalande Banda and Simukonda 1994). But the United Kingdom appears to have had especially high rates of trainee nonreturn. Many people suggested that in the Banda era—and some people say into the twenty-first century—more Malawian doctors lived in Manchester, England, than in Malawi. The reasons for not returning home were complex. Pay and conditions of work were both much better abroad, and the length of medical training in the United Kingdom increased the odds that doctors there would marry locally and become entrenched in the community. In addition, repressive political conditions at home made doctors fear the repercussions of being educated and high-profile citizens in Malawi.

It was less risky for non-Malawians to work in the country. Banda was no fool. He knew that the world would pay more attention if expatriate academics and doctors—especially white ones—went missing than if Malawian ones did. By 1992, when the political repression in Malawi was at its worst, 175 doctors were in the country, only 25 of whom were Malawian (King and King 1992).[39] Most senior medical posts were staffed by clinical officers, nurses, or medical assistants.

For roughly the first two decades after independence, government leaders rejected the establishment of a medical school as economically impossible.[40] Senior clinicians and University of Malawi faculty persisted, however, in part by pursuing outside allies. In 1981, the Africa Regional Director of WHO was invited to conduct a feasibility study; his report made a strong case for a medical school. Two years later, a working group from the Royal College of Surgeons in Edinburgh did a second feasibility study, invited by the University of Malawi, but recommended only phased introduction of one or two clinical years in Malawi to follow several years of out-of-the-country medical training. A third medical delegation, from the University of Munich, then concluded during a short visit in 1984 that a medical school was both possible and desirable (Planning Unit 1984). Several of the crucial foreign donors remained cautious, however, and some refused any participation in the project. Not only were many concerned about whether a medical school was an appropriate use of scarce funds, but some of the students whom foreigners had sponsored through medical training overseas were suffering in Malawian jails without trial, suspected of sedition.

As the population multiplied and sickened, even while doctors and

other members of the educated elite fled the increasing repression of the
Banda government in greater numbers, the shortage of health care providers grew ever more acute. Ultimately, the argument that domestic medical training was the best way to alleviate this shortage prevailed. In 1986,
after twenty-five years of discussion and debate, plans for a medical school
moved forward slowly under the guidance of a "tripartite commission"
with representatives from the United Kingdom, Germany, and the government of Malawi (Broadhead 1998; Dahlenburg 1993).

Once the building of a medical school had been approved, decisions
about how to design the curriculum and recruit the teachers remained.
E. Q. Archampong, a Ghanaian surgeon and medical school dean, has
summed up the difficult choices faced by the first postcolonial generation
of African medical educators:

> The perennial dilemma that dominated their deliberations continues to-
> day, namely: the desire to produce a large number of practitioners who
> were, on the one hand, fully oriented and adapted to the environment,
> and on the other, completely on a par, and on terms of reciprocity, with
> their colleagues on the international scene, that is, Europe and America.
> (Archampong 1990:5)

A medical school gains its prestige, maintains its accreditation, and recruits and retains its faculty by meeting "international" standards. Papers
produced in scholarly journals, student prizes won, outside examiners impressed, research grants received, all count toward these standards; practically relevant matters like numbers of graduates working as district health
officers, or percentage able to treat septic shock competently in the absence
of most essential antibiotics, do not.[41] The obligation to produce physicians
of "international" caliber—and to fund their production—has often in practice meant continuing colonial traditions, relying heavily on external examiners from European countries, and promoting medical research "col-
laborations" that follow the interests of transnational funders rather than
domestic needs. In Ghana and in Nigeria, attempts to craft training programs free of expatriate control ultimately collapsed under pressure from
physicians and policymakers who sought international status (Archampong 1990; Gusau 1994).[42] In Malawi, it is not clear that such an attempt
was ever considered at all.

The college officially opened its doors in 1991 with fifteen academic
staff members and four new brick teaching units attached to the medical,
surgical, pediatrics, and obstetrics and gynecology wards at Blantyre's larg-

est public hospital. An additional teaching unit for community health was located in the town of Mangochi, hours away in a poor and primarily rural community at the lakeshore. During its first few years, the college followed a phase-in process. At first, only the final year of medical school and the newly required eighteen-month internship took place in Malawi, with all training in basic medical sciences in Scotland or London, and the bulk of clinical teaching in London's teaching hospitals. Later, students were sent to do basic science in the United Kingdom, Australia, or South Africa and returned to Malawi for all of their clinical training. Once enough basic science teachers had been recruited, however, by 1994 Malawi's College of Medicine was ready to offer the complete curriculum at home.

Sometimes foreigners characterized the College of Medicine dismissively as yet another expatriate project, fueled by a combination of misplaced missionary fervor and personal desires for glory on the part of its founders. More than one non-Malawian suggested to me that those who couldn't "make a go of it" in their home countries could be very big fish in the small pond of Malawian medicine. Such ideas about expatriate motives are common.[43] But no Malawian I met suggested that the school was an expatriate prestige project, and, in fact, the college's history does not really fit such a characterization.

Dr. John Chiphangwi, a Malawian who studied medicine in Aberdeen and returned to Malawi at independence, was the central figure in the establishment of the college and director of the fledgling "medical school project," as it was called in its earliest days. By all accounts, Chiphangwi was a nearly fearless agitator for better hospital standards, better funding for public health, and better medical education for Malawians. In one famous story, he stood up to the powerful and vindictive head of state by refusing to clean up the labor ward at Queen Elizabeth Central Hospital for "Life President" Banda's annual hospital Christmas tour. Banda would come with fanfare to give holiday cheer, and in preparation for his visit, clinicians habitually "cleared" the overflowing wards by sending home patients who were sleeping on the floor or in the hallways. Chiphangwi, then head of obstetrics, refused to perform the usual flattering falsifications and ensured that Banda would encounter the reality of the wards: he kept all sick and laboring women in the hospital. The other staff were so frightened by this decision that they fled the ward and left him alone to conduct the tour. "Everyone was convinced beyond any reasonable doubt that Dr. Banda would definitely get angry, and that John Chiphangwi was not going to see his relatives again. Everyone feared for his life. He was like a lamb led to the slaughter" (Mulwafu and Muula 2001:114–15). In fact, after a tense few moments as the two doctors faced off over who was responsible for the appalling conditions, Banda agreed to fund construction of a new maternity wing for the hospital.

Students, interns, and graduates who knew Chiphangwi still talk about the medical school as his "baby," and many hold him up as a model for the Malawian doctor. I find it interesting that people who opposed the medical school project frequently minimize or dismiss his central role in the College of Medicine's creation and early operation, the better to characterize it as an expatriate project. I will come back to this issue in the discussion of the college's "Malawianization" or lack of it in chapter 6.

❧

The first students to begin their medical-school training in Malawi walked through the doors of the new college during a time of national jubilation, only four months after Banda's regime was finally defeated in 1994. Several students and doctors I interviewed were the children of political refugees. Some described uneventful homecomings when Banda's regime was crushed at last, but others had darker stories: a father who was never the same physically or emotionally after being jailed for years, a relative who died in mysterious circumstances after protesting against the regime. Many had reasons to fear politics, but they also inherited a rich tradition of activism. They knew the names of Hastings Banda, David Livingstone, Robert Laws, Daniel Malekebu, John Chiphangwi—and they knew that Malawi's history of religious and political activist doctors was deep and ambiguous. The first of the new doctors to be entirely domestically trained completed their internships in December 2000 as the bloom was fading off the rose of multiparty democracy. At the time I worked among them, both the health-sector infrastructure and the health indicators of Malawi's people continued to erode—from bad to unspeakably bad.

Malawi's doctors-to-be, then, decided to attend medical school in a region where the power to heal was a force for both good and harm, where healers propped up but perhaps more often threatened state authority. They learned at the intersection of global curricula and local exigencies, the intersection of poverty and technology. They became doctors in a part of the world where biomedicine was a colonial tool, sometimes even a weapon—but also a force wielded by Africans moving toward independence and self-regulation. They began their practices in a setting in which the "physician" as signifier was unusually multivalent and even contradictory: social and political elite, humanitarian, authoritarian, colonizing influence, activist, dictator. In the chapters ahead, I examine the paths they followed and the ways they came to think about their work.

꩜

Serving Our Nation
Joe Phoya

It was Martyrs' Day when Joe Phoya poked his head into the door of my office for an interview, asking with a grin "Am I welcome?" The March 3 holiday commemorates protesters who were killed in a 1959 demonstration against the unwanted federation with Northern and Southern Rhodesia. In the Banda era, labor and pleasure were both strictly forbidden on Martyrs' Day. Foreigners could be ousted and Malawians jailed on real or trumped-up charges of having a drink or a party, or of unnecessarily working. The ethos began to change in 1992 when underground letters suggested that citizens also remember the "new martyrs," those activists executed under Banda, on this day. Nowadays most businesses still close, but one may go to work if one wishes. In 2002, it still felt slightly transgressive to do so, though, and the campus was very quiet on the third of March. We had plenty of privacy even with the door of my tiny converted-storeroom office open. It was malaria season, but the fresh, damp air allowed the heavy scent of the burning Chinese mosquito coil to dissipate; as Joe told me his story, the coil's glowing ember curved very slowly inward, leaving on my desktop a perfect gray shadow-spiral of ash.

Joe grew up not far from John Chilembwe's old church, Providence Industrial Mission, in what is now a densely settled and mostly poor neighborhood in southern Malawi. His mother farmed their family's maize and vegetable plot; his father, in Joe's words, was a small-scale businessman. He clarified with a laugh, "I call it small-scale, but it's *really* small-scale! Just to enable the family, you know, to eat—breakfast, supper." Both parents had attended primary school but had dropped out somewhere around the equivalent of fourth grade. For his mother, Joe explained, this was partly about family pressure. "In those days in Malawi, education for a female was like—once one knew how to read and write, they would say, 'Ah, we want you to go have children, we want you to have children!'" His parents had just enough resources to keep their own children in school and just enough faith in the educational sector to believe doing so might be worthwhile.

I had met Joe for the first time when he was a premedical hopeful. By our Martyrs' Day interview, he was a few months into his first year of medical school proper. In his early thirties, he was one of the oldest new students on campus, and he was nearly giddy with the pleasure of having made it this far on his journey to become a doctor. "I started as a clinical officer and then progressed into this program. I have worked before, I have had experience with patients before. But when I finished school, I did not have an opportunity to go straight into medicine, so I had to use other channels in order to meet my objective." He broke into a wide smile. "So, yeah—now here I am! Studying medicine!"

I asked him why he wanted to study medicine. "Sometimes, as children, you just have ambitions for things," he said.

> When my mom would take me to a clinic, when I was sick, I could see those people clad in white attire. Apart from being scared of injections, I would say, "Ah! When I recover, I should become somebody who puts on the white coat." Because, you know, the white attire looked so appealing to me. And they had this thing, which I never knew was a stethoscope. . . . And then as I grew up, I looked at the health care system in Malawi, too. And I saw the sick, and I had that passion to assist. But then how could I do it? How could I help? That's when I said, "Ah—let me go do this training." So the real drive started way back. But the secondary motivator was the fact that I had that passion: I would love to help.

But, Joe said, he met with some setbacks when he set out to fulfill this passion.

> I loved medicine, I wanted to study medicine, and in school I thought I was capable enough to study medicine. When I wrote my MSCE [national exams taken at the end of secondary school], I managed to do well, but I was not chosen for college. I was very disappointed and discouraged. I never thought I would do anything; all my dreams I thought were shattered. And there came this pastor and said, "Ah, boy, you still have a chance actually to do well. You can have your dreams realized. You never know how God is trying to do it. So why don't you try this clinical officer program?"

Following the advice of his pastor, Joe trained first as a clinical officer at a mission hospital. He practiced for a time at the mission, but when he applied for a public-sector post, he learned that his degree was not recognized by the government. Joe retook the clinical officer's course at Malawi College of Health Sciences, another three-year training program. His first government posting was in a remote district. He described his arrival there as "a shock"—particularly in the operating theater.

> I don't want you to think that the mission had so many supplies, so much equipment—but when I got to the district, there was no equipment, no proper supplies. It was difficult to know what to do there when we had cases that needed to be operated. By the end of the day, you are quite frustrated. Because you know what you want to do for your patient, but then you don't have the resources, the materials to use.

In the district and mission hospitals where he'd worked, the physicians Joe had encountered were mostly expatriates. The majority of them had not actually wanted to come to Malawi, he believed, but felt obliged because the country had so few doctors of its own. He read their unwillingness to be there from their behavior: a few were overtly racist, most just standoffish, erecting a huge social distance between themselves and their patients and coworkers. Some of these doctors were afraid of operating—in some cases terminating their contracts early—because of the high local HIV rates. More than one refused to touch patients altogether. Others, though, were exemplary. Speaking of two doctors who had worked over a decade in a rural location, he drew a sharp contrast with other expatriates:

> They love the work; it's the spirit that they have. And the people love them. The reason is they have no boundaries: they are not Malawian, but they treat each and every patient equally. And they are really hardworking. These two characteristics that I am talking about, loving and hardworking, are what occur to me. My initial idea to become a doctor was actually further boosted when I saw these guys, saying, "Why can't I become like them? I think I see what it is to be a doctor." It's going beyond what you yourself can realize that you are doing.

But why should he become a doctor when he was already a clinical officer? "I feel if I should qualify as a doctor, definitely I should be proud to serve our nation and be called Dr. Phoya. Dr. Phoya!" He laughed at the sound of it. "That gives me satisfaction." I pressed him: the satisfaction of status?

> Exactly, that's right. People who you might meet on the way, in buses or whatever, right? When they learn you are studying at the College of Medicine, they have their pupils dilated. Because one thing that I must tell you is that people consider the medical college as one of the most difficult. The most difficult! So when you tell them, "I'm at the College of Medicine," they look at you, they say "Eeh!" They consider you as someone who is extremely wise.

The status of physician was higher than that of the clinical officer, and so was the authority—in the hospital and beyond.

> As a doctor, you have command. But also, you know, a general feeling for the nation. Malawi is one of those developing countries, and you will discover that it has very few doctors. One of the reasons why it is important to do this training is actually to boost up the number of doctors in Malawi: join the field, and then at the end of the day we'll have a lot of doctors. One of the reasons why a clinical officer would want to switch and to become a doctor is to actually try to *fill up* the country, to where we have a patient/doctor ratio being very, very good. As we grow, Malawi as a nation. . . . it's pretty difficult, of course, to talk about the future, but sometimes you just imagine. You just imagine. After working for a year or so, God willing, I would wish to do a specialty. That is if—if God still gives me life. I would love to be at a place where I feel my services would really be needed and recognized. I feel I have that obligation to serve my nation.

Even after specialty training, however, Joe hoped to be posted back in a district hospital.

> Coming to a central hospital where you already have maybe two, three, four, five consultants, it would be a bit—it doesn't really [*trails off*]. . . . Then you talk of a district hospital, or a mission hospital which does not even have a doctor. So I feel it would be much better to go to a place where your services can be fully utilized. You can be fully utilized. My love is to serve the people out there. To serve them.

The interview went on for some time. As it drew to a close, I asked Joe if there was anything else he would want me to pass on to people in the United States.

> It's nice to have our own medical school. But these guys should real-
> ize that training as a doctor in an African country is not easy. What
> it needs is that the world out there should recognize us and give us
> help, you know? We are a developing country, especially in the medi-
> cal field. Medical work is quite demanding. It needs a lot of equipment,
> resources, those kind of things. So my request is: Guys, assist us! Maybe
> with learning equipment or resources. Especially now that the school
> has increased the number of students, no longer ten per year—it's now
> over sixty. I know that right now the college is struggling financially.
> And if you guys out there cannot assist us, then progress cannot be ours.
> It may be there, but it will be so sluggish. We want things to move fast!
> We want at least to be closer to other places out there. We know we
> cannot get close enough, we cannot be like them, but at least we can
> strive toward that goal. So my last plea to our friends out there, wher-
> ever you'll be presenting, you can maybe tell them that Malawi College
> of Medicine students would love if they could assist us.

Last time I saw Joe, he was only a few months from graduation. It was a happy but brief reunion, with little time to talk; he was on his surgery clerkship and working very hard with the interns on this busy service. He continued to hope for specialty training but knew he would likely be posted as a generalist in a district hospital first. And he once again asked me to pass on the plea for assistance.

⚇

In the District
Evelyn Kazembe

Evelyn Kazembe was an only child, the daughter of two primary school teachers who worked in a rural part of central Malawi, "not a rich family, and not very poor." She had fond childhood memories of the three of them sitting around a table in the evenings, both parents working over their les-

son plans while Evelyn read her schoolbooks and asked questions. As she
grew older, she found that she did particularly well in the sciences.

> And I said, "I'm going to do anything that is quite challenging! Any-
> thing to do with science that is challenging." I thought of engineering.
> I said, "Ah, engineering is not good enough." Because I think I just had
> this heart for people. To serve. Just to deal with people rather than to
> deal with machines or whatever.

To get into the medical school, she first had to study for a science degree at
the university. It was a particularly difficult place for girls, Evelyn recalled.
"When we first got to Chancellor College, people were like intimidating
us. '*You* cannot easily go to College of Medicine. They want people who
perform very well'—and all that. But just because I had this desire to really
do it, I prayed that I should really do it."

She really did it. At the time I spoke with her, Evelyn was a fourth-year
student. She had learned enough diagnosis and management to feel she
could be useful, and with several other students had badgered the administration to be allowed to spend holidays in hospitals in their home districts.
"At the end of the year, we have two months of vacation. So instead of just
roaming around during those two months, or going to do some other things
that are not medical-oriented, we just thought we could have an opportunity to be exposed to clinical work." The students' arguments must have
been persuasive. Armed with letters of introduction, each student who
wished to headed off to one of the districts.

> That attachment wasn't paying, but the clinical experience and that
> satisfaction that I had after managing people—it was quite challenging,
> but when people stand up on their feet, get well, and go home, it was
> *very* satisfying. I think it's just the satisfaction that you get after treat-
> ing people. If somebody comes, they are very sick, you manage them,
> and they go home well, it just satisfies!

I asked for clarification: she actually treated patients, as (then) a third-year
student?

> Yeah! I remember, I was supervised by the district health officer [the
> hospital's sole physician] just one week. That's when he was available;
> the other times he was busy with workshops and all that. And the ward
> that he attached me to, I was usually alone or with a clinical officer.

The thing is, I did not pose as someone who is more knowledgeable than anyone else. Because apart from the DHO, the others are clinical officers who have not done the MBBS program that I have done. But they are clinicians. They have been trained in health sciences. I benefited quite a lot from them, because I made sure my relationship with them was good—otherwise, if I posed as someone who is higher than they are, they wouldn't help me.

Evelyn found it especially pleasing to be working in her own home district, where "most of the patients were people I knew, or some of them were just people who heard that, oh, so-and-so is at the hospital."

When they came, they were so free and comfortable! And they were actually more open to me, because they knew I was somebody from there and I would help them. And for me, I was just happy to help them because I knew I was helping my own people. Yeah, and—the other thing is, I know after finishing, chances of working in such a place, or chances of working in my home district are very slim. You know? There are so many things that I want to do after. I will do internship in the referral centers. After that, I may want to upgrade, to specialize and all that. And who knows, maybe I will get married and my husband will be in the city! So it was, it was just a good opportunity to work in the rural area, one. Two, to work among my own people. Many others went to their home areas. There were people all over the nation, students working in their home districts.

It was a good experience, but it left her with some concerns. Evelyn had seen how poorly the clinicians were paid at the district hospital. The district health officer was off at workshops because they supplemented his income, while many of the clinical officers had private practices where they worked in their off-duty hours, often following a shift at the hospital with a shift at their own small *chipatala*. Evelyn worried about these financial constraints and other difficulties as she speculated on her own future.

Being a physician is—yeah, there are such things that we have talked of, the status and the reward of satisfaction—but when it comes to monetary reward, it is very difficult. We've heard, we've seen our friends who have finished here who are leaving and now are working, but—it's really pathetic. The salaries, the money that they get is pathetic. And you can just imagine if you have your own family. You have children and

all that. How can you survive? How can your family survive on such
an amount of money? And the other thing is the workload. Apart from
the long working hours, even during your normal working hours, there
is so much workload in the hospital. . . . people really get overworked.
And sometimes instead of offering or delivering the best you can, you
end up just doing what you can do, to make sure that everyone is being
managed. There are so many patients waiting for your care and all that.
So instead of managing one patient in the best way you could, you don't
do that, and I think that's difficult. Especially when you know you are
supposed to do something and you can't do it.

Despite the challenges, Evelyn felt that working in medicine was slowly
making her a better person: more grateful, more humble, and more skilled.

> Now the ward is part of my life. Seeing people suffering every day is
> like, at least I can appreciate that I am alive and I am not sick! And the
> other thing I think is just attitude toward people. I am learning to—to
> work with them. The ones who are less privileged, the vulnerable peo-
> ple, those who are sick, who really need help and all that. And seeing
> the way that different doctors handle people, I think I am learning to
> also create that positivity.

A year and a half after this interview, Evelyn graduated from the College of Medicine. She spent the eighteen months of her internship at a referral center, as planned. She was not selected for a specialty training program, however, and instead secured a placement at a rural district hospital
about six hours' drive (or an all-day minibus trip) from her home district.
The place has become one of the finest district hospitals in Malawi, and
by all accounts a substantial reason is its DHO, Evelyn Kazembe. She is
well known for being there in the district, managing the hospital and seeing patients rather than spending all her time off at workshops. She has
forged a collegial working relationship with a powerful transnational medical organization that runs a local clinic, one that previously functioned in
complete independence from the government health services. Midwives
who work there told me the alliance has made both programs stronger and
has led locals to trust both the government and the NGO more than they
once did.

CHAPTER THREE

Paths to Medicine

W
ho got the opportunity to become a doctor in Malawi, why, and at what cost? How did gender, class, and religion intersect on the paths to medicine? The answers are important because they make clear that, even before they began their medical training, these students were no generic "us" elsewhere. They brought with them to school social distinctions, personal histories, and motivations for medical work that mattered for their trajectories through training. They positioned themselves in stories of their nation's advancement in ways that help us to understand both the pleasures and frustrations they would feel in the years ahead.

In some respects, the College of Medicine student body reflected the polyglot, multiethnic, culturally pluralistic population that results from Malawi's position as an African crossroads. Students hailed from all regions of the country and a wide variety of ethnicities; Malawi's tiny but economically prominent Asian minority was represented, and a small contingent of foreigners from nearby African countries added to the ethnic and linguistic diversity.[1] Some students had grown up in two-parent households and some in polygynous families, some with guardians after the death of one or both parents, plenty with one parent while the other migrated for work.

In other respects, the students were substantially different from their Malawian age-mates. They were overwhelmingly urban, although about four-fifths of Malawi's population is still rural. In a society that stresses early marriage, most were unmarried.[2] Two-thirds were men. Almost all were Christian. Many had spent years abroad as children of an elite class. And, of course, all were very highly educated—even before they began their medical training.

Routes through School

When the students I knew were children, even primary education was not available to all who wished to enroll. Not until 1995, under the new government, was "free" primary education guaranteed; even then, it was neither compulsory nor universal. Uniform fees, costs of educational materials, and travel distances presented significant obstacles to entering and regularly attending primary school. Women were Malawi's primary farmers, cooks, and tenders of the sick, so girls' labor in the home and fields was especially hard to do without. Poorer and more rural families often needed their children's labor and were particularly likely to withdraw girls from school. By completing primary school, these students already differed from most of their age-mates (Davison 1993).

Secondary school differentiated them more sharply. Secondary education was never guaranteed by the state, places were quite limited, and families had to pay.[3] Doing well on the primary school–leaving exams did not ensure selection. In the Banda era, regional quotas for secondary enrollment were instituted openly; popular anti-north sentiment supported the life president's sharp restriction of higher-education slots for Malawians from the northern region. The end of Banda's rule meant the end of official regional quotas. Still, students who had struggled to find secondary school placements believed that classmates from politically important districts or families were more likely to be selected for further education, no matter what their examination scores. Indeed, students from more privileged homes tended to confirm that impression: many had stories of family members exploiting connections to secure them coveted spots at government schools, temporarily adopting them out to kin in less competitive districts, or gathering funds to get students into mission schools. Failing funds or connections, students had very limited prospects, although a few did come in through a back door such as the perennially troubled Malawi College of Distance Education.[4]

Both educated and uneducated Malawians commented frequently on the poor and deteriorating quality of public education.[5] Even when a student made it to—and through—secondary school, success in proceeding to the next level was increasingly likely to elude her. By 2000, only about 13 percent of public-school students actually passed the Malawi School Certificate of Education (MSCE) examination needed to be eligible for further education. The chances that any young Malawian would make it through the eight standards (equivalent to grades one to eight), the four forms (equivalent to grades nine through twelve), and the school-leaving examinations were slim.

The chances for young women were slimmer (see table 3.1). At each level, girls from poorer families were likelier to drop out than wealthier ones, so that by the time students reached the medical school, differences based on gender were difficult to disentangle from differences based on socioeconomic status. Female students were substantially and significantly younger than males, they came from more educated families, and their parents were more likely to be professionals.[6] I knew a few female students who had come up through the public school system, but in the small cohort of women, a disproportionate number were the daughters of politicians and business magnates.

Not all students had to navigate the difficult paths to and through the public school system, of course; many came from families wealthy and powerful enough to ensure that no such maneuvering was necessary. One described failing at one prestigious international school, only to be whisked into another by her well-connected father: "All my life I've been an A student, only it has never really happened because small things affect me and I stop working at it because I get depressed, so I get Bs and Cs or even Ds and Es" (Thokozani Sokela, second-year student). Several such privileged students had years of education abroad; nearly a fifth of the students I interviewed were children of diplomats who had traveled extensively, their school fees subsidized by the Malawi government.

Students needed at least some postsecondary training in the sciences as

TABLE 3.1. Educational attrition and gender in Malawi

| | Malawians age 20–29 (%) | |
Highest level of education attended	Males	Females
None	10.8	23.9
Any of standards 1–4 (grades 1–4 equivalent)	24.1	31.1
Any of standards 5–8 (grades 5–8 equivalent)	35.0	30.5
Any of forms 1–4 (grades 9–12 equivalent)	29.4	14.3
Any postsecondary education	0.6	0.2
Median number of years total education	6	3

Source: Data calculated from National Statistical Office (Malawi) and ORC Macro (2001), table 2.4, using the age cohort (20–29) to which most medical students belonged; the survey published in 2005 no longer contains data on postsecondary education.
Note: Numbers do not total 100% due to rounding.

well. One of the few places to get that training was at a prestigious prepara-
tory school: Kamuzu Academy, or "KA," as the students called it. In the
college's earliest days, nearly all the medical students were KA graduates.
To enter the College of Medicine, one had to have taken A-levels (topi-
cal examinations that in Malawi follow two years of college-level work);
KA was one of only two places in the country such exams were offered.
The academy, a prestige project built and funded by Life President Kamuzu
Banda, was a compound of gracious brick buildings on a lush green lawn set
outside the dusty town of Kasungu in a relatively remote area of Malawi.
From its opening in 1981 until the late 1990s, it was unquestionably the pre-
mier spot for secondary education in the country. The highest-performing
students from each district in Malawi were sent to KA on full scholarship
to be drilled by expatriates—Malawian teachers were prohibited—in a rigorous British-public-school-style curriculum.[7] Some of the students came
from wealthy urban families, some were the academic stars of remote village schools. Whatever their origins, at the end of four years together in this
"Eton in the bush" (Carroll 2002), they sounded alike, walked alike, dressed
alike. Medical student Kamwachale Mandala called the process "blending"
and saw graduates as sharing not just behaviors but character: "Actually,
you can pick out: *this* guy is from the Kamuzu Academy, *this* guy is from
the Kamuzu Academy." Although he had not attended KA, Kamwachale
spoke not with scorn but in a tone of envious admiration. It was a highly
prestigious education, and graduates of the academy who did not enter the
medical school often went on to fill major government posts or to advanced
studies outside the country.

Originally, the other pathway to entry into the College of Medicine
was through science studies at the University of Malawi's Chancellor College. One still had to be academically solid to enter Chancellor College,
capable of passing university entrance examinations, but because fees
were high and scholarships rare, students taking this path tended to be less
socioeconomically diverse. Students who successfully completed two years
(earlier, three years) of the science curriculum were eligible to compete for
positions at the College of Medicine.[8]

Unlike the decorous Kamuzu Academy, Chancellor College had a reputation for rowdiness and partying that followed some of the students to the
medical school. It could be a particularly hard place for women; some of
those who talked to me described pervasive harassment of female students
there.[9] Many had worried that the atmosphere would distract them from
academic success and saw Chancellor as an option "if the worst come to
the worst," as clinical student Florence Assani said:

I looked at myself and I thought that I was weak-minded, so with a period there of peer pressure and everything, I thought that maybe I could be taken up by such things and forget about my school. So I wanted to be in an environment where I can be able to control myself and study very hard.

Not many of the students who entered the Bachelor of Science program with the intent to study medicine ultimately did so, whether because of the environment or for other reasons. Chancellor College professors estimated that fewer than one in ten first-year aspirants actually made it to the medical-school interview stage by their second or third years.

Recruiting from Chancellor College and Kamuzu Academy consistently produced entering class sizes of fifteen to twenty-five—and typically, after failures and withdrawals, fifteen graduates a year. In 2002, under intense government pressure to step up production of doctors, the College of Medicine took measures to increase enrollment dramatically by instituting an intensive one-year residential premedical program during which the entire two-year A-level curriculum in biology, chemistry, physics, mathematics, and English was taught. Students who passed the premedical program were to be "considered for admission" to the MBBS program; in fact, successful completion of the premed program essentially guaranteed one's acceptance to the medical school. The program proved immensely popular, attracting eight to ten times as many applicants as there were available spots. It made it possible—in theory—for students to complete any secondary school, spend one year in premedical training, and enter the college. The low passing rate for MSCEs in the public schools meant that in practice, students in the premedical program were overwhelmingly either those from elite families who were able to attend the private and expensive "international" high schools in Blantyre and Lilongwe, or students with prior clinical experience who sought to upgrade their basic science knowledge and improve their chances of admission to medical school.

These clinically experienced students made up about a fifth of the student body (more in recent years) and were a group quite different from the others: older, all male, more likely to be married or have children, well versed in the realities of medical practice in Malawi, and in general from considerably less privileged backgrounds. Although a few laboratory technicians, nurses, and others were part of this group, the great majority were clinical officers who had either completed their training and come directly to the College of Medicine or, more often, practiced for a few years before returning to school. A diploma in clinical medicine, the credential for clinical officers, made one eligible to interview for admission to the college, and some clinical officers had been admitted directly. But because the first few to enter did not do well academically and were withdrawn from the school, direct entry became stigmatized (even though clinical officers in later years performed well). By 2003, it was more common for clinical officers to do a year's premedical training first, to improve their chances of entry into—and success once in—the medical program. This group of experienced clinicians was set apart in some ways from the clinically inexperienced majority of students, as readers will note in the following chapters; the differences went beyond demographics, but their generally lower social-class origins were part of what shaped their experiences.

Many students, graduates, and others were suspicious of the academic qualifications of the new matriculants, claiming that the push to increase class sizes fast meant risking the quality of Malawi's doctors by admitting "every Jack and Jim," as disgruntled intern Duncan Kasinja put it. Some went further, hinting that under pressure from the government, the college might even be falsifying student qualifications. As one second-year student suggested, "There are stories that some of the students did not pass [the premedical program], yet they are found in the first year. This dilutes the medical career—furthermore, it will make bad doctors in future."[10]

Some of these concerns about low standards probably reflected discomfort over class and gender. Many students and faculty members felt that academic and social differences were increasing rapidly as the new premedical program and increasing inequality in Malawian society affected the makeup of the entering classes.[11] Some faculty members looked back a little wistfully to the days when the school attracted only "the academic cream," as several of them phrased it, while defending what they saw as a move to attract students from a broader spectrum of Malawian society. Others saw the admission of clinical officers, who were generally from less privileged families and were assumed by many faculty members to be less intelligent, as a sign of falling social and academic standards. It is difficult to be certain about these changes, as the college collects almost no demographic data on its students. However, there were more women in the new classes and probably also more economic elites. Kamuzu Academy had once been a source of socioeconomically diverse students. Since the new government swept into power in 1994, in part on a promise of universal free primary education, the formerly generous state budget of Kamuzu Academy was diverted to fund basic education. The merit scholarships were gone, and KA became a private school for the children of the rich—as were the schools that sent most students to the premedical program. Chancellor College, experiencing severe financial difficulties, had been forced to close for months at a time "for renovations and repairs," a phrase widely translated among Malawians to mean an inability to pay teachers or utility bills. The enrollment from Chancellor slowed to a trickle. In the meantime, enrollment by clinical officers and medical technicians, generally not from wealthy families, rose. These students made up a small proportion of the College of Medicine's total enrollment, but unlike the students from poor families who had been trained into the habits of the elite through Kamuzu Academy, they were a visible minority.

These distinctions mattered to the students and shaped their experiences of training to some extent. But it is important to remember that whether they came from the one-year premedical program, entered with diplomas in clinical medicine, or had bachelor's degrees in biochemistry, these students were all part of Malawi's tiny educational elite. Of their agemates, only 1 in 169 men and 1 in 529 women had any schooling beyond secondary level. Whatever the collective identities they brought with them to school—in years past, perhaps KA scholars or Chancellor rowdies, but recently a somewhat more diverse set of group identities—they were all in that fraction of a percent. By the time the new medical recruits stepped between the painted metal gates and entered the medical school, and to an extent far greater than their North American or European counterparts, they were already exceptional.

This exceptional status, of which students were well aware, was the quotient of a very small numerator of postsecondary-educated and moderately wealthy Malawians and a very large denominator of extremely poor Malawians with scanty educational or occupational options. Both the privation of the many and the privilege of the few were evident in the accounts students gave about how they came to medicine.

One consequence of the nation's poverty was the paucity of options for the few people who did make it into tertiary education. For many students, medicine felt less like a choice than an inevitability, the direction in which teachers steered African students with science aptitude. Postgraduate programs were very limited in number. No doctoral programs of any kind were available in country, and the few master's-level programs were offered erratically. As clinical student Dumbisyani Zinyemba explained, "In Malawi, we don't have diverse courses where you can go, for example, through to do science, pure science—you end up just teaching in secondary school—so that's not more attractive, it's less attractive than medical work." (Teachers' pay and working conditions were poor; science teaching without laboratory equipment was a matter of giving rote lectures that students had to take on faith, an unappealing prospect to many with a true passion for science. Many students, including plenty whose parents were teachers, agreed with Dumbisyani that teaching was an unattractive proposition.)

In addition, some of the other options that were available on paper were unreliable in reality. Students often took into account the relative instability of Malawi's other tertiary schools when compared to the College of Medicine. The Polytechnic and Chancellor College were closed on and off for financial reasons; the College of Medicine had once opened two weeks late but had never actually closed, and for that reason, as a group of second-year students concluded, "If you want a serious education, this is the only place you can go." Students counterbalanced the long years of training at the College of Medicine with the likelihood of interruptions to training at the other constituent colleges of the University of Malawi. Tuntufye Chihana, a fifth-year student, had chosen medicine for this reason:

> The way the tertiary education system is in Malawi, you will find—by the time I was finishing high school, this college was the one that was, like, stable. Because the others, they would be closing all the time. So I'm wanting to go somewhere I knew I would finish when [and] as I expected, so this seemed to be the best choice.

The College of Medicine was stable, well funded, and offered a usable degree for a tuition no higher than that at any other tertiary educational site in Malawi, and lower than some.[12] These were advantages many of the students took into serious consideration.

Pragmatic reasons pushed many students to train as doctors, then. Most, however, understood medicine as a vocation, a duty, or an opportunity to "uplift our nation."

A Mission to Help: Medicine as Vocation

Students often felt called to medicine as a mission, or a vocation, and many first experienced this mission after an encounter with poverty or suffering. (Mkume Lifa, whose story preceded chapter 2, was one such student.) Occasionally, they were guided by dreams to this calling.[13] More often it was an encounter with illness—their own or others'—that showed them what their mission must be: the connection they felt with medical personnel who aided them through illness and recovery sparked their own desires to become doctors.[14] Arthur Kamkwamba had suffered from a badly infected leg wound as a child. An uncle who was a medical assistant gave him such meticulous care that he was saved from a proposed amputation. Going into medicine, Arthur said, was "the only way I can respect the good job he did for my leg."

I heard similar fond reflections on many a childhood fascination with medical professionals, whether kin or strangers, Malawians or expatriates— their status, their power, and their accoutrements. The mysterious stethoscope made its appearance in these stories: what *was* that thing the doctor (or clinical officer) put on one's chest as one sat in the crowded outpatient department with a bout of childhood fever and cough? About a third of the students I spoke with at some point in the interview described the mesmerizing grandeur of the white coat, whether espied on someone else when they were children or worn by themselves today. One student's term for the white coat, *whitements*, with its echo of religious vestments, directly invoked the image of a priesthood of science. The doctor's long white coat, emblematic of status, purity, cleanliness, laboratory science, seemed an unchallenged and much-desired metonym of biomedical glory. Students often felt called to wear that coat.

The language of the call curiously combines a sense of moral rightness and certitude with a sense of passivity. A vocation is felt, experienced, imposed upon one by the supernatural. One's choice is simply to accept or resist.[15] This experience of vocation was especially common among students for whom the calling to medicine took an explicitly religious form, those who heard God calling them to become doctors, perhaps in a dream or through the intermediary of another person. A preclinical student described the intercession of a stranger, who had experienced a vision of the student and told her that God had an important purpose for her. An intern described his Christian mother's steady urgings that he live in such a way that he could help others, until he gradually felt directed by God to medicine as a way to serve. Others described their own scholastic performance as revealing divine purpose: "The way things were working out, I just thought that maybe God wants me to do this" (Saul Kaleso, first-year student).

The language of mission and calling was also a very Christianized one and reflected another way that students differed from Malawians as a whole: although Malawi's population is often estimated as one-fifth Muslim, nearly all the students identified as Christians.[16] Students frequently volunteered their church affiliations (and asked about mine) in interviews and casual conversations. God's will and guidance were common themes of discussion, although far more so among the basic science and premedical students than among those who were already in the hospital. *Mission* and *calling*, then, were part of a vocabulary that lay ready at hand.

Students often depicted medicine as a choice that felt right, even when they did not use the language of calling, mission, or vocation. Some hoped to "die knowing that I made a difference," as a preclinical student put it. It would be easy to dismiss this sort of comment as morbid romanticism were it not that nearly all of these students actually had intimate experience with death. Given infectious disease and poverty, Malawi has never been a place one would seek out if one wished to have a long and healthy life, but the HIV/AIDS pandemic has dramatically worsened the situation: by age eighteen, more than one in five children had lost one or both parents, and the babies that students and I caught on the labor ward were expected to average a life span of thirty-six years (National Statistical Office [Malawi] and ORC Macro 2005). Students I interviewed were typically in their early to midtwenties, but most had already lost parents or siblings. In fact, *not* losing family was viewed as an exception worth comment, as intern Diana Kondowe made clear: "I was raised so strictly that all of us are still alive in my family."

The context of unpredictably short lives may give some urgency to choosing the right course. Alex Mkweu, a thoughtful and quiet student about to finish his MBBS degree[17] and begin internship, described "the satisfaction I will get afterward" as the most rewarding aspect of medical practice. He had heard that people sometimes got to their forties or fifties and wished they had another chance to do something different with their lives, or made money but felt unsatisfied. "But I believe, if I can do something, if I can continue with the medical profession, and do what I am supposed to do—I think that at the end of my life, I will be able to say I have really utilized my life to the best, to the *best* I could have done." Young doctors for whom medicine was a calling, a mission, what they were "supposed to do," could feel sure they were using their limited time on earth well.

Short lives could cut both ways, however, for the training was long, an investment of many years necessary before one could be working. Families often urged students to try for careers in which they could earn more, as the pay for doctors was known to be poor, and earn sooner. Alex Mkweu's relatives were among this latter group. They had hoped until the last possible moment (partway through a clinical officer's training course) that he would change his mind about a medical career. His family was disappointed, he said, but ultimately, they understood he was doing what he felt he must do. Bridget Nyasulu, a second-year student, explained how the length of training factored in: "So many Malawian families can't afford to have a child at my age going to a college for five years. Graduating at twenty-three? Doesn't help them much. They need you as soon as you've finished form four [secondary school]."

Short lives might also be made shorter by medical work. Teachers and family members feared a difficult future—or a short one—for the would-be doctor. Davies Msiska got blunt advice from his teacher: stay out of that career if you value your life.

> DAVIES: Already since form three [grade eleven equivalent], I had somehow known that I wanted to do medicine, only I told my teacher, and he said, "If you want to die quickly, you can do medicine," and so I was a bit discouraged. And when I told my parents, they also were discouraging me. They said, "You are doing well in school. Why not law, why not education?" . . . So when the letter came that I was accepted, I talked to my dad, and Dad told me not to go. And I really wanted to go, but I wanted to please Dad, too. And they gave a two-week grace period, and in the second week of classes, I was still in Ntchisi,[18] but finally I said, "I want to do this," and my parents, they accepted, so I began. . . .
>
> CLAIRE: Why do you think they were discouraging you, and why did you want to do it?
>
> DAVIES: Ah, yes! My teacher especially, I will always remember when we are preparing for MSCE exams, he says, "You will be dying quickly if you can do medicine." He said unless, maybe, I could go and practice outside the country. "But as soon as you come back and open your clinic here, you will be gone, dead." I was a bit, you know, down. Downcast.

I was often told stories of doctors, nurses, and clinical officers who had died from infections caught on the wards. Davies's teacher had particularly feared HIV, although no good evidence confirms that doctors working in Africa are at higher risk for contracting HIV than those in other professions. (The data are inadequate, however, and the risks are real; I will return to this topic in chapter 5.) HIV was not the only risk. Most of the students were aware that a colleague of theirs had contracted multidrug-resistant tuberculosis from patients during clinical training on the medical ward. Zaithwa Mthindi, an intern, became very ill with diarrhea while working on the pediatrics ward as a medical student. It was the rainy season, and the ward was full of children with cholera. Zaithwa's mother, who took care of him during his illness, was afraid he would die. He used this experience to explain to me why he would never encourage a child of his own to do medicine, even though he loved his work and would be proud to see his own child become a doctor.

> Just thinking back, if she had been overencouraging me into medicine and then I ended up in that situation—I mean, thank God I am alive, but what if I had died of that? And then it was her overenthusiasm that "Oh, I want my son to be a doctor"? Yeah. . . . So I think medicine is not something you would want to—in a way—overencourage or force anybody into.

Family Matters: Status, Access, and Social Capital

If families sometimes opposed medical training, more often they were neutral or encouraging. Students and interns often mentioned family members involved in medical work, most commonly nurses,[19] who asked them to consider medical careers. Four women whose mothers or guardians were nurses, and who were themselves drawn to nursing as a profession, reported that their relatives urged them to become doctors instead. Fourth-year student Evelyn Kazembe remembered watching her aunt, a nurse, at work.

> Seeing her work in that field was just, for me, something! OK, maybe it's because I've always had a heart for people. I *liked* it, to see her work for people and do this and do that. And I remember asking her what medical field was like. But she was, like, "If you want to do this, because you have this potential, you can do much better than I did. Please, do medicine. Become a doctor, not just a nurse." And she told me the advantages and the disadvantages. Unfortunately, she just practiced for two years, and she died. . . . And when she died, I was really struck. And I think then I was more, you know, like *more*. . . . I think that was something that pushed me more toward that field. Because my auntie studied this and I want to continue it. I don't want just to do what she did but rather to—to *continue*.

Students and family members used explicitly spatial metaphors to describe a hierarchy of medical personnel that put doctors (mostly male) at the apex, clinical officers (also mostly male) midway down, and nurses (mostly female) below that. (Health surveillance assistants, medical assistants, and other auxiliary personnel were lower yet.) Those relatives who saw their own status as lower on the hierarchy inevitably encouraged students, female or male, to aim for the apex.

> My mother was a nurse, and it just interested me. I actually wanted to do nursing. And then, I had a talk with her, and she was, like, "Come on, you're capable. Why don't you do medicine? You can just try to give it a try. Go to the top, instead of just being a nurse, actually make it to the top." (Chikondi Gomani, preclinical student)

Why did relatives, especially those in more educated families,[20] encourage these young Malawians to become doctors? Some explanations will be recognizable to readers from wealthier countries, while others take on a distinctly Malawian cast.

Status was an obvious factor. Duncan Kasinja, an intern, had scored too low on a crucial exam to apply to medical school.

> To me, this was not a problem. I said, oh, OK, then I will just do accounting. And I was happy with that. But my dad wanted me to repeat, and take the exam again. I said no, I don't want to, and we argued a lot, we had a lot of quarrels. But I still said no, I don't want to repeat. It finally took the intervention of a friend of my dad. He came over and he talked to me for quite some time. He said, "You are the firstborn, and it is important that you do something quite all right, something that people will really look up to. We want you to do something big in your life, your father especially." So, at last, I just said, "OK."

Many students reported that their families, like Duncan's father, wanted to be able to say, "We have a doctor in the family." Some students were living out the lost dreams of their parents: nurses who did not have the opportunity to become doctors, erstwhile academic stars working mundane jobs while their "less intelligent" old friends reaped the glory of medical careers.

No one described medicine as a way to get wealthy, and some explicitly reported that they and their families knew that the salary wouldn't be high. In fact, some students' families pushed them away from medicine because of the cost of training and the famously low pay. Every student but one— and all the interns, all the graduates, and most of the faculty and staff—at some point in their interviews mentioned the low salaries awaiting Malawian physicians. Even students early in their training were generally well aware of the financial difficulties they were likely to face working for the public health sector in Malawi, although the details were often hazy to them at these early stages. The relatively low salaries in medicine probably explain why men and students from backgrounds of lower socioeconomic status, both more likely to be financially responsible for an extended family, were less often encouraged by their families to enter medicine.

Paying for school could also be a major worry for many students. The Ministry of Education subsidized the medical college heavily, so that although the real costs of their education were greater, medical students paid the same fees as students at the other constituent colleges of the University of Malawi: US$263. This cost may appear ridiculously low, but at about 165 percent of Malawi's annual per capita income, it was still daunting for many students.[21] Very few could anticipate defraying their expenses by holding down a job, given the unpredictable hours and crushing workload of medical school. Particularly for the older students, many of whom were from less wealthy families, securing this fee each year was a major challenge.[22]

Other perquisites of medicine in Malawi, however, could offset the long and expensive training, low salaries, and physical risks. Doctors had extensive social capital in their communities that could facilitate a good standard of living and ready opportunities for their kin. If they did not have a high income, at least they had a more or less guaranteed one. Thokozani Sokela, the student whose father moved her from school to school until she passed her exams, reported that he gave job security the highest priority:

> It wasn't the thing I wanted to do. I said, "Dad, I can't stand the sight of blood, I'm afraid to see people all broken and bloody, I don't think I will handle it." But he said, "Being a doctor, you will always find full employment. You will get used to the blood and all."

Full employment, social capital, job security: some families saw these benefits as reason to overcome a distaste for the profession, and sufficient compensation for the financial and physical risks of medicine.

Another crucial benefit was medical access for the relatives. Doctors' families had not only a ready entrée to medical care but also some supervision while getting it. Access to care came up again and again in various permutations during interviews and on the wards. Theoretically, medical care in Malawi was free and available to all. Only a very small initial fee of forty kwacha (about forty-five cents at that time) was necessary to get the mandatory "Health Passport," a small medical records booklet carried around by the patient in which all clinical encounters, from medications given to major operations hazarded to children delivered, were scribbled down. Practically, negotiating the maze of medicine required tenacity, patience, transportation, and resources. Best of all resources were the human ones.[23] Neighbors or acquaintances were potentially useful, but a family member in medicine was even more obligated to help the sick person. Florence Assani, a preclinical student whose siblings were often ill, explained that "I had to fight hard so at least one day I should treat my younger sisters so that they don't suffer." Phillip Tembenu, a clinical officer from a well-educated and prosperous family, saw a brother in medicine as a backup plan:

> There are not many doctors in Malawi. So if I advise my brother not to become a doctor, and I become ill or my relatives become ill, I will need, they will need someone to look after them. So if I advise my brother not to become a doctor, it is like I am giving myself—I am putting my other friends and relatives at risk.

A medical relative was a valuable asset in the bewildering world of Malawian medicine. From their first days at school, these students were serving as medical liaisons for their families, a role that quickly became both privilege and burden and that factored into later career decisions.[24]

Nationalism: Healing the Body Politic

When students talked about their own journeys into the medical profession, or when they proffered advice to others, they often spoke of "healing Malawi" as a reason to become a doctor. Students who had suffered through serious illnesses, or found themselves drawn to medical work as they cared for ill relatives, sometimes remembered their experiences less fondly than the stories given earlier in this chapter suggest; many chafed at the inadequate care available in local hospitals and vowed to make a difference in Malawi's medical system.

Comments about improving the doctor-patient ratio came up in a surprising one of five interviews and half of the focus groups, and clinical officers were especially likely to want to improve the doctor-patient ratio. Simply by becoming doctors, they felt, they would act as agents of development and help lift Malawi out of poverty. Joe Phoya was one of the clinical officers who exemplified this thinking:

> I will make at least a change, you know? In the health system. Because definitely I will in the first place increase the number of doctors in Ma-

lawi. And I am very sure that, for example, if I happen to go back to
Zomba[25]—I know that Zomba does not have enough doctors now. It actually relies on expatriate doctors. I can say 90 percent of the doctors
there are expatriate doctors. I can say there are what, two? Only one
Malawian doctor. The rest are expatriates. Which I feel is not really—
it's not that the expatriates, it's not that they *want* to come. It's that
we don't have enough doctors. So I feel if I should qualify as a doctor,
definitely I should be proud to serve our nation.

As a clinical officer, Joe was already doing surgical cases at Zomba, seeing patients, in most respects performing the work of a doctor without
the title. Why would he and his fellow clinical officers feel that changing
their knowledge bases and their titles—without, they agreed, significantly
changing the nature of their work—would be a stride forward for Malawi as
a nation?

The first clue may be that these students actually knew the doctor-
patient ratios in their country: best estimate 2:100,000—as with many
other indicators in Malawi, one of the lowest in the world. I suspect that
not many British or American medical students could estimate the doctor-
patient ratio in their home countries (230:100,000 and 256:100,000, respectively) within even a decimal place of accuracy.[26] But as a "developing"
or "least-developed" country, Malawi is the target of surveillance by international lending agencies, by donor groups and NGOs, by churches, by
supranational organizations like WHO and UNICEF and UNAIDS. Malawi's statistical rankings in one category or another, nearly always awful,
make the front page of the local news on a regular basis: the *Daily Nation*
headline had proclaimed "Malawi Poorest Peaceful Nation on Earth" a few
weeks before I interviewed Joe. Educated Malawians with access to media
know their country by its statistical measures and understand its degree of
development as a function of those measures: doctor-patient ratio, nurse-
patient ratio, births attended by trained personnel, hospital beds per population, per capita health care expenditure. Statistics like these are often
used to assess a country's medical development—and sometimes, without
documentation of a cause-and-effect relationship, and with no attention to
the problem of maldistribution that makes national-level statistics so misleading, a country's health. In these statistics, clinical officers and their ilk
are invisible, but doctors make a big splash.

Another factor may be crucial to understanding why nationalism often
went hand in hand with the desire to become a physician and why this link

should be particularly notable for clinical officers. Throughout the colonial era, most opportunities for black Africans to receive medical training involved limited and heavily practical curricula leading to a midlevel degree like that of the clinical officer. The midlevel clinicians would have many of the practical capabilities of doctors but more limited basic science educations. They would usually work, at least nominally, under the supervision of a physician. Even when these degrees allowed for independent practice, they were rarely useful outside the bounds of the nation or region—unlike a physician's credentials. These training programs persisted after independence, with many politicians and donors championing midlevel clinicians as appropriate technology for an impoverished continent disproportionately afflicted by disease. But Africans often saw such midlevel training as part of a colonial system designed to keep them subordinate to white "experts."[27] Certainly in South Africa at least, a two-tiered medical education system was a deliberate stratagem of apartheid racism. For many postcolonial educators and policymakers, Africanization of medical schools and medical practice has come to be seen as a crucial component of decolonization (Archampong 1990; van Niekerk 1999). Joe was the only student I interviewed who openly addressed—in another context—the issue of racism. But many students, especially clinical officers, felt the opportunity to become doctors to be a validation of their intellectual capacities and a step toward development for themselves and for their country.

The issue of nationalism, of helping Malawi the country, was not an impetus only for clinical officers. Other students also spoke of medicine as a way to improve the health of their nation. Mirriam Kamanga, a preclinical student, had returned to her country after years abroad just as the famine of 2001–2 hit. With other students at her private secondary school, she bought *ufa* flour and dried fish. Every afternoon during the height of the famine, the students cooked *nsima* and *ndiwo* and distributed these staple foods in nearby villages. Seeing wasted children whose mothers were too malnourished to breast-feed them, she said, "Reality hit and all, and I saw how much children suffered in Africa, Malawi in particular. . . . If I'm a physician here, I hope and I pray that I make a difference to the suffering of children."

The nationalist impulses that drove students like Mirriam and Joe into medicine would have a profound impact on their experience of medical training and their ultimate career choices.

Students came from diverse backgrounds and took diverse paths to join the College of Medicine. By the day they began their medical training, however, they were already members of a small Malawian elite, all by virtue of their advanced education, and many also by virtue of wealthy and well-educated families. Students anticipated an even higher status as doctors yet at the same time acknowledged some economic and physical risks of medical practice—medical practice *in Malawi*, that is. Those who spoke about such risks accepted them for the sake of their calling to medicine.

In their retrospective retellings of their journeys to medicine, students were crafting what historian Steven Shapin (1993) has called "realization stories," narratives that describe how people come to be who they are. These narratives are imperfect guides to historical reality, as Shapin warns; they typically minimize the impact of coincidence and circumstance while exaggerating the agency of the narrator.

> We tell "realization stories" about ourselves, and those who approve of us help us tell them, as a way of stressing the intrinsic springs of our actions and as a way of pouring value on those actions. Because such narratives are storehouses of value, their plausibilities are highly protected by a wide range of everyday and academic practices. (Shapin 1993:338)

Precisely because these narratives are "storehouses of value," however, they are invaluable for understanding cultural meaning-making and the crafting of identity. We can think of identity itself as made up of locations within various stories.[28] As people tell and retell stories of their lives, diminishing—or even omitting—certain salient experiences and amplifying others, and as those stories change and intersect in novel ways, listeners can come to a clearer understanding of how the narrators understand their purposes and trajectories.

In the realization stories that appeared in this chapter, many of these students positioned themselves in relation not only to their profession but also to their religion and to their nation. Medicine was not always a choice: some saw it as the only realistic option available for a Malawian with science aptitude. But most accepted medicine as a vocation or chose it more actively, out of religious or nationalist impulses. Simply by becoming doctors, some assumed identities as conduits for God's healing power. Many saw themselves as agents of development for the country as a whole. This issue of national development was particularly important when students contrasted their future roles as doctors with those of clinical officers. Clinical officers were reminders of a colonial past. Doctors, by virtue of their deep scientific knowledge and the international recognition of their professional role, were evidence of Malawi's modernity. In the many stories students told in which they planned to "uplift the nation," that uplifting would be accomplished not necessarily through the specific day-to-day work of clinical medicine but by the very existence of the new doctors.

ᘉᘏᘆ

Welcome to the College of Medicine

January of 2003 was unseasonably hot.[29] If you were a newly admitted medical student coming from Chancellor College in Zomba to begin at the College of Medicine, and if you traveled packed into a minibus with fifteen other passengers, you would have been drenched with sweat by the time you reached Thondwe a few kilometers along the way. On hot days in this sugar-producing country, workers sometimes sprayed the roads with molasses to keep the dust down; your scent and that of your fellow passengers mingled with the smell of burned sugar. All this heat had most people worried. With the rainy season a month late, everyone's newly planted maize fields were at risk, and after last year's poor harvest, the stakes were especially high.

Most of the passengers chatted quietly or dozed on the hour-plus ride from Zomba town to the big city and through the rich agricultural lands between. Excited and anxious at the start of the momentous journey, perhaps you scanned the familiar landscape instead, newly alert to the signs of affliction and healing along the way. Just as the road left Zomba, a dirt track led east to the compound of a famous herbalist. Africans, Asians, and *azungu* all sought her out for fertility treatments, you had heard: her *mankhwala achikuda* (African medicine) was strong, stronger than *mankhwala achizungu* (European medicine). In the rural stretch that followed, as the road wound among fields thirsty for rainfall, here and there a triangular flag hovering high on a pole marked the business premises of a *sing'anga*, tucked into a clump of trees.

The medicines on offer proliferated suddenly as farmland gave way to the outskirts of the city and the minibus honked and jostled its way through crowds of people. The signs were less subtle, too. Many of the brick structures packing the sloping hills here were half built, abandoned as the builders fell ill or ran out of money. Not functional as dwellings, they did service as billboards, their crumbling walls bright with hand-painted signs. By your rough count, about half the advertisements were more or less medical, touting Novidar SP single-dose malaria tablets, Chishango condoms, or Thanzi oral rehydration salts. Many of the buildings in more active use also offered medical help. As the bus stopped to let off a few passengers and jam a new lot in, you caught a glimpse of Bangwe Health Centre at the top of a hill. The road to it was not marked; anyone who needed it would know where it was. In one- or two-room private clinics lower on the slope, the slightly less poor paid minor fees for minor medical treatments. Many a little *chipatala* like this, you knew, was a money-making enterprise where off-duty nurses or medical assistants supplemented their government wages. A coffin-maker had placed his establishment strategically between the health center and the paved road. Workers planed boards in back while coffins ranging from infant-sized to adult lay displayed on the ground in front.

Western medicine and Malawian carpentry were not the only services on offer to the suffering. Nailed to a tree at the stop where you changed buses to go to the College of Medicine, a signboard claimed in bold black letters that Dr. Mkango used spirit wisdom from Mozambique to treat a long list of complaints, including asthma, infertility, weakness of body, too fat, too thin, business problems, AIDS, and jealousy. It ended with a warning: "Witches Beware!" Posted on an adjacent tree was an offer for a competing service. Apostle Dr. Felix Zalimba would be at the Malawi College of Health Sciences auditorium on Sunday, where he promised deliverance from family curses, disease, and poverty: "Bring All the Bewitched & the Sick."[30] As the bus pulled away, it passed street vendors selling small plastic bags of antibiotics and dewormers. You wondered how many were cheap Nigerian counterfeits and how many were pilfered, perhaps even from the central hospital where you would be learning your trade in the years ahead.

That hospital was close now. Trying to see as a doctor might, you noted the signs of its approach in the bodies of the people thronging the roadside. Beggars, many of them missing limbs, worked the intersection at Ginnery Corner where Queens Hospital sat. Patients learning to use their hand-crank wheelchairs labored slowly up and down the roadside from the nearby orthopedic rehabilitation center. An albino woman rounded the corner as your minibus waited at the "robot" (the stoplight). Nearly every inch of her skin was covered, long sleeves and gloves protecting her from the sun—she must have been sweltering on a day like this one. Her red eyes met yours indifferently as she glanced up from under the shade of a floppy-brimmed hat. Now she saw you as just another traveler, but not long and you might be one of the white-coated doctors excising her skin cancers at a Queens clinic. Perhaps you felt a flush of pride at this thought, perhaps a surge of anxiety.

The minibus turned left when the light turned green, and pulled over at the stop on Mahatma Gandhi Road. Anyone going to the College of Medicine compound had to get off here, retrieve luggage strapped behind the backseat, and walk the packed orange dirt path the remaining hundred meters or so. At the college gate, bougainvillea draped over a white plastered wall where neat metal letters spelled out "University of Malawi College of Medicine."

Here you were at last.

Traffic crowded the gate that day. Some students were brought right up to the compound in the family "saloon car" (sedan), shiny suitcases in hand. Others walked from nearby bus stops, carrying cardboard boxes of clothes and books tied up with sisal twine. Some were boisterous, shouting out to classmates in Chichewa or English—not their first year here, probably. Others looked around them uncertainly, perhaps wondering who would be their friends, not sure where to check in or how to get their class schedules.

The campus spread over a few hectares of sloping land between Mahatma Gandhi Road and the foothills of Mount Soche, the college itself a compact cluster of buildings at the western end. In your parents' youth, this area had been forested, but by now the graceful *mopani* trees had gone to make charcoal, and the cleared areas just beyond the edge of campus were planted with maize, groundnuts, cassava, pumpkins.[31] As you slipped in through the narrow pedestrian passage next to the main gate, to your left was the small medical library, blue tin roof dazzling in the hot sun. Farther down on the left were two modest laboratory and research blocks, one still under construction, and then the main teaching building. You made note of the cafeteria across the way to the right, and the student hostels gathered behind that. All were tidy, blocky brick constructions, plastered and painted white, with gray stripes where the water of rainy seasons past had discolored the walls.

In the main teaching building, where you walked in search of a place to register, two stories of classrooms and offices faced inward onto a small square courtyard. The hallways were lined with tall bulletin boards, on which notices to students were posted: the microbiology lab schedule has changed as follows; there shall be absolutely *no* removal of dishes or cutlery from the cafeteria; Reverend Ngwira will be speaking to the Christian

Medical and Dental Society Tuesday; the following five students must see the dean immediately. Not so different from Chancellor College: all the usual paper indicators of student life.

The lights were all out and the windows all open, for there was no power this morning. The whole country was on rotating blackouts while the power station repaired damage to two of its three hydroelectric turbines; the school's allocated five hours of power were scheduled for the afternoon, though these things often failed to happen as scheduled. You had been assured that minor problems like that would not stop this school. The lecture rooms, designed with such power outages in mind, all had high windows that allowed natural light to filter in. Even on a gray day, the light was good enough to see the blackboard and to take notes. The business of making doctors could carry on largely as usual, and only visiting lecturers who had counted on their computers and projectors were sometimes at a loss.

If you were a new student at Malawi's College of Medicine, you would find the assistant registrar's office and check in, unpack your clothes and hang up your white coat, place your notebook and pen on the desk in your shared room at the hostel, and wait for the breaking of the next day—the day you would begin to learn to be a doctor, the drizzly and foggy day when classes started and the rains came at last.[32]

CHAPTER FOUR

Seeing Deeply and Seeing Through in the Basic Science Years

Malawi's medical course, like that of most Northern schools, began with two years of basic science training before students had extensive contact with patients. The major task set out formally before students was to gain an intimate knowledge of the anatomy, physiology, and pathological processes of the human body. In the same years, less formally but to some extent consciously, students began to learn the bodily dispositions and practical senses they would use as physicians: how to use their own bodies to diagnose pathology. As they learned on themselves, their bodies became models of the universal and hence models of their future patients' bodies. The self that had already stood in for the nation now stood in also for the sick patients they hoped to treat, or served as a measure of the normal for purpose of comparison.

They also trained their bodies to convey medical authority, to show the gravity and constraint they believed was expected of them as doctors. This, too, was in part a conscious process. They became citizen-doctors, or doctor-citizens, members of a worldwide community of scientific doctors, Malawian healers who were sharply distinguished from both the clinical officers and the traditional healers of an African past—even while they accentuated some features of Malawian linguistic and nationalist identity.

During these preclinical years, dissecting cadavers and examining blood smears under microscopes, students willingly took on an identity of "doctor as scientist" very similar to that found in the many North American studies. Negotiating social divisions among their classmates, they experienced strong homogenizing pressures and spoke of them approvingly as part of what made them real doctors. Most took for granted, and many rejoiced in, the high status, reductionistic empiricism, and markers of separateness (such as the white coat) that were becoming part of their professional armamentarium. Conditioned into ways of being and seeing, they gave every evidence of embracing both as paths to full membership in a community of medicine.

Studying the Body

The College of Medicine's curriculum would look familiar to an American or European student. In their first and second years, students studied anatomy, biochemistry, physiology, and community health (the latter something of a grab bag of epidemiology, ethics, psychology, and other topics). Administrators intended courses to be organized by human organ systems, so that as students learned the structure of the gastrointestinal tract in anatomy, they learned the mechanics of digestion in physiology and the metabolism of proteins and carbohydrates in biochemistry. In practice, this coordination did not always happen.[1]

The amount of material to be learned in these first two years of school was enormous, the resources suboptimal, and the stakes very high. Year one ended with a "barrier" exam: if a student didn't pass, he or she had one try at retaking the exams ("sitting supplementals") and, if unsuccessful, had to leave school. Students referred to leaving as "being weeded." Being weeded was more than just the end of one's medical career. The student who failed barrier exams, or flunked out later for any reason, was also barred from the entire University of Malawi system: students got one shot at Malawi's scarce tertiary education resources. If your family could afford to send you outside Malawi to get further education, you might be able to go on. If not, it was time to look for a job. Students rarely talked about classmates who had been "weeded," and then always in respectful there-but-for-the-grace-of-God-go-I terms. Typically, weeding was the fate of roughly 20 percent of the first-year class; of the eleven first-year students I interviewed, three were later weeded. Students with money had a significant advantage, especially after the sudden increase in enrollment stretched already-thin resources. At one point, eighty-seven students were sharing a single embryology textbook that circulated on two-hour loan in the library. (This book-to-student ratio was particularly bad. It was more common to have at least five or ten copies of key textbooks in the library.)[2] The student with money to photocopy essential pages, or better yet to buy the book in South Africa, was one step further from being weeded.

Coursework was heavily didactic. Students sat at long rows of tables in the drafty John Chiphangwi Lecture Theatre, listening for hours to lectures and scribbling down notes on the processes of the human body and the pathogens that can afflict it. When there was electricity, they might have overhead transparencies or slides. When the electricity was out, the blackboard did the job. A typical day included six hours of lecture and two hours of laboratory work, followed by long hours of study in the library or dormitories. Students learned a great deal by rote, in lectures, or from textbooks, but even this knowledge inculcated various bodily practices of concentration and attention. They learned to study on a patch of lawn with a soccer game going on around them, shirts and skins shouting for the ball and pounding up and down the tilted grass field, or in the school library hunched over their textbooks, oblivious to the racket of a monsoon rain on the small building's corrugated iron roof. The capacity to exclude outside attractions and distractions would be helpful to them later in the heat of the operating theater or as they examined one patient at a time in a crowded ward.

Learning continued in the laboratories. In gross anatomy lab, teams of medical students examined the structures of the human body firsthand. The cadavers they studied were laid out on steel trolleys in a white-tiled room that smelled of formalin and where the chattering and laughter of the students echoed off the walls. Here the students, wearing for the first time their white coats and latex gloves (intended by the manufacturers to be disposable but instead carefully washed and hung out to dry between lab sessions), sawed off limbs for closer inspection, dissected out the courses of arteries, nerves, and muscles. They traced the intricate folds and curves of the abdominal and thoracic cavities, glistening internal organs tucked compactly into place yet able to slide around enough to avoid getting stuck or pinched. In the dissection theater, too, their knowledge was embodied. They learned the feel of a scalpel on human flesh, the different depths of pressure needed to cut through skin, fat, fascia. In contrast to some anatomy labs in Northern countries, there were plenty of cadavers—one student mentioned this as a plus of doing training in Malawi—but not enough anatomy atlases or proctors. Students relied on their classmates for guidance and often did dissections without being certain they were finding the structures they were supposed to see.

Bodies are variable, and medical students who use cadavers to learn anatomy quickly come to understand how different bodies are from one another, and from the atlas.[3] When I learned anatomy on the donated bodies of the elderly, many had cancerous growths somewhere. Surgical interventions over their life spans made most of them unlike the pictures in our textbook: several were missing gallbladders or prostates, and we had difficulty finding a female body with a uterus in place. The Malawian students' cadavers were differently different. Relatively few had undergone surgery. They were short, dark, young, heavily muscled or badly wasted, visibly shaped by a social world of very hard work and not enough to eat. They tended to have far less body fat than the anatomy books showed. Cadaveric dissection is supposed to be about learning the normal, but of course every dissected body was a person who had died of something: students quickly learned to suspect AIDS in the thin woman with telltale white deposits of candidiasis in her throat, and to recognize the ravages of malaria in the red-spotted gray of a child's brain matter and in his grossly swollen spleen.

While in anatomy these students dismembered actual bodies, in the rest of their labs they learned to doctor completely disembodied organ systems. In biochemistry and physiology, their teachers taught them the chemical processes of parts of the human body and how to test such processes clinically: how a urinalysis reflects renal function, or what chemical alterations hepatic disorders produce in the serum. A precipitous drop in college funding that coincided with the sudden flood of new student enrollment altered the teaching of biochemistry and physiology. Shortages of staff and of laboratory reagents meant many of their "practicals"—laboratory projects meant to demonstrate the didactic teachings—simply never happened. Even when practicals did take place, scarce supplies made them difficult. I often walked by classrooms in which clusters of eight or ten students huddled around a single microscope (a scene captured, oddly enough, in the College of Medicine's recruitment brochure). In practice, this equipment scarcity meant that each student had only a short time to see and sketch out the tissues they were supposed to examine microscopically. First-year students noted that because of the large enrollment in their class, some students simply could not get close enough to the remaining practicals to see what was happening at all and copied results from other students instead. The student with no results got a failing grade on the practical; it was better to cheat than to fail, and the students considered it justified when circumstances made it impossible to perform in the way expected of them.[4]

Scientific practice and learning are supposed to be about direct observation and experimentation; the test of a theory is the replicability of experimental results. Even where resources are relatively plentiful, however, experiments are rarely repeated unless the results have been called into question for some reason. As historians have pointed out, scientific discovery becomes in part a matter of forming intellectual community: if a trustworthy member of the collective of scientists makes an observation or conducts an experiment, and reports it according to agreed-upon standards, that is adequate grounding to consider it scientific knowledge that belongs to the collective (Shapin and Schaffer 1985:90). In Malawi's College of Medicine, learning scientific medicine in a situation of scarcity worked rapidly toward cementing students' sense of professional community. If one of this group of would-be doctors observed the sickle-shaped red blood cell of a child with joint pain under the microscope, or saw parasitic ova in the stool sample from a patient with diarrhea, that individual's observation could be converted to collective knowledge. The knowledge of doctors was theirs for the use, and the "science" of medicine, founded on precepts of observation and experimentation, was also about setting the boundaries of community. (Perhaps this is why basic science students at the College of Medicine often grumbled about being taught by clinical officers, chemists, or microbiologists rather than doctors, and why medical students in many other places have found lectures given by PhDs or nurses suspect in a way that those by physicians are not.)

As students learned physiology and anatomy in the laboratories, they learned to see—or at least to visualize—the muscles and nerves within their own bodies and those of their (at this point imagined) patients. They spoke of the metabolic processes and embryologic development of their own bodies with awe: as one student described his long hours studying, when learning to see deeper and deeper into the human body, "the greatest thing is that you find your *self* more interesting."

Sight was not the only sense they used. Rachel Prentice (2007) has rightly pointed out that studies of medical training tend to overemphasize the visual: the dominance of sight is especially notable for those theorists who draw heavily on Foucault's concept of the clinical gaze.[5] These students, like medical students around the world, also used their senses of smell, hearing, and touch. Some of this sensory learning happened in the labs, as when students learned that the sweet odor of ketones in a urine sample could indicate uncontrolled diabetes, but it accelerated once they began to encounter living patients. On the wards, they learned the metallic rotten-meat smell of a gastrointestinal bleed and the foul stench of an infection caused by anaerobic bacteria. They learned the sounds of normal and abnormal heartbeats, gut noises, and lung sounds. They came to recognize the high-pitched whistling breath of a child with epiglottitis whose airway was closing. They started to accumulate the palpable knowledge they would need, too. Students began to feel the difference between a hard and gritty cancerous lump beneath the skin of a woman's breast and the rubbery resilience of a fibroadenoma. They learned to place the flats of their hands against a patient's rib cage as he spoke in order to assess the vibrations of "tactile fremitus"—abnormally strong when the patient's lung is consolidated by pneumonia or absent if his lung has collapsed.

In addition, they sometimes used their own bodies as normal controls and as mnemonics. To assess a patient's strength when a muscle-wasting disorder was suspected, they learned to have her resist against their own muscles, measuring the force of her limbs against their own exertion and against their embodied memories of other patients' responses. To test peripheral vision, abnormal in certain neurological problems, they locked eyes with the patient while moving one hand slowly from the periphery toward the center of a vertical plane between them. If the patient and the student doctor saw the hand at the same time, the exam was normal.

Acting Like Doctors

French social theorist Marcel Mauss (1973) described "techniques of the body" as products of imitation and education. We may think of the ways we sit, stand, speak, eat, etcetera, as "natural," but in fact we are educated into how we use our bodies. Some of the bodily practices that doctors learn are explicitly taught; many more are learned (and taught) without ever being formally articulated. Pierre Bourdieu (1977), building on the work of Mauss, further developed the concept of "habitus" to include mundane bodily practices and social actions or "dispositions" that become our ways of interpreting and interacting with the world. One's habitus is in part consciously acquired, in larger part learned through unconscious imitation. It reflects one's membership in certain class, family, educational, and other social categories, but varies among individuals and also in response to external conditions. It is *structured*, then, a product of the individual and collective past, and *structuring*, a mode of perception that reproduces groups and classes.[6] One's habitus is durable but not fixed, culture and society encoded on the body but never simply a conscious product of adherence to rules. It sets the conditions for one's perceptions of and actions in the world, including perceptions and actions that are genuinely innovative.

Brenda Beagan (1998; 2000) and Simon Sinclair (1997) have shown that powerful homogenizing influences in medical school (in Canada and the United Kingdom, respectively) shape for doctors a consistent medical habitus.[7] Time pressures, isolation from those outside medicine, shared experiences, and overt encouragement of conformity work together to mold students into professionals who share a collective identity. Some of these influences also worked among the Malawian students described here. Their nascent doctor habitus seemed especially molded by three major forces, often observable in action and sometimes reflected upon consciously by the students: the active negotiation and resolution of social tensions, which resulted in a welcome homogenization of the student body; the increased status granted them by the community; and especially their own growing medical expertise in the esoteric workings of the corporeal human.

The attentive reader may be struck by how embodied these students' descriptions of becoming doctors were. Male students talked about learning to speak more quietly, females about speaking more forcefully. Donning the white coat took on an outsized prominence. Students felt the respect of fellow Malawians, as Joe Phoya had said, by seeing "their eyes dilate." Modes of dressing, speaking, and interacting became emblems of their new status. Even their new knowledge was embodied: many traced out the lines of muscles and nerves on their own bodies, half consciously, as they talked about what they were learning.[8]

Social Tensions and Homogenization

Living conditions forced students together and accelerated the process of social homogenization. All College of Medicine students, married or unmarried, with or without homes elsewhere, lived in the hostels attached to the college. They worked together, ate three meals and tea together daily in the "caf," quizzed one another on the difficult metabolic pathways of biochemistry in the dorm rooms at night, started and ended game tournaments and romances and feuds, and in general got to know one another very well. Some students chafed at the peer pressure, degree of surveillance, and lack of privacy involved with living in such a small community. "You do something, and the whole campus is talking about it by the next day," said Medson Namanja, "and suddenly, you feel very claustrophobic." Or as Gift Mkango put it, "Sometimes I think, goodness me! Am I in college, or am I in prison?" Most students, however, enjoyed the camaraderie of the hostels. They described themselves as having improved social skills from mixing with "all sorts of people," and as growing more alike despite initial differences. Sometimes this "blending," as a few called it, was a deliberate process; students watched their neighbors and learned to emulate desirable characteristics—and efface undesirable ones.

> [Here] we have a group of people, and you actually sort out *what is a good person*. . . . Either you tend to adapt, or tend to *copy* somebody's character, or in a way, you also *discard* your own characters, if they are

uncomfortable. Yeah. So that has really shaped my understanding, and overall my character. (Kamwachale Mandala, third-year student)

Kamwachale explained that this process of copying and discarding was especially important as a future physician. "With our profession, you and me—because we judge a person by character, and if you are a doctor, a doctor is seen as having the *same* character." Patients and the public expect a consistent self-presentation of doctors:

> So, to me, it is basically a good thing to *blend* the people to do the same. I think I have also blended into the same situation, whereby we have to—we have to *walk* in the same direction. Have the same qualities, yeah. To me, I don't have any problem with that. I don't have any problems with that. Because we are doing the same profession!

To walk in the same direction, to demonstrate the same character, one had to move beyond differences of class, gender, and previous training, as well as those of character.

Class differences were the most visually striking. Among the first- and second-year students, it was easy to distinguish between students from wealthier families and those from humbler backgrounds:

> Now recently we have had this change. . . . [The private-school students] are from a very high class, a high social class. Their families are quite rich. And the difference between these students and the Chancellor students who are basically from the middle class is very large, very striking. The way they interact, the way they dress, the way they speak—it seems even just looking at them, you can tell there is that difference. . . . It was a difficult adjustment for the teachers, because you know we are more used to traditional Malawian style. (Dr. Gregory Wathu, faculty member)

Male students from wealthy families might wear baggy pants and casual shirts, affecting the rolling gait of hip-hop stars as they crossed the campus.[9] Meanwhile, their middle-class colleagues showed up for class in suits and neckties, and those students most strapped for funds wore whatever they had, one I knew alternating all year between two carefully mended shirts. In 2002, a few upper-level female medical students and faculty and most women outside the medical school wore the Malawian women's style called "national wear," consisting of an ankle-length dress, or a *chitenji*, and (sometimes) a head wrap. In contrast, some of the wealthiest first- and second-year women students wore skin-tight pants and belly shirts that their lecturers found shockingly immodest.[10] Women from middle-class families tended to be very quiet and kept to single-sex groups. Women from more privileged backgrounds might be outspoken to the point of being loud, interacting freely with men, rather than conforming to the traditional expectation that women be self-effacing, keeping out of the way—or quietly serving food and drinks—while the men talked. Over time, however, these styles changed. Loud behavior got more subdued. Instead of resembling either American music video stars or traditional Malawians, most students ended up with a more muted sober-young-Western-professional style, although some of the poorest did not have the budgets to carry off this style as effectively as their classmates.[11]

Language was another signifier of difference, one that created tension, and one of many in which students managed an eventual homogenization. The school was a polyglot place; groups of entering students were native speakers of at least nine different regional languages. English was the official language of teaching and the accepted language of laboratories and classrooms. Initially, however, students from the prestigious private academies spoke English not just in class but in the hostel and on the soccer field. Students from the public schools interpreted the English as snobbery. By acting as if they didn't understand the private-school students, they set the linguistic terms on which the student body would interact.

> We found that [English speaking] tough—like, "Is this how we are going to stay here?" But after two, three weeks, some of them now started speaking Chichewa. So we were like, "Ah, now, these people *also* can speak Chichewa!" Yeah [*laughs*]. . . . So it's like when they were speaking to us in English, most of the time it's hard for us to reply. "*Sindikumva*, 'I don't hear [understand] you.' Can you please come again?" So maybe you keep saying and they give up! "Pardon, pardon?" like that. . . . So they were like [*laughing*], "Ah, I think with this man, I should just speak Chichewa." (Dalton Chupa, second-year student)

This linguistic shift might have been more difficult to accomplish had the students not been aware they would need to be facile with Chichewa soon. In the hospitals and community settings where they would do their clinical training, few patients spoke English and most could speak Chichewa. Even the expatriate students tried to speak Chichewa with one another as much as possible, although it sometimes made communication difficult, both to prepare for the hospital and to engage socially with their fellow students.

One of the social divides most difficult to bridge was that between clinically experienced students and the rest. Many of the clinical officers felt strongly that they had to prove their intelligence and capability—again and again—to their fellow students, and even more so to their teachers. They reported that classmates and lecturers assumed that students who were clinical officers simply weren't smart enough to make it through college or A-level exams. Arthur Kamkwamba, a clinical officer and medical student, saw the clinical officer as an artifact of government policy:

> They came to train clinical officers just because, after they sent people to study [medicine] abroad, not many of them came back. So they said, "OK. We need to train somebody who is above a medical assistant, but who is below a doctor, but who can do most of the things that a doctor can do. But this particular person should *not* be able to have the access to travel out." You see?

Continuing to train clinical officers now that the country was producing doctors, Arthur contended, was a bad mistake: "Really, you know, you are just a fly in your own market." The stigma was greater now that a higher tier was open to Malawians, he felt. "If you didn't understand the whole [policy] thing, you would just say, 'Ah. These people, they are *dull* people. They are not *supposed* to be trained.' But that's not the situation. That's *not* the situation."

When compared to students without clinical experience, clinical officers, laboratory technicians, and other clinically experienced students were older (by an average of seven years) and came from families with a lower educational status.[12] Many had strong regional accents and less fluid English than their privately schooled classmates. I never saw one wearing the hip-hop-style garb of the urban elite. Pierre Bourdieu (1974) has analyzed how the cultural and aesthetic styles, tastes, and practices exhibited among the ruling class were taken for signs of "intelligence"—and rewarded with scholastic successes that reproduced class privilege—in the French public schools. For these Malawian clinical officers, it seems likely that a similar process was at work, and that class divisions were at the root of some of the pressures they experienced. There is no reason to think that the clinical officers entering Malawi's College of Medicine would be any less intelligent than their classmates, but plenty of reason to suspect that their mistakes and failures might be seen in a different light than those of their colleagues, more readily attributed to an essential intellectual lack rather than inadequate studying or a fluke bad performance.

Gender also posed differences difficult to resolve. Female students often felt they were treated differently by lecturers and classmates because they were women.[13] A few women reported being taunted by male classmates: "Girls are not supposed to do medicine. You are supposed to do nursing." Others felt they were accepted as women, but only if they behaved in an appropriately subservient fashion. The all-female second-year focus group, members of a class with an unusually high proportion of women, commented on the expectations of male faculty and students.

> MUKONDWA NDIUZANI: They want to secure that we'll be lower than them or something. . . .
>
> DOROTHY KAMANGA: They want us to just curl up and be silent!
>
> ALICE MATEBULE: Like the other classes. The other classes of girls aren't that, weren't that, aren't that loud—but our class, you know, when a guy stands up and wants to tell us, we say, "No! [*two other students chime in* "No!"] We're not like that, we don't want that," so they are not used to that.

A student near the end of her training agreed and described herself as ostracized because she refused either to be "submissive" or to cultivate romantic liaisons with male faculty.[14]

> Most girls here are more submissive than the boys. And they tend to be favored in that way. Well, that's a bit strong, but they tend to be, things tend to be easier for them one way or the other. And like I told you, I grew up a bit independent. And I don't need to—don't *like* to beg for attention from a lecturer. That I don't like to do. Or to draw their attention deliberately, so that I develop a relationship that will put me at an advantage. I don't like to do that. Now I haven't learned to do it, but it has put me into trouble. . . . Most females won't talk, they will just keep quiet. Whether they agree or they don't! If they don't agree, they can become very uncooperative, they don't show up for meetings or things like that. But they never comment, they never say what they feel. And I'm usually there. I say my feelings, so I think some of them label me as a rebel. (Patricia Zembere, clinical student)

Women felt strong pressures to be passive, but as the numbers of women in the college grew, they appeared to be able to resist these pressures more effectively. The only students who described themselves as becoming more vocal and outspoken during their medical training were women—and women described such changes consistently. My observations corroborate their self-descriptions. In the earlier and smaller cohorts, the few female students rarely spoke in lectures or on ward rounds. By 2007, women on clinical clerkships or internships were no longer noticeably quieter than men.

In general, women students felt that their presence and outspokenness were slowly becoming more acceptable to their male colleagues and supervisors. Some saw their own medical training as a step toward "lifting up" *all* Malawian women from a subordinate status that happened "naturally" but could be changed.[15] "Like right now women do not have much voice here in this country," Thokozani Sokela said.

> And maybe when there is only one woman in a group of men, she will not say much and the men will say a lot—it's not trying to suppress us or anything, it just happens naturally. But if we have more and more women, then there are two or three women in any group and they will find a voice. Like it has happened in our class!

It is worth noting, however, that the changes women saw among themselves could also be understood to reflect the "neutralization" toward male norms seen in other studies of medical socialization (Beagan 2000; Dufort and Maheux 1995). Changes in gendered behaviors can be read in ways similar to those that marked class and linguistic affiliations; students created public selves that submerged those markers into a "doctor" identity, even while their class and gender and other social locations continued to affect their experiences.

In their early training, then, these Malawian students moved more or less consciously toward a common way of behaving. Their language, dress, and patterns of interaction converged around a norm. When students themselves spoke about this norm, they described some policing. If a lecturer saw one out at a bar, or even just shopping in the city, it could mean trouble—one risked being marked as a student who was "not serious enough" simply by having fun off campus. Mostly, however, they felt strong internal drives to attain the neat appearance, quiet (but not too quiet) manner, good social skills, and character traits that they saw as essential to being a doctor. If anything, these issues of presentation took on a new significance once students finally reached the hospital. Esther Bvumbwe, a clinical student, commented on interacting with patients: "So it's also helped me think about—how presentable am I? You know? And am I mature? Do I look like someone who can be trusted or not? Not just talking or thinking about it, but actually *being* that person." Being that person, that mature and responsible doctor, became one of the highest priorities for medical students.[16]

A serious demeanor (or, as some put it, "acting elderly") was high on the list of desirable traits, and restraint and constraint figured prominently: not "overdoing things," not drinking enough to stumble, not having too many girlfriends (as several men mentioned). "Learning to stop yourself, you know? From having too much fun. Where you stop. Where you get serious." Students feared that people might see doctors doing dangerous things—examples they gave included everything from casual sex to opening bottles with one's teeth—and decide such behaviors must be all right. The degree of social authority involved in this assumption is impressive, but no one openly questioned it, even though some rebelled against the idea that they had to behave carefully all the time.

Citizen-Doctors in the Community

Even in their basic science years, a sense of their citizenship began to frame these students' experience of medical training. As they faced engagement with communities in school, students sometimes talked about "learning to be Malawians" as part of learning to be doctors. Understanding Malawian poverty was integral to becoming a citizen-doctor. This theme has appeared already in the nationalist motivations some students took with them into medical school; as discussed earlier, for some students, encounters with their country's poverty led them to medicine as a career choice. For others, the order was reversed: they first seriously encountered poverty through their medical training, often specifically in an experience called "Learning by Living."

> I have also learned that—like in Malawi, in general, that it's a really poor country. Because from where my mother comes, the village that I go to—while I knew that, yes, the people they are poorer there, but then they are not as poor as the rest of Malawi. Because almost every house there you get corrugated iron sheets [for roofing—a marker of relative wealth when compared to thatch]. Maybe no electricity, but they are better off, you know. So when I was thinking of the villages, I was thinking really in *that* way. That you know, people are not really so

bad off. But then ever since I got here, I really understood how poor, how *poor* people really are. . . . Mainly, it's our community health—the Learning by Living. That's like, that was like the first time I really got to know that, gosh, there are people—when people say Malawi is poor, *this* is what they mean. You get people maybe having one meal a day. That's when, for them those are the *good* times. And then, for the worst times, you find that maybe they are eating, they are eating grass. Like just pounding seed. . . . That's expanded—broadened my view of the situation in the country. (Tuntufye Chihana, clinical student)

The Department of Community Health was the pride of the College of Medicine's curriculum, what faculty pointed to as making the school distinctively Malawian (Bandawe 2005; Broadhead 1998). In community health in the first two years of medical training, students learned basic principles of epidemiology, biostatistics, and preventive medicine. Their ethics course was a part of this curriculum, as were the lectures on patient interviewing and basic psychology. In addition to all this material, however, the hours spent in community health were times when students learned about specific health conditions and concerns in their own country. The community health practicals were constantly evolving; in 2002 and 2003, they included a tour of one of Malawi's jails to learn about prison conditions and prisoner health, and home visits in the company of a community-outreach nurse to terminally ill residents of the poor and crowded Blantyre township called Bangwe.

Learning by Living was the centerpiece of the preclinical community health curriculum. The entire first-year class took a bus to the district hospital in Mangochi, a dusty town near Lake Malawi. From there, the students traveled in pairs to more rural areas where they stayed with families for a week. The pairs chose various projects they were to complete during that week (for instance, assessing local nutritional patterns), but they agreed that the best part of Learning by Living was the living: working, eating, relaxing, sleeping side by side with poor and rural Malawians. Even much later in their training, students often reflected back on this experience as a formative one.[17]

For most of these students, it was their first time staying at any length in a rural setting. Many of the College of Medicine faculty members I spoke with imagined their students as coming from "the village"—a widely used name for rural Malawi, where over 80 percent of Malawians still lived at the time. In fact, the great majority of the college's current students were urban. An upper-level student commented that he was the only one in his class to have a village background (which he felt gave him helpful insight into his patients' realities); of the class I talked with as they returned from their Learning by Living experience, not one had lived in a village before. Although their urban origins surprised their teachers, they make sense in light of the country's pronounced urban-rural educational disparities.[18]

Their urban backgrounds had important implications for students' ideas of what it meant to be Malawian doctors, and implications also for their understanding of the rural lives many of their patients led. Their own remoteness from "the village" allowed them to romanticize it or demonize it as an imagined (and generic) place. In Chichewa, the term for village is *mudzi*, a word that also means community or, loosely, home. In general, students, faculty, and other urban Malawians talked about "the village" as a community defined, positively or negatively, by its opposition to modernity. This opposition was typically depicted in one of two ways: the village was either a recalcitrant site of ignorance and superstition, waiting for redemption by the teachings and techniques of the modern/urban world, or—less commonly—a romantic site of resistance in which the "true" values of Malawi stayed pure despite encroachment by the outside world.

Immediately on returning from their village stay, students often deplored the backwardness of the villages. When I spent time with a group who had just returned, most seemed very happy to be back in town. Sitting around a pair of battered wooden tables pushed together in a room at the back of Mangochi District Hospital, they traded stories from the week. Through the windows drifted the sounds of bleating goats and, from a little farther away, the wailing of women near the mortuary. Public health posters, some new and some faded from years of the African sunshine, exhorted us from the wall on the virtues of cleanliness, bednets, and child spacing. Students' tales, like the posters, frequently featured themes of ignorance, superstition, sexual pathology, and lack of hygiene. "The girls are having sex in primary school! Boys want it, and girls can get five kwacha [then about six cents] for it." "Men won't use condoms because they say they transmit viruses," one student told the rest. "They say, 'If you fill a condom with water and hang it up in a tree, you can see the virus after three days.'" Another chimed in, "Children don't ever wash with soap—no wonder there's so much diarrhea." But some contested these depictions, too. When Ben Kamwendo argued that people in "his" village didn't build latrines because they were lazy, his classmate Esau Mlanjira corrected him: the villagers had explained that the soil was so sandy that latrines without concrete liners collapsed, and the village had no funds for cement. Two young women coming from another site differed over why the borehole pumps there weren't working: one claimed that women preferred to gather water from the contaminated river because it was easier and it was the custom, so no one was in a hurry to fix the pumps, but another disagreed. The only people who had been trained to repair the pump machinery had left the village, part of the political fallout from a conflict over which of two women should be the chief; besides, to get replacement parts, someone had to travel all the way to Blantyre and back on the minibus, and no one would have the money to do that until the maize harvest was in (if then). Kids weren't attending school regularly because "they don't see that they can be somebody someday," claimed Gift Mkango. Lucy Phiri disagreed: "No, the kids are working out in the maize field keeping monkeys out of the crop. Now that the maize is almost ripe, monkeys are making major raids." When a group of young women students lamented what they saw as the appalling workload of village women whose husbands were not helping as much as they should, Ben Kamwendo, slouched in his seat next to me with a hat half over his eyes, muttered disagreement under his breath. "It's just natural. Even from fertilization, girls [embryonic girls, that is] are more active than boys." In these arguments, no one saw "the village" as a morally pure or romantically appealing place, but a perception of the rural as culturally backward contended with perceptions that this apparent backwardness was either "natural" or, more often, produced by the material conditions of people's lives.

Villagers themselves had quite clearly expected to be the objects of expert surveillance and discipline. One site hosting two medical students had insisted on dragging them around the entire community to count pit latrines. "We don't want to count pit latrines!" the young women protested, to no avail. All outside visitors were concerned with village hygiene, and therefore, these students must want to count pit latrines. (The students eventually gave up and did so.) Students in the villages were consistently cast as outsiders, experts, and people of high status who might have useful connections. Every member of this group reported being approached by villagers for money, school fees, sponsorships, or jobs, an experience most clearly found dismaying.

As time passed, however, and the immediacy of Learning by Living faded, students seemed often to recast the experience of alienation as one of connection: connection as fellow Malawians. In later years looking back on this time, they were likely to describe it as a period in which they had been "true Malawians," or at least learned who true Malawians were. Clinical student Tuntufye Chihana described her village experience as part of maturation into both adulthood and citizenship:

> I feel being here [in the College of Medicine], I have grown up really
> like in the real, real, proper Malawian sense, to say that I really *am*
> Malawian. . . . I mean I used to go down, out to the villages, to my
> grandmother's place, but that is different. Your grandmother practically
> spoils you all the time! [*laughs*] So, now if you're going to the village
> and you're meeting strangers, you actually—now you have to learn to
> be with *people*.

By sitting on the floor to eat, cooking *nsima* with the family, and speaking
only Chichewa through an entire conversation (so as not to give offense by
using English words these unschooled villagers would not understand), she
felt a sort of breakthrough: "I've been the—probably—true, true Malawian,
where people actually expect you to be." Tuntufye, like some others who
spoke about their village experiences, contrasted the responsible and respectful behavior she assumed there favorably with the Westernized values
she had taken on as a privileged urban teenager, and saw it as a transforma-
tive moment.

In fact, it was the most privileged urbanites who were most likely to
identify *as Malawians* with a somewhat generic rural and impoverished
"people" through a village experience, and then only in hindsight. The few
rural students did not comment in this way on "the village" and were more
likely to mark the distance from it that their medical education made possible or necessary. One graduate from a very rural community looked back
on her transformation in these words: "When I came to, to starting studying medicine, of course I didn't know anything. Most of the terms, they
were new. But now, as a medical professional, I think there is a maturity.
That remote girl is now an educated medical doctor." Medical terminology, maturity, knowledge, and urbanity were conflated in this comment
in a way that suggests it would not be possible to be a "remote girl" and
an "educated medical doctor" at the same time. The consumption and ap-
propriation of local styles perceived as traditional, as Jonathan Friedman
(1999) and other anthropologists who write about globalization have noted,
are sometimes processes integral to the construction of a "cosmopolitan"
identity by an elite that seeks to transcend locality.[19] Perhaps only the urban elite had enough social distance to be "true, true" village Malawians
safely; it may have been easier to identify with "the people" when they
were not one's immediate family.

In addition to feeling that they were true Malawians, even before they
began spending time in the hospitals, well over half the students began to
feel that they were really doctors, much earlier than their North American

counterparts tended to do.[20] This feeling was particularly strong when they were in the community—whether the village setting of the Learning by Living attachment or at home over their school holidays.

> They tell you—us—"As long as you are there, in the College of Medicine, you are already a doctor." So it's that kind of feeling that sometimes makes you feel like you are already a doctor. (Joe Phoya, preclinical student)

> OK, you walk into a health center, and as soon as people realize that you're a—that you're in medical school, they suddenly give you a lot more respect than you deserve! Even though I had no clinical knowledge, the fact that I was a medical do—that I was a medical student gave me status in that place. And I guess I like that. Very much. (Medson Namanja, clinical student reflecting on preclinical experience)

Students were called "doctor" from the first day they started medical school, or even before. One student described her whole extended family clustered around the radio on the day the roster of students accepted at the College of Medicine was read out, jumping and shouting "*adokotala, adokotala!*" ("doctor, doctor!") when they heard her name. Many took on the role of family or community doctor from that day forward and shaped their behaviors to match that role.

> Once you are *at* the medical school, when you go home, everybody says, "You are a doctor." If you don't behave like one, you feel you'll disappoint them. So you just adopt the little things which make you—you do those little things which make you fit into the role that society has given you. . . . You are supposed to be concerned primarily with the people's health rather than anything else. And sometimes when someone is in trouble, you've got to help. (Mkume Lifa, first-year student)[21]

Mkume's deliberate adoption of the doctor role and behaviors he perceived to be expected was by no means exceptional. Treated as doctors in their communities, most preclinical students felt like real doctors at least some of the time, even in their first year or two of training.[22]

The new status of doctor could be exhilarating, and students usually rushed to embrace and embody it. It came at some cost, however: they often felt growing separation from friends and families. Students in the West have also described increasing social distance from people outside medicine, although they rarely link it to status. For them, part of the separation is typically a matter of workload, and part is a matter of feeling that they have transgressed important human boundaries by, for instance, dissecting cadavers, asking intimate questions of naked strangers, or watching someone die (Good and Good 1993; Hafferty 1991). Among the Malawians I spoke with, the issue of transgressing normal human boundaries never came up. Several described distance from family and friends as a product of their long working hours, which restricted opportunities to spend time with family. Alice Matebule, a second-year student, explained: "All the year long, when, oh, your uncle died or someone's getting married—you can't come. You know? So you miss out on a lot." Gradually, the family adjusted to the missing medical student. You go home, Alice said, and "things have moved around. They've adapted to being without you. So it's as if you're leaving home slowly."

More important than the long hours, though, was the distance created by status. Friendly arguments stopped when the opinion of "the doctor" came to be the final word on any matter—whether medical or not. Friends outside medicine were sometimes intimidated by the idea or appearance of the soon-to-be doctor.

> Of course, my friends, they see my whitements when I am working. They see my whitements, and they seem to be giving me too much respect. And they put me apart from them in capitals, which I don't like. So—they are free with me, but it seems they are beginning to respect me too early. Or too much, which I don't like it. (Phillip Nkhandwe, second-year student)

Some students visibly gloried in their high status, but for others, particularly those from less privileged backgrounds, this separateness could feel painful. Several described encountering a stiff reserve when they went home, sometimes accompanied by more serious jealousy and alienation. As a bitter joke had it, "In Malawi, *PhD* stands for 'Pull him down.'" In this traditionally communal society, anything that made one person stand out from others could potentially result in jealousy, sometimes with disastrous consequences. Like the newly wealthy, highly educated individuals were at risk both of being subjected to witchcraft and of being subjected to accusations that they themselves used occult powers to achieve or maintain their success. One intern explained that it was very difficult for college-educated Malawians to return home to rural areas for this reason: they could be subject to witchcraft or other forms of violence, if not within their families then from locally powerful chiefs afraid of any threat to their authority. Jealousy could also be particularly problematic for students from polygynous families: two of these students felt that their education as doctors was being used at home to put one wife's family ahead of another's interests.

Besides the dangers from without, students felt their high status could present dangers from within, as it could tempt the doctor or student doctor to feel genuinely superior to other people. Alex Mkweu, a clinical student, described "the honor people give you" as one of the chief rewards of doing medicine in Malawi, but quickly added a caveat: "But I should say, of course, that the honor is also dangerous. Because I think some—you may, you may start to be *proud* and the like. And you look at other people as nothing. And that's very dangerous." Other students agreed: medical status was a moral danger if it made one think of oneself as separate from, better than, other Malawians.

Scientist-Doctors and the Disembodied Body

If their status in the community produced ambivalent feelings for students, another source of professional identity did not. Preclinical students at the University of Malawi's College of Medicine, like their North American counterparts, relished their growing deep knowledge of the human body and saw it as a key component of their "doctor" selves. A preclinical student described the sheer pleasure of coming to understand health and illness by seeing physical structure.

> When you do anatomy, you will understand the whole thing that something will get explained to you and you actually will go out there, do like a practical dissection, and you actually *prove* that it really *is* there— that, that just brings a lot of excitement! That, oh, it *does* exist, it *does* work this way and everything. That. And, even in the disease, when you learn about it, it's, like, now you're looking for something going *wrong*. You're actually looking at an organ that is actually going wrong or whatever, and you as a person have to find a way to *fight* that.

In the imagery of empirical proof, visible structure, and "fighting" against disease, this comment reflected not only growing knowledge but the inculcation of medical values.[23] When students talked about medical knowledge, their emphasis was squarely on individualized curative medicine and not—despite the efforts of community health faculty—on public health and preventative medicine. The fundamentals of bioscience training, its focus on cells and hormones and bones and genes, ensured that students absorbed an underlying model of illness as bounded by the individual body. Their discussion of their own esoteric knowledge also emphasized the visual. If health and disease were located in the individual body, the doctor's job was to *see through* erroneous theories of disease (like those that understood personal suffering to be the product of larger social structures), to *see deeply* into that body to its structure and pathology, the better to correct abnormality.

Traditional Medicine: Seeing Through

Some students understood their ability to "see through" traditional health beliefs, a capacity made possible by their new scientific knowledge, as a benefit of studying medicine. They could no longer be fooled by "those traditional things you hear growing up" and would resist nonbiomedical explanations for illnesses. One student, early in her second year, presented it as an inevitable but impending conversion:

> Like where I am now, I still believe in traditional things, go to the *sing'anga*, the traditional healer. And I believe, maybe by final year, it will all have gone. Maybe knowing stuff that I've learned, all the disease, maybe it changes people who used to believe in traditional culture. (Dorothy Kamanga, preclinical student)

Most who talked about it put their own conversion to the biomedical model in the past. They used to think that one could get sick from not going to the *sing'anga* for *mankhwala* (medicine) to protect against malevolent forces, some said, but now they knew better.

This shift in epistemologies is quite different from the experiences of the vast majority of Northern medical students, for most of whom biomedicine *is* the vernacular belief system—"those traditional things you hear growing up"—or at least a large part of it, and for whom no such conversion is needed. There is some risk of overstating the difference, however, either by overestimating the biomedicalization of lay knowledge in the North[24] or by underestimating the impact of biomedical knowledge in southern Africa. Biomedicine, at least in the form of pharmaceuticals and often in the form of medically trained nurses or health assistants, has been a part of many rural and all urban communities in Malawi for decades. Most of the students with whom I spoke would have grown up with a pluralistic set of resources and epistemologies on which to draw. Unpublished data from urban Malawi (Chipolombwe 2004; Chokani 1998) showed that both lay community members and biomedical professionals consulted herbalists and *asing'anga* as well as hospitals for certain of their own ailments, even when the biomedical professionals were unlikely to recommend outside consultations to patients. What is interesting is that during their training period, students felt a need to reject pluralism for a biomedical orthodoxy, at least in most of their conversations with me. Here, too, there may be some policing of the boundaries of medical community, particularly important at this point when their own membership in that community is new and somewhat tentative, as well as a response to faculty exhortations to "reject superstition for science."[25]

Even when they seemed to feel a twinge of regret for their lost beliefs and protective *mankhwala*, as a few did, students did not question that as doctors they would be capable of understanding the real truth of human health and illness better than traditional healers could. Few medical students spoke about traditional medicine at all, but those who did usually either rejected it entirely or argued that the *truth claims* of traditional medicine should be evaluated through the lens of the *truths* of scientific biomedicine. Occasional senior students and faculty, in contrast to this oppositional schema, believed that as medicine in Malawi "matured," there could be a melding of the best aspects of Western science and the "best" aspects of Malawian medicine (typically the herbal knowledge that fits most easily into a medical paradigm)—subject, of course, to the testing, licensing, and control of scientifically trained doctors.

Medical Science: Seeing Deeply

For preclinical students, deep knowledge of the visible, individual yet universal human body was consistently and—unlike status—unambiguously linked with being a doctor. The knowledge did not need to extend to therapy in order to be legitimating.

> People have got burning questions with regards to medical issues! You discover that even though the questions are burning, it's just basic knowledge, it just requires basic knowledge to answer them. So, yeah. If you are asked questions and you give the right answers, then you feel like a doctor. (Mkume Lifa, first-year student)

> I usually don't know what is really wrong or how to treat, but now I have learned so many systems, I can at least say, "Well, here is this muscle

and here is this bone and the pain is here." So when I know something, I feel like a real doctor. (Thokozani Sokela, second-year student)

I feel like more or less a doctor. Because, in the first year, I have learned many systems. . . . You find that at home people are asking you, "Ah— what happens when someone has this or this?" At least you have an idea. You can tell them, "Basically, this is what I think is happening." (Dalton Chupa, second-year student)

The depth of their scientific knowledge was particularly important to these fledgling physicians because it was the only thing that reliably separated them as doctors from the lower level of practitioners, whose training was more procedurally oriented and less grounded in basic science: clinical officers. "That's what differentiates us from COs and other medical assistants," explained second-year student Mukondwa Ndiuzani. "We have to know almost everything. Compared to them where they just have to know surface issues, and we have to know the depth of everything." This differentiation was even more important for those students who were already experienced clinicians. When I asked how they had changed during their medical training, every clinical officer I interviewed promptly volunteered an increased understanding of the body and its processes as the most significant change. Although the actions they took with patients might not differ, the reasoning behind those actions did. Arthur Kamkwamba explained that in the past when he gave an injection, "*then* maybe I could just do it for the sake of, OK, I am supposed to do—but now I really know, OK, I am supposed to do it *just because of that*." Or as another clinician explained,

I have studied much of this in the past but not with this level of detail, of depth, so my knowledge has been increased. Now I know what protein synthesis means, while in the past, I had never studied protein synthesis. . . . Before, I never knew how a muscle works. But now—how it works, histology, gross, embryology [*finger outlining his quadriceps*]— where does a muscle come from? It's a much greater depth of knowledge. (Anthony Boloweza, clinician and preclinical student)

Medical school is often compared to what Erving Goffman (1961) called a "total institution," an institution that controls every aspect of the lives of those within. Prisons, mental hospitals, and convents are among such institutions. In spaces like these, one becomes a new person, bodily habits and moral orientations and subjectivities attuned to an institutionally specific model of reality (see, for example, Lester 2005). Byron Good and Mary-Jo Delvecchio Good, like other anthropologists who have studied medical education in the North, see the study of the body as a process in which medical language and anatomical knowledge remake the world for students. The Harvard students they interviewed, like the students I studied, learned to imagine the interiors of the bodies they encountered, including their own. Suffering people became patients; illnesses became matters of biology; the only reasonable way to see a human was as a set of interlocking functional organ systems. Ultimately, the Goods concluded, "the intimacy with that body reflects a distinctive perspective, an organized set of perceptions and emotional responses that emerge with the emergence of the body as a site of medical knowledge" (Good and Good 1993:90).

Researchers studying preclinical training among North American students have consistently described a profound emotional detachment that comes with the process of examining the disembodied body. The detachment or "hardening" taking place in the cadaver lab, in much of this research, is the beginning of a process by which doctors become fundamentally different from other humans (including their patients), capable of violating normal mortal boundaries without experiencing mortals' emotional responses. Observers have raised concerns about the effects of such hardening on doctors and their patients since at least the nineteenth century (Imber 1998); recognition of emotional distancing among students themselves has been documented repeatedly since the 1950s (see, for example, Fox 1989; Hafferty 1991).

If talking about the body in terms of organs, muscles, disease processes, and chemical alterations—what Good (1994) calls "the medical body"— signifies detachment, then Malawi's preclinical students demonstrated it as well. Students clearly saw the body as a worksite, distinguishing their responses to illness now from those they had experienced before their medical education began. "Instead of thinking of somebody who's sick, and getting fixated on how nasty that is, you find there is work which you have got to do," said Mkume Lifa. "There is a disorder somewhere, somehow, which can be corrected." Unlike North American students, however, the Malawians did not speak about the shock of dismembering bodies, or reflect— either positively or negatively—on their emotional responses to cadaver labs. One student about to start internship, looking back on his experience of dissection, thought it might have contributed to what he called "a more formal way of grieving," but no preclinical students discussed anatomy with anything other than pleasure in their growing knowledge. In fact, no one discussed detachment at all, and no one ever referred to cadaver lab in terms that evoked a rite of passage.

This is a striking difference from North American and European studies of medical students, in which anatomical dissection takes center stage in students' own descriptions of the "hardening" process that signifies their transition from laypeople to doctors (Hafferty 1991; Sinclair 1997). Some of the difference may have to do with life experience: high death rates and a strong cultural emphasis on funeral attendance give Malawian students a much greater previous exposure to death and corpses than most First World students could be expected to have. It may also be a matter of a difference in familiar narratives. "Cadaver stories," including jokes about cannibalism and hoary (and likely apocryphal) tales of medical student pranks involving cadaver parts, have circulated among Northern medical students for decades. Frederic Hafferty (1988, 1991:59ff.) and others have argued that in such stories, dissection becomes a synecdoche for the emotionally hardening effects of medical training. Cadaver tales convey the ideal of medical detachment—after all, they ask rhetorically, who but a doctor could treat the dead body so cavalierly? In Malawi and much of the rest of southern Africa, this is no rhetorical question, and "cadaver stories" could be expected to have a very different resonance. Everyone knows who treats bodies and body parts this way: not doctors, but witches. It is witches who seek body parts to access occult powers, witches who dismember. Engaging in—not to mention circulating tales of—cadaver pranks would be profoundly problematic, even unthinkable.

The narrative of distancing and detachment, then, was not a notable thread in these students' stories of anatomy lab specifically, nor was it in their discussion of preclinical training more generally. The narrative of seeing in and seeing through was. Looking at blood slides and dead bodies was a part of their training that students believed to be paramount in making them real doctors, through the seeing-and-knowing process itself rather than any affective detachment that accompanied it.

⸱≫⸱

Medical students, as every study of them has shown, learn far more than facts. For these students, the first two years of school were all about the body: studying the body as an object and training the novice's body into that of a doctor. Students seemed to want to see themselves as transformed into someone new by their training. These students often "felt like doctors" earlier than their American counterparts; they were recognized as physicians by their families and in their communities from the day they began medical school. Recognition alone was not quite enough to make them feel secure in their professional identities, however. When they laboriously acquired a deep knowledge of the body, its structures and pathophysiological processes, then they felt they were really physicians—whether or not they knew any measures to help those who came to them with health problems. The depth of their vision, reaching beneath the skin to see the hidden workings of the universal body, justified their authority and became central to their identity.

The neutral, objectifying if not detached, technoscientific content of this doctor-scientist identity was very similar to that described by medical anthropologists and sociologists working in the First World, although it lacked the profound emphasis on "hardening" seen in Northern work. The "commonsense" assumption that empirical science is the ultimate arbiter of truth, the vision of doctors as rational and authoritative agents of science, were parts of a doctor-scientist identity that reflected the hegemony of Northern biomedicine.

In these years, I found no evidence that the students resisted ideas of the body as a biological organism, divided into functional systems and subject to medically knowable pathological alterations. They accepted—indeed, eagerly embraced—the medical science of the body, including the notions of rationality and modernity that go with that science. Biomedicine became the only way to really "know" the body. An apparently neutral and universal biomedical knowledge explained the world in ways that at least sometimes justified social distinctions, as when Ben Kamwendo drew on (a dubious) embryological fact to cast the inequitably hard workload of poor Malawian women as "natural."[26] In fact, the essential perceptual dispositions students learned performed social work for them, too. Their medical habitus cast them as people of very high status, even while their medical knowledge distinguished them from certain potential competitors. They understood themselves as "seeing deeply," in a way that they believed that clinical officers and other workers lower in the medical hierarchy did not, and as "seeing through" the practices and epistemologies of the people they called "traditional" healers.

This was hegemonic knowledge in the making, the exclusion of other possible epistemologies and the elevation of a medical reality in which reductionist empiricism became the only sensible way to see the world. There was perhaps a certain underlying instability to this knowledge, however. Laboratory training was supposed to teach students "how things are everywhere, anywhere, always" (Schaffer 1994:9). Science studies and ethnographic fieldwork, as Simon Schaffer and others have shown, both complicate any such picture of nature speaking in an immediate and timeless fashion to the scientist. Medical knowledge, too, is uncomfortably in between the universal and the irrevocably particular, even in the basic science years in which students first acquire it. Anatomy is supposed to teach students systematically how the body is everywhere, anywhere, always. Yet the Malawian students, like any other medical students who dissect cadavers, encountered bodies that never quite matched the pictures or one another, and the differences among them were very often embodied manifestations of social life.[27] They spent time in villages that were poor in nearly everything but "so, so rich in infectious diseases" (as an intern wryly put it) long controlled elsewhere, and where people pounded their seed to eat in the lean seasons. Some students found themselves compelled to link these problems to political developments or regional poverty, if not yet to larger systems of resource extraction and deprivation, even as others preferred to see individual behaviors or motivations at work. There were, then, some potential fractures in the radically individualist view of the biomedical human these students came to assume, and perhaps some potential fractures as well in their own medical habitus. In general, however, students welcomed their new knowledge and did not appear to challenge it. Their enthusiasm for the science of medicine was palpable in these interviews, and they eagerly anticipated the opportunity to put their scientific theory into medical practice as their training continued.

⚘

Welcome to Queens

Five minutes' brisk walk took you from the quiet white halls of the College of Medicine to the chaotic sprawl of Queen Elizabeth Central Hospital. A sign at the gate of the brick-walled compound directed visitors to the separate entrances for A&E (accident and emergency) or the mortuary. Inside the compound, rusted metal placards pointed the way to X-ray and the outpatient department. A fading blue and white billboard exhorted "Family Planning: Key to a Better Future" and guided visitors to a square brick building where a nurse gave lectures on child-spacing methods to attentive women packed onto long wooden benches.

All the signposts helped, but not enough for students new to the place. Like many hospitals, this one was cobbled together over the decades, growing by bits and pieces from the four hundred–bed original building constructed in the 1950s.[28] Banda allocated money to add an obstetrics wing in the 1980s; new operating theaters were constructed in the early 1990s with funds from the UN High Commission on Refugees, as Queens staff struggled to cope with an influx of Mozambicans injured by land mines and fleeing their civil war; the College of Medicine built four teaching annexes a few years later; Malawians against Polio helped pay for a new orthopedics ward after the old one burned down in 2001; other funders added other bits. One construction project or another always seemed to be ongoing, shirtless, wiry men laying brick or framing windows, balancing on scaffolds of stripped blue-gum poles bound with rope. The hospital was a palimpsest of clinics made into wards, wards into offices, offices into research units, research units into clinics, all nondescript brick one-story buildings with concrete floors and corrugated tin roofs, some partially covered with scabrous tile shingle. Clinics and labs and student hostels and research units were linked by long, sloping hallways, some glassed-in, some open to the air. The whole labyrinth perched on a gentle hill, so if someone dropped a marble on the floor near the casualty ward in the northwest corner, it would ultimately end up somewhere near the malaria project in the southeast corner. (The slope actually helped new students navigate.)

As you walked toward the hospital looking for an entrance, you would pass by brightly colored (if ragged) cloths festooning the walls, shrubs, and occasional clotheslines. Outside each ward was a courtyard with a pair of concrete sinks, where family members washed patients' clothes or blankets. A donated autoclave, broken beyond repair, and a few irreparably damaged bedsteads rusted in these courtyards. These, too, provided places to spread out drying laundry. Patients and their families sat together on the grassy patches or slept in the sun. In the shade of a mango tree, you might see a healing service, the Bible-waving prophet healer and her followers clad in blue and white outfits with white headcloths. Passersby could catch the phrase *dzina laMulungu*—the name of God—as the prophet labored to cast disease out from the patients who clustered around her, while their relatives prayed fervently.

The hospital had many entrances, although some of the grander-looking ones usually stayed locked. A newcomer's best bet was to follow the crowds of visitors and staff to one of the side doors that would actually get you in. You would have to pass by the guards, with their blue uniforms and billy clubs. In a medical student's white coat, though, you would not be challenged even if they didn't know you.[29]

Inside, especially on a steamy day, you would probably be struck first by the smell: a distinctive compound of sickness and sweat, clothes washed without enough soap, dried blood and fresh blood, death and Jik-brand bleach solution. If you walked down a hallway toward one of the wards where you would be working soon, your feet would slide a little on the concrete floors, worn shiny and smooth by thousands upon thousands of feet. Red plastic signs hanging from the ceiling warned *Osalabvula—Osalongolola* (No Spitting, No Making Noise). Relatives and hospital staff filled the long halls. Periodically, everyone crowded respectfully to one side to allow a funeral procession to pass, attendants pushing a trolley on which a body lay under a white cloth with a red cross stitched on top, grieving relatives walking behind wailing or singing. You would stop as one of these processions passed; to keep walking would be an act of disrespect.

Eventually, you would get to one of the wards. Typical wards at Queens were a series of rooms strung along a long central hallway. A nursing station guarded the entrance, with a desk, supply cabinets, stacks of dark blue log-books, and a small locked medicine box on wheels parked where the nurses could keep an eye on it. The sickest patients awaiting admission were tri-aged through a small nearby examining room, while those well enough to sit waited in line on a wooden bench outside the nursing station. In the four small side wards that came next, the most acutely ill patients fit eight to a room. Past the side wards, the hallway entered a large open area, about the size of a basketball court, divided by hip-high concrete walls into six bays. Communal washrooms, shared by the entire ward, were at the far end.

In the open area, iron cots lined each side of the bays, sixty to eighty patients crammed into a space designed—at least according to the place-marking numbers painted on the walls—to be tight quarters for forty. By 2007, Queens had about eleven hundred beds. Because bed occupancy rates tended to range between 150 and 200 percent, there were almost as many patients lying on the floor *between* the cots as there were patients *on* cots. And they were cots: narrow frames welded together out of pipe with wire mesh for springs, some but not all with vinyl mattresses on top. No sheets except in the smaller paying wards—the mats got wiped down with a rag between patients and sometimes set outside in the sun if there was time. There rarely was.

The rooms were lit only by the open windows during the day to save on electric bills. The high ceilings and concrete walls made the space feel cavernous despite the crowding, and amplified the moans of pain, the keens of grieving, the squeak of a medicine trolley, or the conversation and quarrels of families clustered near the beds. Patients—your future patients—were everywhere: not only on the wards but in the hallways, lying under tables or curled on benches in the nurses' stations, outside under the shelters where their "guardians" (the relatives who cared for them in the hospital, fed them, cleaned them, and helped them to the toilets or showers) did their laundry and sometimes cooked their meals. Some patients died in these unlikely places. Others improved and went home.

CHAPTER FIVE

The Word Made Flesh:
Hospital Experience and the Clinical Crisis

Students anticipating the journey from the classroom to the hospital spoke frequently about "the challenge of turning theory into practice." Indeed, the third year of medical school was designed as a transition between basic science theory and mastery of its clinical application. Students spent four days each week on the wards at Queens, attached for two months at a time to medicine, obstetrics and gynecology, surgery, and pediatrics. Every Friday they retreated from the hospital to the basic sciences building, where they continued the pathology studies begun in their second year—hours of lectures, followed by lab time to examine diseased organs. Students spent the last one to two weeks of each attachment on community health (for example, community obstetrics, community pediatrics), which meant working at sites outside the main hospital, and usually outside the city of Blantyre. In the third year, they were expected to learn diagnosis: how to find signs of tissue damage or invading organisms under the microscopes in pathology lab, how to interpret basic laboratory tests and radiographs, how to take a patient's history, how to do a good physical exam.

Once the third year was over, all teaching was in the clinical setting, and nearly all of it was in the hospital. Fourth-year students had brief attachments in subspecialties, mostly at Queens Hospital, but also traveling a few weeks at a time to other places with specialized resources (such as the mental hospital in Zomba). At the end of the year was a summary exam, but not one so difficult that anyone failed. Also in the fourth year, each student was expected to complete an independent community health research project. These projects were taken seriously by the faculty and often cited on teaching rounds or used to craft locally relevant treatment protocols.[1] If third year was about diagnosis, in fourth year the students were beginning to learn about management.

In the fifth and final year of the medical program, students were expected to integrate all they had learned, demonstrating their capacity to diagnose disease, explain its pathophysiology, and recommend appropriate management. Back at Queens for the majority of the year, the students cycled again through the same attachments they had in third year, but now they had to function more independently. They worked side by side with the interns and looked toward the day not far in the future when they would be interns themselves. They also prepared with considerable effort and trepidation for their final exams, during which both internal examiners (from the College of Medicine) and external examiners (from other medical schools in the region and beyond) tested their knowledge and skills. If they failed, they would repeat the year. If they passed, they were doctors.

Students entering the medical school and beginning their training had expressed almost limitless beliefs in their own power to heal. Andrew Kanyenda described what he had expected: "Someone comes in, is completely bedridden, and then within a few minutes or within an hour, that person is a bit relieved and is now *able*, just from a mere stroking of pen on the paper! Just prescribing medicine, a few tablets." In their clinical years, students' narrations of their experiences changed sharply. The pride and exhilaration so evident in the recounting of many basic science students ebbed; pain and anger took their place. Neither change was invariant, but both were common and striking. The conditions students faced on the wards prompted a rise in negative feelings about their work and new doubts about their healing potential, contributing to what I will call a "clinical crisis."

Entering the Hospital

Students beginning their clinical training encountered a hospital that did not much resemble the idealized one in their textbooks. At the turn of the millennium, on the medical and surgical wards of Queens, an estimated 80 to 90 percent of the patients were hospitalized for complications of HIV/AIDS: estimated, because the public sector rarely had the money to buy reagents for HIV testing.[2] It was not just reagents that were unavailable. On a Ministry of Health spot check, the pharmacy stocked only 46 percent of the country's already quite limited list of "essential drugs." Intermittently in 2003, the operating theater had no iodine or "spirits" (methyl alcohol), so surgical site preparation was done without benefit of antiseptics. In 2007, we had spirits and sometimes iodine, but the entire country ran

out of suture for a period of several weeks. Sutures well past their expira-
tion dates that had been saved to teach students surgical knot-tying, emergency donations shipped in by the Red Cross, and sterilized fishing line
stretched the supply chain at Queens, but at more than one outlying hospital, patients died because they could not get necessary operations or have
traumatic injuries repaired. At times, barely adequate equipment could be
patchworked together from donors, government stores, and various multinational research projects. Sometimes we were flush with odd bits of equipment: ostomy bags, for instance, or donated disposable surgical gowns. At
other times, the hospital was without soap, water, "plaster" (surgical tape),
or gauze. When I worked there in 2002 and 2003, the labor and delivery
ward rarely had a thermometer and never had a scissors, although ten to
twelve thousand births took place there in a year. Midwives sometimes
conducted deliveries using as their tools only a bare scalpel blade—without
the handle—and two pieces of string, at the largest tertiary-care referral
center in Malawi.

Staff was stretched just as thin. The pediatrics special care unit, on the
day I spoke with an intern there, had twenty-eight beds, 106 patients, and
one nurse. On wards so poorly staffed, if a nurse failed to show up for work,
there might be no trained clinical staff at all, only students and cleaners.

When I started working at Queens, first as a medical student many
years ago, then returning as a volunteer staff member, I thought the poverty, chaos, and sadness I saw there were products of my Northern vision,
that of a doctor used to abundance, order, and the systematic concealment
of suffering and death in hospital settings. Again and again, my journal recorded a plaintive question: "What kind of a hospital is this?"[3] During this
research, I struggled—mostly successfully, I believe—not to let my shock
and dismay at the clinical conditions leak into the interview setting, lest
they compromise the data. After many interviews and many informal conversations with patients and staff, I came to believe that most Malawians,
including clinicians, also found the hospital overwhelming. As a young
Malawian man who had come from the village to visit a dying friend told
me, "He had TB, and he was on 3B [the male medical ward], and I went to
see him. It was awful. I went in, and I thought—it will be a miracle if *anyone* in this ward survives and goes home." Such comments about Malawi's
public hospitals were common even in casual conversation.

Other than the privileged few, sick people in Malawi faced difficult
choices. The patterns of resort varied, but typically people tried home remedies, often proceeding next to various local healers and choosing hospitals
or clinics either simultaneously or as a last hope (Chokani 1998). Wealth-

ier Malawians seeking biomedical care could afford to go to the better-equipped private hospitals, and the richest could fly to South Africa for top-notch private care. The rest faced a choice between defunded, decrepit, and demoralized public hospitals and health centers, medium-quality mission hospitals, or small and minimally regulated private clinics. The public settings were nominally free, while either of the latter options involved potentially crippling payments.[4] Even a minor illness could plunge a family living on the edge into desperate poverty.

The student doctor assigned to a medical, surgical, or pediatrics ward in a public hospital (for students did not rotate through missions or private hospitals) typically faced sixty to a hundred patients daily, some with relatively minor illnesses and most with very serious ones. In all but a few wards, the great majority were HIV-positive. For each of these patients, the illness represented a complex set of social and economic problems that reached well beyond the sick individual into a web of family and other connections. For the students, there was little if any time to address such complexities and little to be done about many of the problems that brought patients in to the hospital.

On the other hand, the routines of the hospital did not require students to dismiss those complexities. They were not forced to separate "social" facts (assumed to be irrelevant) from "medical" (and therefore relevant) ones, as medical students in the North are painstakingly taught to do (Anspach 1988; Apker and Eggly 2004). The social facts, typically, were all too relevant. When Tom Tayanjah reported the clinical history of a patient referred to the high-risk antenatal clinic with a scrap of paper on which was scrawled "QECH: query twins," the facts that she lived in Ndirande with her four children and that she was widowed two months ago, all of which suggested economic compromise, were just as relevant as Tom's discovery of the suspicious purple spot on her hard palate that suggested immune compromise. A twin pregnancy was going to add trouble to trouble. In most cases, there were similar concerns to consider, and while I saw students chastised for many (real and imagined) lapses, including "irrelevant" social details in case presentations was never one of them.

Jameson Tongole, a loud and confident older student, presented at pediatrics rounds one morning the case of a child admitted with unexplained abdominal and leg swelling. Her parents had brought her to their local health center several times about six months ago until they got "fed up with just always getting Fansidar and aspirin," Jameson said.[5] She improved considerably after a consultation with an herbalist, but two months later began to have diarrhea and vomiting, and soon also developed leg swelling. She had met few developmental milestones; now two and a half, she could sit up but could not crawl, walk, or talk. Her mother had finally brought her all the way to the district hospital, and the district had transferred her to us.

It was the pediatricians' custom to bring patients in for examination at rounds. This one was carried in by her mother. She was tiny and listless, the size of an eight-month-old, very wasted—when Jameson picked her up gently, I could easily count her ribs and could see the origins and insertions of all the muscles in her little shoulders. Her belly was distended, her hair sparse and reddish, her legs puffy, and she had a look of hopeless sadness on her face. She lay curled into her mother, who cradled her protectively and resignedly, tilting her head to one side so she could look into her daughter's face. It was a textbook case of chronic malnutrition: even the look of despair was classic. She could have simply been the unlucky one in this marginally nourished family, unlucky enough to wean off the breast in the first of two famine years. Or she might have been a different sort of canary in a coal mine: sometimes malnutrition and failure to thrive in the youngest child was the first marker of HIV in a family.

No one dismissed as an irrelevancy the mother's thirty-kilometer walk to the hospital with her child slung on her back. Too poor even for a minibus? That was a bad sign: treatment options would be very limited. No one reprimanded Jameson for mentioning that the child's father had stayed with the family maize plot or for explaining which district they lived in. The child of subsistence farmers in a badly drought-stricken district would be especially prone to severe protein deficiency. Her transfer only made sense if you knew that the district hospital's "nutritional rehabilitation unit" (where starving children got fed) was down to providing one meal a day; in most districts, emergency refeeding would not have required a transfer to a central hospital.

An ethical and emotional crisis engulfed many trainees when they reached these wards and encountered their first living patients, when the professional identity and expectations they had taken on during preclinical education came up against the realities of patient suffering and physician helplessness in this extraordinarily resource-poor setting. As the previous chapter showed, these students had come to envision themselves as scientist-doctors whose knowledge of pathophysiology would enable them to heal using global medical technologies. For two years, like the Northern students studied by others, Malawian physicians-in-training had been anticipating this moment with a mixture of attraction and dread: wearing their white coats among patients instead of cadavers; laying hands on the sick; diagnosing and curing; cutting and stitching live flesh. Malawi's medical students faced a clinical reality far different from that of their Northern counterparts, however. "Most of the time we have had to meet patients where you have *zero* thing to offer," fifth-year student Itai Chilenga reflected. "Oh, you are thinking, now that's it—I have nothing to offer them. That hurts a lot." Lacking access to many of the medical tools and technologies their textbooks assumed to be available, faced with the realities of risk, poverty, and an apparently endless workload, they struggled with this transition in ways that ultimately forced many to reevaluate their roles as doctors.

Workload and Compromised Ideals

Workload in the hospital took on a different meaning from workload in the preclinical years. The sheer volume of patients was one factor: wards and clinics were spaces of bottomless need, where desperate family members would drag anyone foolhardy enough to enter wearing a white coat to come and attend to their sick relatives. In the preclinical years, one could master the material given enough diligence and a tolerance for sleep deprivation. In the hospital, time and energy were never enough. Many students quickly learned to avoid going into the wards alone whenever possible.

Students who were *adokotala* in the eyes of those occupying the hospital wards were still students in the eyes of the school. Their actual clinical time was highly fragmented by lectures, observations, rounds, and other obligations. Students were graded in large part on the completion of logbooks in which they recorded procedures witnessed or performed, disease cases they had followed, or "case presentations" they had given in which they summarized a patient's presenting complaint, history, and physical examination for a senior doctor. The logbook's requirements on some attachments meant students spent nearly all their clinical time "chasing for signatures and not knowledge," as one put it. It was not uncommon to see clusters of students rushing to and fro in a sort of medical scavenger hunt, searching for an intrauterine device insertion or a forceps delivery or a radical hysterectomy: "Has the patient for vacuum aspiration come yet? No? But we have class at ten!"

Even on more sensibly organized attachments, however, time and space to do things right—to find a private spot for a medical history or a physical exam, for instance, or to spend time consoling a mother whose baby had just died—were in very short supply. With limited time and limited space, clinical students began to make compromises with which they felt deeply uncomfortable.

We are not able to apply all the ethics that we are supposed to apply. . . . Things like privacy, things like confidentiality—you *need* to apply them. What we learn *here* [at the College of Medicine] we are supposed to be applying *there* [*nods toward the hospital*]. . . . I find it difficult to do, for example, a rectal examination within a ward. There are forty people there, and then I tell someone, "Can you remove [your clothes]"—then I do a rectal examination! In the presence of the rest of the people. (Andrew Kanyenda, third-year student)

Students learning basic sciences had often expressed pride in their ability to manage the heavy work, but clinical students and interns did not. Instead, when they spoke about workload, they talked about compromise. "There is too much to be done, but you can't do it all," a tired intern explained at the end of a day in which he had seen 150 patients in the outpatient department. "All these patients require time in order to be treated, that by the end of the day you can say, 'I have *worked* with the patient.' But sometimes that time is not there. So, you see, sometimes you feel that what you might offer you don't offer, simply because you're alone." Compromise could also involve treating patients with a detachment students had not described earlier in their training. One intern remarked that the workload could produce a dehumanizing effect that he characterized as the hallmark of bad medicine. When I asked him to tell me about a bad doctor, Zaithwa Mthindi described himself on a busy day.

When I'm doing ward rounds, you know. Sometimes you are so immersed in the—you are so concerned about finishing the ward rounds, so you don't really—treat *people*. You are just treating diseases. You are examining bodies, not examining people. For all your good intentions, you get so consumed with the bulk of work, and you lose your human face. And you realize that you have done ten, fifteen patients without even smiling at patients. Without even just giving a kind greeting. . . . I wish I could do better. I wish I could do better.

Fifth-year students, who often worked side by side with the interns, knew both the workload they already faced and what they would be expected to face soon. An intern might be expected to staff a clinic alone, or to round on an entire ward in a half day, making decisions on treatment plans, conducting bedside exams, performing minor diagnostic or therapeutic procedures. Patients had to be seen in two minutes or less, barely enough time to explain what the problem was. Sometimes students and interns just copied the diagnosis from the previous note without reinvestigating. Zaithwa, who described "losing your human face," also told me of a patient who had been admitted for unexplained muteness, a diagnosis repeated in his file for days until one morning a medical student finally greeted him—and he responded.

Students and interns agreed that it was impossible to do an adequate job under these circumstances, but they felt they had no other choice. Many spoke about the work in language that made a generic reality of their individual experiences by using the second person, and that evoked helplessness in the face of inevitable reality: "You have no option." "You must do it." "You get consumed." Intern Brian Msukwa's framing was typical: "You see all the patients that come through the doorway. . . . You forge ahead. You just do it. We don't—we don't have another option, just do it." When students talked about the wards and the clinics, rather than using the battleground metaphors so common in the North, they evoked floundering, wandering, drowning: the wards were "the deep end," "the forest."

Mortal Bodies, Dangerous Bodies

These students, experienced in the embalmed or discursive medical body, in the hospital encountered the real, living, and suffering human bodies with whom they had planned on working for the rest of their lives. This transition could involve reexamining their own priorities or confronting their own mortality.

> The whole process of what death is about—I feel, to me, the view has really changed now. . . . You have to face the realities of life, to say, "Nobody is actually immortal, everybody is going to die one of these days." Death actually is the reality—*I am going to die.* (Zebron Ching'amba, fourth-year student)

Many of the clinical students commented that being in the presence of so much death and suffering had changed them personally. Among other things, sometimes the change involved a less lighthearted view of sexual relationships; a few male students reported that they were less likely to be casual about sex, having seen repeatedly the potentially deadly consequences of both childbearing and HIV.

Students spoke most often of contagion as occupational, however, not sexual. The patient body as site of personal risk was a major theme in these interviews, appearing in a quarter of interviews with preclinical students, a third with clinical students, and two-thirds with interns. Their odds were probably greater of contracting drug-resistant tuberculosis on the wards (Harries 2002), but their major fear was HIV.

At the time I conducted the bulk of the initial interviews, roughly twenty-nine million people in sub-Saharan Africa were estimated to be living with HIV/AIDS (UNAIDS 2003). Malawi was neither the hardest- nor the lightest-hit of African countries, but the impact of the epidemic, visible if insidious elsewhere, was enormous in the hospitals.

> You are very aware now that we have—apart from the many curable diseases—that we have the HIV/AIDS. And this alone is a very big challenge. A very big challenge in the sense that it has actually added to the influx of patients to the hospitals. . . . And at the same time, you talk of the risk of being a physician. If you have to work at a district hospital, you cannot run away from the knife, you know? You have to do some surgeries and those kind of things. And not only surgeries but even in the ward itself. Interacting with HIV/AIDS in your patients is not quite a simple thing. (preclinical student and experienced clinician Joe Phoya)

Their risk of infection was exacerbated by the poverty of Malawi's health sector. Students were not immunized against the few preventable contagions, such as hepatitis B, because there was not enough money. Postexposure prophylaxis for preventing viral disease was unheard of, and reliable protective equipment (such as gloves, masks, sharps-disposal containers) was often unavailable. (By 2007, short-course antiretroviral medications were available for Ministry of Health employees who had "blood-borne exposures" to HIV while at work. They were not offered to students.)

The interaction of poverty-related factors could be synergistic. In the seventy surgical cases I did at Queens in 2002–3, I had five blood-borne exposures, or needle-sticks as clinicians more commonly call them. It was a small number but a high rate, more than twice what would be predicted, and several factors contributed.[6] First, the operating theater usually lacked a working suction machine. When too much blood welled up to see the point of the needle or scalpel—not uncommon in surgery—it had to be dabbed away from the surgical site by hand with sterilized cloths rather than sucked away with a plastic catheter, a catheter that would have kept my fingers far from the needle. Second, there was only one overhead light, instead of the three customary in American operating rooms, further impairing visibility. Third, our needle holders were either used donations from abroad or old Ministry of Health relics. The gripping teeth that should hold a needle in place had worn down long ago, but there were no new replacements, so we kept using them. Fourth, we used the needles that were cheapest for the Ministry of Health to purchase in bulk: round in cross section, these needles were less expensive than the three-sided "cutting" suture needles I often use in the United States, but they were prone to slipping. With a toothless needle holder grasping a round-bodied needle, no matter where one put the needle into the tissue, one couldn't be sure where it would come out as it twisted and torqued in its holder. The interns spoke of them resignedly as "dancing needles," and all of them had plenty of needle-sticks or scalpel lacerations, too.[7] In fact, blood-borne exposures were so common that students and staff often shrugged them off fatalistically. Clinicians saw their exposure as inevitable and were more inclined to worry about their posthumous reputations, as a graduate of the College of Medicine working a public-sector job with a heavy surgical caseload explained:

> It's a very challenging job, because we are being hand in hand with the fluids of the patient, which are contaminated with HIV. But it's part of the job we have. So that is hard. And in the end, when you die of HIV yourself, people may think otherwise. They can't think, "Oh, she is a doctor, she might have had it from a patient." But they think, "No, she was going some other—going outside [having an affair]." I don't know. I think there will be more and more infectious conditions which when— maybe by the time they have been identified, most of us doctors will have acquired them. It will be too late for us. (Ellen Mchenga, graduate)

Did occupational exposure really increase the risk for doctors, nurses, hospital cleaners, and other personnel? The consensus among Malawian students and doctors, all of whom knew colleagues lost to HIV/AIDS, was "of course." However, very little research has been conducted on occupational exposure to HIV in Africa (Akeroyd 2004), except among sex workers. Epidemiologic research in Africa, in marked contrast to studies in Europe or North America, consistently shows that increased levels of education and socioeconomic status are associated with *increased* risk of HIV/AIDS among the general public. (The theory, which fits well with Western assumptions about African sexuality, is that mobility and income increase opportunities for sexual exposure. See World Bank 1999 for a good overview of the data, much of it unpublished.) This pattern makes it very difficult to sort out how much additional risk might be due to occupational exposure.

Some researchers believe occupational exposure to be a negligible risk factor.[8] It is true that, if they were representative of their age and geographical cohorts, two or three in ten of the students should have already been HIV-positive when they began their training. It is also true, however, as Ellen's comment suggests, that Africans have been fairly consistently assumed—by researchers as well as by gossiping relatives—to be victims of their own promiscuity. A recent review (Gisselquist et al. 2002) attributing up to a fifth of African HIV cases to faulty medical procedures and supplies drew enormous criticism, in large part because health policymakers and others feared it would detract from the consensus on behavior change. The fracas over this report suggests that supporting good-quality studies on occupational exposure to HIV was simply not a priority for the major research funders. Malawian doctors and students I knew typically assumed that substantial health care transmission was likely, for both health care workers and patients. I agreed with them. But whether exposure was actually a major risk for students or only a major fear, it affected clinical students and interns negatively.

In 2002 and 2003, students for the most part appeared uninterested in HIV testing, either for themselves or for their patients. Rumor had it that only one College of Medicine graduate applied for a prestigious scholarship for postgraduate education in a country that mandated HIV testing as part of the application process. One preclinical interviewee told me she was appalled when she saw a doctor recommend an HIV test to a patient:

> I was actually shocked. This doctor was seeing a patient and just said plainly, "I think you should get an HIV test." Just like that! Telling someone basically, "I think you have HIV. You should lose all hope." I think that is wrong. One thing people need to have is hope. (Thokozani Sokela, preclinical student)

This situation was very different when I spoke again with students and hospital staff four years later. Many knew their own status, some were on antiretrovirals (although few were open about this with their colleagues), and all whom I asked recommended HIV testing for patients. In 2004, Malawi had begun a public-sector program of antiretroviral therapy that, although it had reached only a fraction of those who needed treatment, was expanding quickly and functioning fairly well. An HIV diagnosis no longer meant "you should lose all hope."

Poverty and Frustration

The numbers and riskiness of patients were sources of concern, then, but a more significant problem for most students was the lack of resources available to help their patients. Patients came in too late to be treated because they lacked funds for transport; once they did arrive, there might be little with which to treat them. Nearly all the textbooks the College of Medicine used came from First World settings and were oriented toward First World technomedicine; many were the same classics—in updated editions—over which I had pored in medical school in Michigan many years earlier. The students' textbook concepts of technological medicine, acquired in preclinical training, crashed headlong into a clinical world of understaffed, underequipped hospitals that frequently lacked basic supplies, not to mention magnetic resonance imaging, fluoroscopy, mechanical ventilator support, or other technologies of "global" biomedicine.

The hospital day in every clinical department began with "handover rounds," in which the overnight on-call team (typically, an intern, a third-year student, a fifth-year student, and the night nurse or nurses) handed over responsibility to the incoming group. Handover rounds nearly always featured tensions between what students and doctors thought should have been possible and what had actually happened. The report began with summary numbers of patients admitted, discharged, transferred, absconded, and died; the ward nurse would read from her report book a summary of any surgical cases, complex problems, or deaths—marked in the report book with a red ink cross and "RIP." These reports were typically very brief: "Chimwemwe Chisale, 22-year-old gravida one para zero admitted with septic abortion around 1 a.m. At 3:30 a.m. patient found to be gasping. At 4:10 a.m. returned to see patient, who was found to have died. Very sorry."[9] Faculty members could then make inquiries into any of these cases, and the team would defend management. Handover had both practical and pedagogical purposes: students and interns were expected to have read up on complex cases in their textbooks to assure faculty they had mastered the knowledge assumed to be important for every doctor. Yet the discrepancy between textbook and ward was often glaring, and available options shaped or foreclosed therapeutic choices.

One steamy morning in the early rainy season, fifth-year student Catherine Gunya gave the handover report; the pied crows squawked through the open hospital windows as they picked at detritus in the courtyards, nearly drowning out her quiet voice. Emergent Cesarean section for fetal distress following a failed forceps extraction had led to a neonatal death, Catherine reported. The infant had come out pink but then breathed in thick meconium, a tarry stool passed in situations of distress that should be promptly suctioned from the newborn's trachea at birth. "Was the infant suctioned?" "No, sir." "Why not?" "The suction machine was not working. We intended to suction manually, but the batteries were stolen from the laryngoscope [a lighted tool used to see the trachea properly], and there were no replacements. We tried to suction without seeing, but the infant died in the operating theater." That same night a twenty-six-year-old woman had died on the gynecology ward of a malignancy that had spread to her lungs. Catherine explained that she had made the diagnosis—the pregnancy-related tumor called choriocarcinoma—a week earlier by seeing the classic round "cannonball lesions" on chest X-ray. A biopsy or blood test would have confirmed it, but there was no histopathologist in the country to read the biopsy, and the appropriate blood test was unavailable. "What is the proper treatment for choriocarcinoma?" "First, you must give methotrexate, but we do not have any. We just gave her oxygen therapy." And so a disease that Catherine's textbook reported to be 95 percent curable with a low-cost drug remained 100 percent fatal for her patients.

In this context, the new would-be doctors often felt they saw little return on their learning and hard work, because they had little to offer patients. Fifth-year student Itai Chilenga had had "a very bad time" on his pediatrics attachment: "Almost all the patients who I was able to see, three-quarters of them passed away, and it—it became stressful." He described fighting the urge to skip his on-call shifts. "It becomes demoralizing. And at times, you always get discouraged. Why should I go to work at night, when obviously the patient maybe who I might see may die two or three days later? But if there were something I could have given the patient—ah." Young doctors often commented on the disjuncture between textbook and clinic: "Sometimes you just read in order to pass your exams, but you can't be able to meet such situations in real life, and that—that, that is quite difficult. . . . So, really, what you learn in medical school is not exactly applicable when you start working." Students learned about diseases of the elderly but had almost no elderly patients. They learned about neuroimaging and fluoroscopy and care of the extremely premature neonate, but had access to none of the equipment necessary.

HIV/AIDS complicated this picture further, for in 2002 and 2003, there was little to offer HIV-positive patients. Many students talked about a sort of helplessness-induced fatigue that set in on the medical wards, where so many of their patients could not be treated effectively: "It's been useless all these years. Studying from first year to third year, fourth year, and, and at the end of the day, people still die." Third-year student Mirriam Kamanga had entered medicine to "make a difference in the suffering of children." She found pediatrics particularly hard: it was "difficult for me to watch these mothers sit there and pray and hope that their child will be all right, yet I know myself that it's—you know, it's going to be really difficult, and that's not gonna be the case." Students and interns quickly grew sick of feeling useless, and bored with the frequency of AIDS-related illnesses they could do little or nothing about.

> You know, you want to help someone, but you can't see a positive result. You don't have enough drugs to offer. Most of your patients are terminally ill, and not everyone is cut out to do that kind of work, working with terminal cases all the time. And then there are the dangers you have with it as well—you know, blood everywhere, exposure. But also in some ways it's hard to see the same things all the time. Someone comes in with a problem, and you know exactly what's going to happen next. There are no surprises. (Diana Kondowe, intern)

> Medicine will not be very much interesting, because all your focus will be on HIV. . . . Really, there's very little that a doctor in a developing country can do in such cases. (Zebron Ching'amba, fourth-year student)

Readers may wonder why their conditions of work were so demoralizing for these young doctors. They were Malawians: had they not seen plenty of death, plenty of HIV, plenty of poverty before? Did they truly not know what to expect? The answer to these questions varied somewhat with the social situation of the entering medical student. It was very common for the most privileged students to report that medical school gave them their first inkling of what life was really like for most Malawians. The group of previously trained clinicians, on the other hand, seemed to be somewhat inoculated against this particular shock. Experienced clinical officers were the only students who spoke about Queen Elizabeth Central Hospital as a site of relative abundance (compared to the smaller Malawi district hospitals in which they had worked). The majority of the students fit neither of these categories, however. For most members of the class, it seemed to be the experience of their own powerlessness in the face of medical need and systemwide breakdown that was demoralizing. They were already aware of the magnitude of poverty and suffering in their country, but they were not used to facing it as those charged to heal yet unable to do so.

Encounters with the International: Medical Tourism

While students struggled under the conditions of their work, they also struggled with competing images of what medicine could be. In Malawi as elsewhere in Africa, expatriate doctors and medical students flowed south on the same ideological and technical currents that brought biomedical techniques and curricula to the region. Where biomedical education was relatively new, as at the College of Medicine, expatriates often made up a substantial proportion of the teaching staff. (In Malawi, roughly a third of the faculty was Malawian, a third expatriates from other African countries, and a third expatriates from other continents.) In those same places, visiting medical students from wealthier countries came and went in a constant stream of what were usually called foreign short-term medical volunteers but could just as legitimately be termed medical tourists: health care providers and trainees eager to see how medicine was practiced in parts of the world far from home.

At Queens Hospital, at any given time there were thirty to sixty Malawian medical students in their third, fourth, or fifth years, plus midwifery students, nursing students, clinical officer students, and other Malawian trainees. There were also typically five to ten foreign students, usually near the end of their own medical-school coursework and widely dispersed through the wards. The hospital and medical school had long-standing relationships with several research universities in the United States, the United Kingdom, Western Europe, and Australia. In Malawi, most visiting medical trainees came from one of these institutions; none that I met hailed from elsewhere in Africa, and all were white. Foreign students stayed as briefly as two weeks or as long as three months. In general, they were quite informally supervised, and their commitment to work in the hospital varied widely. Some put in token appearances and then spent the bulk of their time at Malawi's well-known and expensive lakeside resorts. Some, with the blessings of their home institutions, excused themselves from all procedures involving blood or body fluids because of the HIV risk and simply watched.[10] Others worked as hard as their Malawian colleagues, side by side.

For Malawian students and interns, at least those in their hospital training, contact with short-term foreign visitors was an everyday affair. The visitors were topics of conversation in enough interviews and focus groups to suggest that part of how students formed their ideas of what it meant to be doctors was through reflection on what it seemed to mean elsewhere. Like the figure of the clinical officer, that of the "international doctor" became something of a foil for them: an identity to embrace or to alter. Their comments suggested that students' experiences with medical tourists led them to contrast medicine in Malawi with medicine in an unmarked international "elsewhere." Thus, encounters with foreign medical trainees became another site in which these students struggled over what "real medicine" was. Cross-cultural tourism often raises questions about authenticity and identity. In the case of medical tourism in Malawi, it was the *visitor* who was assumed to be the authentic representative of global biomedicine. Malawian medical students and their fellow Africans became the marked impoverished Other, while visiting Northern student physicians became unmarked global doctors.

Some of the few Malawi graduates who had spent time abroad felt that this very transformation was the most important part of their experience and used it to argue for increased exposure to electives abroad. One explicitly argued that students who went on electives "would be trained as *international* doctors, not just as *national* doctors." Another spoke of his own enlightenment during advanced training in London, and how he felt coming back to Queens Hospital: "The conditions there are terrible—it's hard to work like that. But the students may not know any better. You need to be exposed to the other situation. If you haven't had the experience, you can't know what should be changed, what is needed."

Malawian students often referred to the foreign students who came to Queen Elizabeth Hospital for electives as their friends, their colleagues, their brothers or sisters. Sometimes simply working together made the Malawians feel more like international doctors. But while they clearly identified with the expatriate medical tourists, they also noticed differences. Nearly a third of the comments students and interns made about medical tourists focused on the relative riches—in both equipment and opportunity—available to the tourists and the relative poverty of resources for Malawian doctors. Several noted wistfully how well equipped their fellow students were, draped with stethoscopes, white coat pockets bulging with reflex hammers, pocket medical guides, blood pressure cuffs, and the usual diagnostic accoutrements of Northern students. Often these medical tourists and their Malawian colleagues had used the same textbooks, but the tourist students had inevitably also seen in action Swann-Ganz catheters, laparoscopic procedures, radiation and chemotherapy, and other expensive technologies of Northern medicine—things their Malawian counterparts had only read about. An intern recalled hearing touring students talking about using MRIs to image the brain.

> We don't have that here, so you just read about it. . . . We admire our friends when they come over here and do something in our hospital. They have so much advanced technology, and medicine is quite a field which *requires* quite a big advancement in technology. And we look at our friends as being so fortunate to have all those technological advances at their disposal.

Encounters with medical tourists, clearly, could reinforce a sense that real medicine was what happened elsewhere.

Tourists inevitably take more than photographs and leave more than footprints. They leave behind images, ideas of what other places and other cultures are like. In Malawi, medical tourists left behind them an image of the international doctor, the real doctors without borders—but with plenty of advanced technologies and a comfortable life to go home to when their travels were done. In the case of Malawi, students' exposure to "medical tourists" from Europe and America became one mechanism by which they created a concept of the doctor as unmarked global citizen. From there, it was a short step to seeing real medicine as a necessarily expensive and high-technology endeavor, and Malawian medicine as somehow less than real, or second-rate. It was a short step, and one many students took—but not an inevitable one.[11] For other student doctors, encounters with medical tourism became prompts to reflect on their own strengths as clinicians: flexibility, understanding of the underlying causes of disease, commitment to the health of the nation. I will explore these issues in chapter 7.

In the Deep End

Students were not paralyzed in the face of their working difficulties. No one quit in dismay, although some students reported that they had seriously considered doing so. Instead, they used various combinations of avoidance and improvisation to cope. The clinical officer group already knew how to function on scant resources. By their fifth year, many of the previously inexperienced students were learning this lesson, too. They learned to improvise on the wards: they made urinary catheters from used intravenous saline bags, saved and resterilized suture, put together sharps-disposal containers from plastic buckets or nested cardboard boxes. In the absence of nursing staff, they handed off tasks to family members or student nurses or junior medical students.[12] Several reported that they were happy when they found ways to help patients "even with the minimal resources we have." But most seemed saddened by their experiences, "drained," as more than one student put it.

Toward the beginning of my fieldwork, I sat one day in the small operating theater office with Aubrey Nkhandwe, an intern. We each had post-surgical orders to write on our patients' files—a few sheets of histopathology forms or other useless requisitions, the clean sides and blank spaces serving as places for orders and notes. Our patients lay side by side in the hallway. There was no recovery room or recovery nurse, and many of the trolleys on which patients lay had no side rails. If they were packed closely together, though, no one could fall, and this close to the office, if blood began to drip on the floor, someone would probably hear it. Once finished with orders, Aubrey and I chatted as we drank cups of sweet, milky tea and waited for our next cases. When I told him what my research was about, he grinned and announced that I did not need to interview anyone. He could tell me what I would find:

> Someone starts at the College of Medicine, he has been getting very good grades in his secondary school, probably he is top of the class. The first year or two in the college, he is still working very hard, mostly making good grades. Then, by the clinical years, he realizes how hard this work is, how he will not make a very good salary. . . . Soon he is mostly doing as little work as possible just to pass, just to survive, and taking alcohol. Maybe even being alcoholic.

The trajectory Aubrey outlined was one other students alluded to as well, and the use of alcohol as a coping strategy came up frequently in interviews and in casual conversation (although I never asked students directly about alcohol use and never saw a student drunk).[13] Preclinical students sometimes worried about the heavy drinking they saw among students in the third to fifth years and puzzled over "how to combat stress without destroying yourself." Medson Namanja, a third-year student, explained: "I think we have several methods of relieving stress. Mainly it's alcohol, that's a big one, especially for the guys. It's effective. At least for a couple of hours, because that way you forget for a while."

There was much to forget. These students had been the academic stars of their secondary schools, they had survived the intense pressure of their basic science training, but now they found themselves unable to perform the way they had hoped.

When you are coming from maybe from doing A-levels, O-levels, you
have very high marks. And you come to medicine, and somehow you
are *not satisfactory*. I thought I was very brilliant! [*He laughs.*] That's
the only thing maybe which makes me sad. Does it mean, yeah, I am
not all that, what I thought I would be? Yeah, that's the only thing.
(Dumbisyani Zinyemba, fifth-year student)

At some point in the interview, nearly a third of the clinical students and
interns volunteered that they felt worse about themselves since beginning
medical training: inadequate, ethically compromised, disillusioned about
their own capabilities. Not one preclinical student had reported such a
change.

Losing Faith

Several of the inexperienced preclinical students spoke at length about
their religious faith as sustaining. They anticipated that this faith would
help them through difficult clinical situations and sometimes characterized God as the ultimate consultant:

We are God's creation, and even though we get a PhD in anatomy, we
can't totally understand the body of a person. You still meet a strange
disease that you have never encountered in your entire life, maybe
you've been practicing for more than twenty years, but you still find
something strange ahead of you. So if you know God, then you can be
able to consult God. I am sure you will be able to cope with such a situation. (Clement Chafunya, first-year student)

Like many of the other preclinical students, when Clement described a
good doctor, that doctor's strong Christian faith was an important characteristic. In fact, three preclinical students described the good doctor as
one for whom no surgery ever went badly, because of the power of the doctor's faith and prayers. And four preclinical students looked forward to the
chance to use spiritual healing and counseling to help patients' lives improve and bring them back to paths of righteousness.[14]
Once in the hospital, clinical students rarely brought up religion in interviews. None spoke of a crisis of faith, but social pressures would have
worked against any such disclosure.[15] The perception among many students was that one's perceived religious fervor correlated positively with
one's grades on certain clinical attachments; some students joined cam-

pus religious groups at strategic times to take advantage of the potential grade boost. Students seemed to feel free to discuss their beliefs with me. They may have felt less free to discuss doubts. Still, there is some evidence that the clinical transition diminished student certainty about the medical utility of faith, if not faith itself. Clinical students no longer spoke about God the consultant or about prayer as the key to surgical success, never described good doctors they knew in terms of religious faith, and never discussed spiritual counseling with patients. On questionnaires, they were much less likely to believe that a strong spiritual life made a better doctor. If God was not missing from the medical world they had entered, he was certainly—and newly—missing from their conversations about it.[16] This absence echoed other absences, as previous certainties fell away and new doubts entered students' reflections on their work.

Where Is the Government?

Many of these students had described entering medicine with a dream of uplifting Malawi, healing the nation as part of a coalition of doctors. The "Learning by Living" experience had helped to cement their feelings of being true Malawians, and they were ready to help their fellow citizens. This dream hit reality hard in the clinical years. Although clinical students were no different from others in the way they spoke about Malawian people in general, they began to speak with much more anger and cynicism about their national government. A notable exception was the group of students with prior hospital experience: even in the preclinical years, they already spoke with anger and cynicism about the government.

At Queen Elizabeth Central Hospital, students saw the effects of national and supranational policies—which they interpreted as policies of deliberate neglect and tended to attribute specifically to the Malawian government—upon facilities, patients, and workers. They became well acquainted with the low salaries they could look forward to receiving, and with the effects of low salaries and missing paychecks on other health personnel. They also saw the lack of other resources, like drugs and equipment, as a government failure. They came to believe that Malawi's politicians were out of touch, hypocritical, and uncaring.

> I feel sometimes that the government, and even the people in authority who look to—who, who, who are looking after the local hospitals like Queens, they *don't have the heart for the people*. It's like, they *pretend*

and *announce* that they care. But in reality? They are doing nothing. Ah. Of course, other people can go to the private practitioners. [*in a sarcastic voice*] That's very good. But then the majority, the poor Malawian cannot afford to go there. And even those who are actually deciding for the fate of those who are at Queens and the other hospitals, they themselves *do not come to Queens.* They go to the private hospitals! So I think that's a very big problem. (Alex Mkweu, fifth-year student)

In many ways, students and interns felt they were treated with enormous social respect as doctors. They frequently reported that they felt a lack of respect and commitment from the government, however, and described themselves as "disillusioned" or "disgusted."[17] Widespread resentment of government failure surfaced: foreign students talked about going home and spoke contemptuously of Malawi's government, which they saw as "turning a deaf ear to the problems of the people," while Malawians' sense of anger and betrayal was palpable.

Much of the anger focused on the waste of money that resulted from corrupt practices, and students' comments echoed a larger nationwide unrest over corruption during those years. On the day I interviewed Graham Mapundula, a clinical student, antigovernment protests had broken out at the nearby Polytechnic. Cronies of then president Bakili Muluzi were seeking to amend the constitution to allow him a third term in office, against great resistance from a populace mindful of longtime dictator Kamuzu Banda's similar early strategies. In the operating theater, the interns and nurses were referring to Muluzi mockingly as "His Excellency," a chilling reference to the Banda reign of intimidation. Despite vocal opposition from constituents, many members of Parliament (MPs) had recently voted to allow a third term. Malawians I spoke to believed that these votes had been bought—with cash or, even more controversially, with international food aid given preferentially to compliant MPs to distribute in their districts during a famine year.

On this day, the police were trying to break up an anti-third-term rally at the college with batons and tear gas. Truckloads of "Young Democrats," members of a militant youth arm of the ruling United Democratic Front Party known for beating and intimidating the opposition, were bused in for a pro-third-term demonstration and brawled with protesters. Wafts of tear gas drifted through the open window as Graham talked, making us both cough. At the end of the interview, I asked Graham whether he had anything he wished to add. His amiable face tightened into a scowl, and he spoke with vehemence.

Just a comment. I feel that to achieve the basic health standards in Malawi is a—I mean, at the moment, we should *forget*. At the moment, in
these two years, we should *forget*. I say this because the guy, the president that is our president at the moment, does not have the people of
Malawi at heart. He doesn't have the vision for this country. And maybe
it will be the duty of most of us that will be graduating that will make
that dream a reality.

The policies and budgets "on paper" were reasonable, said Graham, who
knew about budgets from his years running a hospital unit as a clinical
officer. But the designated staff resources, the supplies, and especially the
money never seemed actually to arrive. Graham believed that it was buying votes instead and that these votes were very costly.

You talk of *one* person? Twenty-five million kwacha. And that is just an
MP. . . . So if you spend money to have somebody in power, definitely
you will not have money to keep the health sector running. Yeah? If we
had kept all, each and every penny that we had received from donors,
I tell you that we wouldn't be where we are at the moment. If we had
committed *each and every* penny that we received from the donors, we
wouldn't be where we are. Yeah? I mean, we have squandered a *lot* of
resources.

Corruption not only diverted resources away from the health sector
but also could divert resources within the health sector toward certain
favored constituencies or patients. Clinical students and interns often described the political pressures they would face as district health officers,
sometimes illustrating with stories they had heard from graduates working
out in the districts. One tale widely circulated at the College of Medicine,
for instance, was that of a recent graduate transferred by the Ministry of
Health to a famously undesirable post in an exceptionally remote, exceptionally poor, and exceptionally hot part of the country. While working as
a district health officer in a first posting near his family home, this young
doctor had noticed that only a small fraction of the medications allocated
to his district ever arrived at the hospital. He tracked the lost medications
to the local MP, whose relatives were selling the hospital's scarce supplies
in the public market, and he lodged a formal complaint. Nothing happened
to the MP, people told me, but the doctor was punished.[18]
    It was not all just rumor and secondhand stories. Clinical students also
encountered examples of this sort of political pressure and internal diver-

sion of funds at the hospital. Four clinical students, demonstrating considerable courage, wrote and signed a letter in the *Malawi Medical Journal* protesting the abuse of a special program intended to help children with cardiac anomalies (see Masambo et al. 2004). Another student, Dumbisyani Zinyemba, explained the problem to me:

> DUMBISYANI: The MP will send family to use up scarce resources. For instance, their family member may have something that is very easily treated, that you can just treat at the district, and they will say, "No, you must transport them to Queens." Even for something simple, they will force the doctor to write a referral to the central hospital. Or—have you heard about this program from South Africa, for heart surgery?
>
> CLAIRE: A little bit, but tell me. I don't know much about it.
>
> DUMBISYANI: OK. So, the government of South Africa decided they would take ten patients from Malawi each year to have heart surgery in South Africa, because there are not the resources to do it here. And it would be free. Malawi would have to pay transport and housing, but all the hospital, medical costs would be at no cost. You know we have many children here with congenital cardiac problems who could benefit from this program, who could have their surgeries and live. Well, what happened was the MPs forced the doctors to send their relatives instead—who didn't even have heart problems, who didn't even need surgery, who maybe had some other disease entirely! They forced the doctors to select these people for the program, so then they could fly to South Africa and stay for free. But then, when they got to South Africa, those people at the hospital said, "This program is not working—these people do not even need heart surgery," and in the end, they canceled the whole program.

Students lodged the blame for Malawi's miserable health-sector situation squarely on the national government, and particularly on political corruption.

Some Africanists (see, for example, Burke 2003; Kitching 2000) believe that scholarship on African poverty has typically underplayed the role of state misrule, a role seen clearly by those on the ground. However, it would be difficult to defend an argument that all of Malawi's trouble was of its own making. Macroeconomic factors related to North–South capital flows affected the health sector as well, in ways that the students perhaps did not fully see or acknowledge; students rarely discussed supranational factors except occasionally to mention donors, and then nearly always in positive terms.[19] Like most other countries in sub-Saharan Africa, Malawi had contracted major debt in the early postindependence era. Debt service had been among the country's top exports for decades, and continued to be even after some loans were forgiven as part of the HIPC Initiative. As discussed in chapter 2, the terms of loans probably had effects as profound as the debt service itself. The effects of international lending policies, along with the steep rises in drug prices brought about by world trade agreements, were felt keenly in Malawi. With little military or other expenditures to trim, the "fat" of the state budget had to come in large part out of the health sector even as prices for essential drugs and numbers of sick patients were escalating rapidly.[20] Some of the deterioration in the health sector that shocked these clinical students was attributable to policies and capital flows out of the hands of Malawi's government. Nonetheless, it was clear that both corruption and lack of political will to improve the health sector were indeed significant problems. Students consistently argued that politicians worked the system so their own relatives had other options for health care, relieving them of any pressure to improve conditions at the public hospitals.

Bad Medicine

As they lost faith in their government, and as their religious faith offered less support, clinical students also started to lose faith in medicine—both as a career and as a force for good. Clinical students were the only people I interviewed who sometimes could not think of anything good about being a doctor in Malawi. A notable wavering of faith in medicine can be read in students' advice to a hypothetical sibling wanting a medical career (table 5.1). When I asked students in the first two years of their training what advice they would give a brother or sister who told them, "I want to be a doctor in Malawi, too," they all gave positive responses. Most preclinical students were unequivocally supportive of the idea. First-year student Gift Mkango's response was typical: "I think medicine is a very exciting field, and I would say, 'Hey—if you want to try it, go ahead. I think you'll enjoy it. It's hard work, all right, but at the end of the day, you enjoy it, and there's always satisfaction.'" Those preclinical students who weren't unhesitatingly positive wanted to examine the motivations of the aspiring doctor and would be supportive if these motivations were "right." Usually, this meant if the sibling truly wanted to help rather than to make a fat salary.

Clinical students less often gave either of these responses. When they

TABLE 5.1. Should a sibling become a doctor in Malawi? (% giving each response)

Advice type	Preclinical students	Clinical students	Interns[a]
Yes	59	25	0
Yes, if sibling's motivations are good	35	8	20
"Informed consent" response	6	50	40
No	0	17	40

[a]I have included interns here to demonstrate the overall trends, but the number I asked this question of (5) was very small.

did, they were more cautious. One of the students I have coded in table 5.1 as answering "yes," for instance, wanted a sibling to do medicine only because one could always find a job even in Malawi's shaky economy. It was a *secure* job, he said, although it was not a very *good* job. Another, after thinking for a while, decided, "Well, it's not a terrible idea." Instead of encouragement, clinical students most often gave a response I came to think of as "informed consent," talking about the pros and cons of working as a doctor and then leaving siblings to make up their own minds.

> I think I would tell him the truth in that how I see it. You know, if you want to be a doctor in Malawi, this is what you will face. And let him make the decision, the final decision, himself. But I wouldn't lie to him that, you know, it's great, he should do it—no. I would let him know. This is what happens. (Tuntufye Chihana, clinical student)

Some clinical students and interns flatly discouraged others from entering medicine. Brian Msukwa, an intern, gave an incredulous laugh when I asked the question. "I would guide them to do some other courses," he said when he was done laughing. "Let me suffer—I have suffered already—let them do something else." Another intern, in 2007, recalled her interview as a naïve preclinical student with embarrassment: "I probably said, oh, medicine is a great career or something like that. If [you] asked me now, I would say differently!"

Much of this disenchantment with medicine seemed to be about salary, workload, and working conditions. Another component of the students' disillusionment related to some of the doctors with whom they worked. Once they had experienced medical work in the hospital, students often spoke of witnessing hypocrisy, discrimination, and disdain for patients. Some students had worked with doctors whom they saw as prejudiced against poor patients in general or against Malawians specifically. Three students described doctors who actually refused to touch patients, two of them telling me the same story of a doctor (probably the same doctor) who would position his stethoscope in his ears and ask a nurse to place the stethoscope diaphragm on the patient, considering it beneath him to touch patients himself. Complaints about doctors who were harsh with patients, or would not listen to patients or subordinate staff, were very common.

Clinical students and interns spoke most bitterly about consultants who were absent when needed, however. Some consultants were Ministry of Health employees or part-time volunteers. Most were faculty (primarily expatriate) who accepted salaries from the College of Medicine in return for supervising and teaching medical students and contributing to the college's research agenda. Sometimes they could be very hard to find.

> There are times when you're in the hospital. You have an emergency, and to actually find a consultant is impossible, pretty much impossible. Because they are off doing their private practice, while their main aim for them to be *in* this country is so that they may improve the—or so that they may impart knowledge on us. (Medson Namanja, clinical student)

Many students felt that absent consultants weakened their training, leaving them to learn as they could from nurses, clinical officers, interns, and one another.

Consultant absence was more than just an educational problem, however. Students saw the unavailability of consultants as an ethical failure among the doctors with whom they worked. In interviews, clinically experienced students consistently listed availability as one of the most important characteristics of doctors they admired.[21] When asked to describe bad doctors, they were much more likely than clinically inexperienced students to talk about doctors who weren't there when needed, and to talk about them in terms of dishonesty or hypocrisy. Tuntufye Chihana said she hated those doctors who lectured about being good but then "they don't practice what they preach. You look at them, you see that they don't care about the patients at all."

> And when they are on call, they don't come. And then the next day, say maybe in report, people are saying, "You know, such and such a thing happened," and then you know that maybe that thing couldn't have happened if a senior person had seen that patient, and then they're,

"Oh, no, I wasn't called," but then you know they were, they are just covering it up. That's what I hate.

Students judged absent consultants very harshly, as "hypocrites" or "brutes." The severity of their judgments was likely related to the real terror of being left alone when one did not know what to do, an experience common to clinical students and interns and one they dreaded.

Early one morning, I walked onto the antenatal ward to evaluate a patient scheduled for surgery. At the nurses' station sat Frazer Makano, a normally irrepressible intern I knew well, slowly writing a note in the report book with his head drooped over the battered desk. I asked him how he was, knowing he had been on call, and he got out, "I am a little bit, a little bit . . . not fine." Around midnight, a young pregnant woman had been brought in, hemorrhaging vaginally, he told me. She was "paper-white" when she hit the door, and Frazer had rushed her to the operating theater with one pint begged off the blood bank. With a rapid emergency Cesarean, he and the theater nurse delivered a live newborn, also paper-white, who that morning was still gasping in the nursery but not looking likely to survive. As he sewed the uterine incision closed, Frazer saw that his patient was oozing blood steadily from every spot where the needle had gone in. He and I had practiced a surgical technique for dealing with hemorrhage a few weeks before, while doing some scheduled Cesarean sections together, and he tried that.

> I thought perhaps she was getting into trouble, so I tried to remember what you had taught me about the uterine artery ligation, but I could not palpate the uterine arteries, perhaps because she was in shock. I think I should have, maybe it would have helped. Because after she was closed, as I massaged the uterus and blood was just gushing out, not even clotting, so I saw she was in DIC.[22] And I called the consultant, and the consultant—the consultant chose to manage it over the phone.

He choked, eyes filled with tears, and looked away. After a few seconds' silence, he resumed the story. As dawn broke, one of the hospital staff drove to the home of another consultant, banging on the door to wake him and bring him in. This doctor "came in to my rescue," Frazer said, "but as we took her to the theater for emergency hysterectomy—we were just going to do a very rapid one, you know—we were even in our gowns, we had blood all ready—she died."

Most consultants, like the one who tried to rescue Frazer and his pa-

tient, were too responsible to manage dire cases over the phone. Yet with
the workload as high as it was, the human resources for dealing with it
stretched to the breaking point, and a small handful of consultants notori-
ous for refusing to come in on call, nearly all clinical students and interns
had experienced the terror of facing a true emergency alone and unprepared.
The impact of these experiences was devastating, and felt beyond the individual. Those who had not yet faced such traumatic situations themselves
often told me stories of their friends' experiences.

Students interacted with clinicians they considered to be good doctors,
too. But their descriptions of good doctors did not change as much from
preclinical to clinical training as their descriptions of bad doctors. Their
experience of doctors in the hospital may not have been what they had
expected.

Clinical students reflected critically on their own experience of preclinical training at this point as well. All of the stories I was told about corruption or incompetence within the College of Medicine itself came from
clinical students—even when the events they described took place during
the basic medical sciences years. One student discussed the anatomy professor who insisted that students purchase "his" book—mostly material
plagiarized from a well-known textbook, mixed with photocopied lecture
notes and without pictures. Students were downgraded for using the picto-
rial atlases many found essential for learning anatomy: "You are in danger of failing if you learn from another source, and also in danger if you
are discovered learning from another source." Students talked about lecturers who told them, "It doesn't matter whether you learn. I still get my
paycheck." One reflected on a formative experience during the first year,
when one of the faculty members published a student group project as his
own. When the students discovered the publication and confronted him,
he threatened them: "Wherever you go, I can find you!" Knowing he had
the power to make sure their careers were stillborn, the students backed
down—but never put effort into a group project again and were labeled as
an indolent and poorly motivated class as a result.

Not only were they critical of their teachers, but students also became
more critical of their own motivations during the clinical years. Almost
half the clinical students spoke regretfully about "cramming" for exams
and forgetting everything afterward, a problem preclinical students did not
acknowledge in themselves (although they did sometimes critique their
fellow students for this behavior). Alex Mkweu, a final-year student, said
he would know he was a real doctor "when I will *exert my mind to know
things*, not because of the exams but to know them so that I can help some-

body." Alex's comment illustrated both a shift toward a physician identity based on application more than knowledge, and a negative judgment of his own behavior. Students saw cramming as the only way to cope with their heavy workload but thought less of themselves for doing it.

In chapter 4, I described how students' bodies became sites for medical knowledge and medical feeling, and for knowing *by* feeling—by practical and physical senses, dispositions of perception and action that came together into a medical habitus. In their clinical years, students continued to know by feeling, but their reflections on the experience of clinical work made it clear that the feeling was often one of pain. Surrounded by risky bodies, by suffering and death for which they—at least initially—believed they could do little, many of them expressed grief and anger, even betrayal.

The gaze of medicine looks in order to know, and this visual knowing, according to Michel Foucault (1975), is a form of tacit violence. His insight has given rise to a fruitful body of scholarship on biomedicine as a set of knowledges and practices that can dismember the individual body into a collection of organs and molecules, or the individual self into an assemblage of risk factors. Foucault-inspired work on the violence of medical knowing tends to omit the emotional experience of the knower, however. Here the work of philosopher Martha Nussbaum is very helpful. When Nussbaum (2001:45) writes that "knowing can be violent, given the truths that are there to be known," she is writing of a violence that is exerted *upon the knower*. At the moment one learns a terrible truth, emotion and cognition happen simultaneously, "putting the world's nail into [one's] own insides" and thus demanding both passionate attention and moral appraisal. Emotions, as Nussbaum and other scholars have argued, are forms of engagement and of moral judgment, ways of measuring the world and oneself (see, for example, Hawkins 2002; Lutz 1992; Robichaud 2003).

The Malawian students' stories, as they retold their experiences, tended to turn in the clinical years from what they knew to what they felt. In their narratives, the judgments those feelings entailed are evident: how what should have been was not; how their consultants or their government failed them and their patients; how workload or crowding or staffing prevented the exercise of a good and ethical medicine. I will argue in the pages ahead that these feelings gave them access to an understanding of the social and political forces underlying their patients' illnesses and deaths. Northern students at this point in training learn to experience their own emotional responses as distractions, as threats to the practice of scientific medicine. For these Malawian students, such responses did not seem to be perceived as distractions. Their emotions were doing ethical work. They were neither threats to objectivity nor threats to a real understanding of what was happening; instead, they were in some cases the mechanism by which that understanding happened.

Not every student described the clinical transition as a devastating one. Medson Namanja, the student who discussed drinking as a way to "forget for a while," also explained that he was proud of the increased responsibility and confidence he got from being left alone on the ward so often, and occasionally other students and interns made such comments. The few clinically experienced students in these years, as I discussed briefly above, also did not demonstrate the sense of shock or crisis so often present in other interviews, although their anger and cynicism about the government seemed particularly profound. Nonetheless, as should be clear from the excerpts given in this chapter, the majority of comments about hospital experiences supported the idea that a significant transition was taking place. The realities of sickness and healing in a very poor place were painful to encounter and began to force a rethinking of medicine that continued into clinical practice.

Complications
Johnson Chisale

Johnson Chisale was a tailor.[23] An energetic man with nimble hands, he could copy any item of clothing brought to him, running up a replica in the fabric of his customer's choice on a trusty treadle Singer sewing machine. In recent years, Malawi, like most other African countries, has been inundated with used clothing from the United States: usually intended as donations to Goodwill or the Salvation Army, it ends up sold at markets all across Africa. This abundance of cheap clothing has been a boon for poor Africans in many ways.[24] It has been disastrous for tailors, however. Johnson's nearly manic energy, high-quality work, and impeccably honest business practices, plus a few lucky contacts that led him to a network of potential clients, just barely kept his family afloat.

In the rainy season, Johnson, normally a healthy man, got a bad case of diarrhea that left him dehydrated. Such infections were common in the crowded neighborhood where his family lived in a mud-brick house; there was no public sewage system, outhouses drained into open ditches running down the steep hill between ramshackle dwellings and shops, and the only clean water came from a public tap several houses away from his. The diarrhea left him weakened, and one day, after walking several miles to a customer's home and back without having eaten anything, he fainted on the path just outside his house. His neighbors were alarmed when he failed to awaken immediately. Reluctant to relegate him to the free public hospital, they took him to a nearby mission instead.

When Johnson awoke, he was lying between sheets on a mattress, with an intravenous drip in one arm. The mattress and sheets told him instantly he was not in a public hospital, and he leapt out of bed in a panic. Mission hospitals are not fully subsidized either by the government or by their affiliated churches, and Johnson knew he would be required to pay for his treatment. Dragging his IV pole, he searched the hospital until he found the doctor—who sternly commanded him to get back in bed, insisting that he absolutely could not be discharged until he had been observed for at least a week.

After three days, Johnson managed to convince the doctor that he was well enough to go home by demonstrating (repeatedly) that he could run full tilt down the hospital corridor. Feeling well and dressed again in his neat suit, he went to the hospital accounting office to pay his bill, where he found the sum was even worse than he had feared: thirty-eight hundred kwacha (US$40). They would not let him leave the hospital grounds before he paid, so he told his wife where their hidden savings were, cached behind a loose brick in one wall of their house. This was the money he had been putting away over the years whenever he could, hoping to get his clever oldest daughter into medical school. But even after Mrs. Chisale brought the family's entire savings to the office, Johnson still owed eight hundred kwacha. The clerk gave him two choices. Either he could become a groundskeeper for the hospital for over a month until his debt was paid off, or they would confiscate his sewing machine (his only possession of any monetary value) and hold it as collateral until he could pay. Either way, his family's sole source of income would be gone until the debt was paid.

Johnson at least got better, although he wished desperately that his well-intentioned neighbors had bought him some oral rehydration solution instead of taking him to the hospital. He was ultimately able to pay his debts, and keep his sewing machine, only by soliciting pay-in-advance orders from his network of customers. He knew he was lucky to have such a network. But his painstakingly accumulated savings were gone, and with them his dream for his daughter's education. Not only that, but there was no more safety net should anyone else in the family become ill.

On the Ward
Enelesi Nyirenda

Enelesi Nyirenda had left her mother's farm near the small town of Ntcheu to find work in the city ten years ago. Elegant, educated (she had completed junior secondary school), and with good English skills, she landed a job as a "shopgirl" in downtown Blantyre. She continued to work for some time after she became ill. Her coworkers and family had noticed that she was getting thin and seemed fatigued, but silently hoped for the best until one day Enelesi collapsed in the shop where she sold mobile phones. Her legs could no longer hold her weight. A fellow shopgirl helped her in a minibus to the Queens outpatient department (a trip that cost the coworker her day's wages), left her in the long queue of patients waiting in the dark and cramped hallways, and on the way back to the shop stopped at the house where Enelesi's older sister Loveness worked as cook and maid to let her know what had happened.

When Loveness arrived at the hospital hours later after work, Enelesi had been admitted to the medical ward for female patients. She could barely move her legs. She did not know her diagnosis but told Loveness that the ward's clinical officer had said she might have to stay for some time. Loveness called a Catholic mission near their home village, where one of the nuns had a student take a message to Enelesi's mother at her house half an hour's walk from the mission. The next day Enelesi had an X-ray of her spine, and the nurse began to bring her daily medication she said was for treatment of spinal tuberculosis. The nurse also told her that this treatment would need to be directly observed in the hospital for at least two weeks. Enelesi's mother arrived to take care of her, helping her up to the communal bathroom, bringing *nsima* she cooked in the courtyard (although Enelesi had no appetite and could get little of it down), sometimes sleeping under Enelesi's metal cot on a woven mat during the hours that "guardians" were allowed in the hospital.

A month passed, then six weeks, and Enelesi was no better. In fact, she was much thinner, hardly speaking, spending most of her day staring at the wall. She had developed a sore where her leg lay pressed to the interlaced wires that served as springs on her metal bed. Although the sore had a piece of gauze over it that was changed every few days, it never seemed to get better. There was only paracetamol—the nonnarcotic pain reliever Americans call acetaminophen or Tylenol—to treat it, and she got little relief. The nurses, and the clinical officers and medical students who sometimes came by on rounds, seemed unable to tell the family what to expect or when Enelesi would begin to improve. No one mentioned HIV, although the majority of southern Africa's spinal TB cases are HIV-related.

The family was growing increasingly anxious. Enelesi's mother had spent nearly all the money she had. The hospitalization and medications were free, but not all food and supplies were, and prices in the city—especially near the hospital's captive market—were high. Worse, she was running out of time to plant the maize at home that would be the family's major income and food source for next year. In desperation, older sister Loveness contacted two acquaintances, friends of her employer, who worked elsewhere in the hospital: my partner and me. Could we come see Enelesi and advise the family on what to do?

We first came to see Enelesi at the lunch hour, when families come to visit and feed patients, and in addition to the patients, at least a hundred other people packed the ward. Most poor Malawians are short, and I was a head taller than anyone else, looking out over a sea of round brown heads, some colorfully wrapped and others bare. The sickest patients are supposed to be in the side wards near the nurses' station, but in the women's medical ward, most patients were very sick indeed, and plenty of those in the open bay with Enelesi looked near death. Three beds were surrounded by groups of women all dressed alike; two of the groups prayed aloud over the beds, while the third group sang in a keening harmony with a refrain calling down the power of Jesus: faith healings. In each of the three beds around which the faith healers clustered, skeletal patients with glazed eyes stared up at the ceiling. They looked as if they needed miracles, desperately and immediately.

So did Enelesi. When we first met her, she weighed thirty-five kilograms (seventy-seven pounds), down nine kilos since admission. She lay curled in a fetal position, not speaking or making eye contact with anyone. Her emaciated body lay on a *chitenji* cloth atop a reed mat, leaving her little protection from the metal webbing of the bed. There were too few mattresses to go around. When my partner peeled the filthy gauze away from her bedsore, she did not flinch. The wound was dreadful, foul-smelling, and deep; I could see bone at the bottom of it.

The nurse said she had continued to give TB medication because there was nothing else to do. There were no new orders, because no one could find Enelesi's file (her medical chart—two or three pieces of paper threaded together by a string of raveled and knotted gauze), so they had been continuing to give her the same medication in the hope that it would help. The clinical officer in charge of the ward seemed well meaning, although harried and exhausted by the enormous number of patients in his care. His white coat was sharply pressed but already spattered with blood and other body fluids. He explained that because this was not a surgical ward, the nurses did not have the supplies necessary for adequate wound cleaning or dressing changes. They also lacked expertise: two nurses were out sick and had been for some time, several others had recently quit, and the ward was functioning primarily with students and new trainees. If we could find some gauze to bring in, that would certainly help a little. Perhaps we could help push for a transfer, too? The clinical officer had been trying to transfer Enelesi to the orthopedic unit, where at least the nurses had wound-dressing supplies, but that unit would not accept her because she had no file and therefore no real diagnosis, and besides, it, too, was already operating at over double capacity.

A week of pulling strings, exploiting connections, tracking down medical and orthopedic consultants and badgering them into taking a look at Enelesi, cleaning her wound, and bringing in supplies made little difference. Orders were written, transfers approved, consultation forms filled out, dressings changed, the few medications available in Queens given. But she looked worse, and somehow even sadder. Despite the care, her bedsore had grown from six to ten centimeters wide in a week, and deeper than before; it was eating into the bone itself now. No HIV tests had been available for months, but that seemed unimportant; there were no antiretroviral medications to be had even if she had been given a diagnosis. (Loveness didn't see the point of testing her sister anyway. How could she have HIV? She had never even been married.)

Enelesi's family decided to take her home. No one—including my partner or me—said the word *dying*, but it hung in the air, and there seemed little point in keeping Enelesi in the hospital. She could not uncurl enough now to get into a minibus, however, and neither the extended family nor any of their friends had access to a car. More string-pulling and exploiting of expatriate connections got us an under-the-table loan of a vehicle owned by a transnationally funded research project, which we could use on a Sunday when the project didn't run if we came up with the money for petrol. We took Enelesi, her mother, and Loveness home to their village, four hours of bumping over dirt roads in an ancient Land Rover ambulance. It must have been excruciating, but she only cried out once or twice. At the house, a cluster of family members waited to carry her gently out of the ambulance and settle her in on a pallet on the floor. We left her with more paracetamol, more gauze, and a bottle of expired codeine my partner had brought from the United States in case of dental emergencies. She died about two weeks later, in her small brick house under a spreading mango tree. Her mother cared for her to the end.

CHAPTER SIX

Resource Is a Verb:
Realities and Responses

Malawian doctors-in-training understood that the difficulties they faced during their initiations into clinical work would continue into their practice lives. The clinical crisis had made clear that some options for "turning theory into practice" were limited, others altogether unavailable. As they became more familiar with the hospital world, and as they approached the time when they would be expected to work independently, they learned to improvise new options from the resources available—material and cultural. In Malawi, *resource* is also a verb. Just as Malawi's sick and their families resourced care from whatever people and goods they could mobilize, their doctors resourced medicines, money, and practical assistance: for themselves and for their patients. They cobbled together social networks, material goods, short-term opportunities, and ideas to craft ad hoc solutions to the problems they faced.

In order to understand their responses to the clinical crisis, and the practical ethics they forged from the pain and anger of working under very difficult conditions, we must first step back briefly from the world of the teaching hospital to consider the various destinations medical trainees saw ahead. This chapter considers those destinations, the paths that had to be taken to get there, and the examples set by working doctors students knew (as real senior colleagues and teachers, and as figures of rumor). With the possibilities laid out, we can then return to the ways students tried to reconfigure the work of the doctor, their attempts to make a Malawian medicine both possible and worthwhile.

The Northern studies that examine medical students' transitions into clinical practice focus on specialty selection, a selection that involves relative prestige, personality match, income opportunities, and especially the possibilities for creating balance between work and the rest of life.[1] Con-

siderations for new Malawian graduates were much different. "Balancing" work and life, a central concern for Northern trainees, rarely came up
among the students I knew. Most did not expect or experience boundaries
between work lives and home lives. In addition, specialty "choice" was sel-
dom a choice: real-life options rarely matched up with student aspirations.
Instead of dwelling on specialty selection, these trainees tended to muse
over whether or not to emigrate. Considerations about family weighed into
those decisions, sometimes in complex and surprising ways, as did political
concerns. Trainees expected severe financial pressures, and their expectations were colored by a sense of injustice. They also expected to be able
to "work" the system—at least sometimes—to access funds and resources
they, their families, and their patients needed.

Although I present these issues separately for clarity, they were tangled up together, both in students' discussions and in the lives of working
doctors. New Malawian doctors faced difficult choices in which their perceived obligations to their patients, to the state, to their profession, and to
their families often clashed with one another and with their more individual ambitions. In the first part of this chapter, I explore the ways in which
new doctors considered their choices and the ways in which they coped
with the politics of practice and the ethics of scarce resources in a setting
in which no course of action was morally unambiguous.

Internship and Beyond

Every College of Medicine graduate had to complete an eighteen-month
internship to be eligible for medical licensure. Most interns stayed based at
Queens Hospital; some worked at Kamuzu Central Hospital in Lilongwe,
the nation's capital.[2] Interns managed the hospitals, especially at night: on
each major service, one or two on-call interns would cover admissions and
emergencies for roughly two to three hundred patients. A backup consultant was available, at least in theory, to be called in for complex cases.[3] After sixteen grueling hospital months, internship ended with a two-month
district-management course, in which interns listened to lectures on handling personnel problems, drug procurement, and other bureaucratic concerns relevant to their future postings.

The new doctors were licensed as general practitioners by the Malawi
Medical Council as soon as their internships were successfully completed.
Most were then assigned posts as district health officers (DHOs), working
out of the hospitals and health offices of the country's thirty-one administrative districts. It was never completely clear to me or to the interns how

the assignments were made or how much weight the new doctors' own requests were given. Most interns believed they were likely to be posted in the regions they wanted. Some of those who had seemed most certain about where they were going, however, were unhappily surprised at their actual assignments when the list of postings finally came out, a few weeks before their new jobs were to begin. Everyone agreed that a new doctor could turn down a position and ask for a reassignment without negative consequence, as long as he or she had a good reason.[4]

For a few, becoming a general practitioner was not the only option. Although no formal specialty training was possible within Malawi, those doctors with good contacts and stellar academic performance could sometimes find sponsorships that would allow them to go on to postgraduate specialty studies abroad. In the early days of the College of Medicine, as part of an agenda to "Malawianize" the school, these opportunities had been more plentiful. Pediatricians, obstetricians, internists, orthopedic surgeons, and others were to be trained elsewhere, then come back to Malawi and teach future doctors. By 2003, sponsorships for specialty training were very rare. Students and interns I knew often talked about the specialties they would have ideally liked to pursue, but they understood that their decisions would probably be more pragmatic. Those few who had any opportunities for advanced training typically found their options dictated by donor or sponsor interests (as when a radiologists' professional society offered scholarships to study radiology in Taiwan, or an American infectious-disease-research consortium sponsored a training program in microbiology). A superb student, or one with good connections, would typically compete for whatever training opportunity was available.

Interns could also compete for the opportunity to stay in one of the central hospitals as a "registrar"—a trainee doctor assigned indefinitely to a single department. In theory, registrars were to learn the essentials of their specialties while preparing for exams. Once they passed the exams, they would be eligible to apply for the formal training abroad (usually in South Africa) required for specialist licensure. Becoming a registrar was a gamble, however. Registrars typically labored in their assigned departments for years with poor pay and high workloads; some never got the opportunity to go abroad or the teaching and study time required to succeed on their exams.

Occasionally, new doctors were able to find work in other places, either without serving as district health officers or after brief stints in the districts. A few graduates were employed by Malawi-based nongovernmental organizations, and several more worked at the Ministry of Health above the district level, either in the central bureaucracy or in vertical (disease-specific) public health programs such as the National AIDS Council or the National TB Control Program. Others worked in the mission hospitals scattered throughout Malawi.

Flight Plans

Emigration figured prominently in students' talk, in interview settings and casual discussion, from their premedical years through internship. Salaries were a major issue and an especially sore point, but brain drain was about much more than money. Students were very aware that medicine in Malawi was not what it could be elsewhere, and neither was the life of the doctor. They made these distinctions clear from the beginning of training.

> MKUME LIFA: Another frustration will be the working conditions themselves. You know we have a lot of HIV/AIDS and TB here. The chance of contracting disease is high. The working environment is nasty, unhygienic, not clean. You don't have even basic equipment and drugs. . . .
>
> PHILLIP TEMBENU: What you earn is not the only thing pushing doctors out of the country. If you are a doctor who wants to operate on complex cases but there is no equipment, if it is a cancer, there is no chemotherapy—it's difficult. (first-year focus group)

When I asked them specifically, one in three medical students and nearly all the interns thought they would be gone from Malawi within ten years.

The question of where graduates actually ended up working was a contentious one. College of Medicine faculty and administrators often told me that nearly all graduates stayed in Malawi and worked in the public health sector. Students, on the other hand, commonly claimed that most graduates either had already emigrated or were attempting to leave. People who saw the College of Medicine as an expensive white elephant, including many expatriate doctors, tended to share the students' view. Physician brain drain, some contended, was one reason the school should be seen as an inappropriate investment for Malawi.

In a retrospective of the first ten years of the University of Malawi College of Medicine, two faculty members took on the critics by reporting that two-thirds of graduates were actually working in Malawi, with another quarter about to return from postgraduate specialty training (Muula and Broadhead 2001). The numbers they provided are summarized in table 6.1. Several students and interns brought up this article when talking about

TABLE 6.1. Disposition of College of Medicine graduates

Work status	Number (%)	
Specialists		
In postgraduate training abroad	38	(28)
In Malawi after postgraduate training abroad	19	(14)
Generalists		
In internship in Malawi	20	(15)
In district or mission hospitals	18	(13)
Left Malawi	4	(3)
Died	4	(3)
Other: "either working in COM or other government or NGOs"	31	(23)
Total graduates 1992–2001	134	

Source: Muula and Broadhead 2001.
Note: Those listed as graduates include students from the early "hybrid" years of the college, in which most of the medical-school training took place abroad.

their own futures, but none believed the data presented there. They usually questioned whether the graduates listed as receiving postgraduate training abroad had any intention of coming back to Malawi, as it was far easier for a specialist to find work abroad than for a general practitioner. Many wondered where the thirty-one "other" graduates actually were. Interns and students were well aware both that the college was under pressure to make it appear that graduates stayed in the country and that physician shortages remained acute. Joe Phoya was one of the skeptics: "Honestly speaking, on paper it can be made to look that way, but practically, I don't think that is right. Because right now you talk of some districts in Malawi who don't have doctors. So, what, what are we talking about? Where *are* those people?"

Although my own inquiries tended on the whole to corroborate the results given in Muula and Broadhead's article,[5] many trainees and some faculty strongly believed that most graduates of their college either had already gone abroad or were waiting for the earliest opportunity to do so. Students and interns consistently alluded to large numbers of graduates abroad, but none could name more than a few. The émigré-doctor archetype seemed to acquire an importance for students out of proportion to the actual number of doctors who had left the country for good.

Conditions of practice and other obligations—to family, to community, to nation—preyed on trainees' minds and came up in their conversations as they imagined emigration. I found no demographic differences that correlated reliably with plans to leave Malawi.[6] Other differences surfaced, however. Students who said they hoped to stay in Malawi were more likely than their peers to express nationalist sentiments, were more impressed with the social status of doctors, and were more likely to describe medicine as a calling. Students likely to want to emigrate, in contrast, expressed more strongly a desire for jobs in which the tools and technologies of medicine would be available to them. In addition, for this group, the issue of work-life balance sometimes did come up. Although no one actually used the word *balance*, students who wanted to emigrate were more concerned about being able to set limits on working hours and more desirous of private lives.

Whether they planned to get out of Malawi as soon as possible or hoped to stay, those discussing it very often characterized emigration as "human nature" or "only human." The tendency to characterize emigration as inevitable, a natural human desire, may explain why students insisted that "most" doctors had left the country even when evidence suggested otherwise. This characterization allowed those who wished to leave to feel normal and highlighted the sacrifice of those who chose (or had) to stay. Their choice of words suggested that many saw patient care in Malawi as a superhuman—or perhaps inhuman—endeavor.

Indeed, *most* students felt that they were being held to high standards of self-sacrifice by donor countries, by the college administration, and by their own government: they were expected to practice in very poor conditions, for long hours, and with little remuneration. Some accepted this call to altruism as part of the job, describing it as a sacrifice but voicing no complaint. Others expressed resentment at the expectation that they would "be saints." One student asked me to take a message to Americans who believed a medical school was the solution to Malawi's health problems:

> Tell them what you really deal with, what you really have. 'Cause that's like—in developed countries, what they have, they are *advanced*. They have advanced medicines. All we have are basics. We don't even *have* the basics sometimes. And maybe they should try to imagine if they were in this place, where they don't have many opportunities, many medications—what would *they* do? Would they still follow the same path? Because they say, "Train doctors, train doctors." Yes! Train doctors. But if *they* had to come here and they'd do this, would they go through with it? Or would they choose other careers? (Bridget Nyasulu, clinical student)

The bitterness of Bridget's comment, like those of others, had much to do with the anticipated frustrations of medical work. The clinical poverty, personal risk, and heavy workload discussed in the previous chapter remained central concerns, but they were not the only issues. As students graduated and became doctors, other features of their working lives also daunted them.

Money and Sacrifice

No subject was as ubiquitous when students and interns discussed actual practice as money, and no subject elicited as much agreement in interviews and on questionnaires.[7] Their comments did not demonstrate the increasing focus on money with the passage of years in training that is often noted in the North; even Malawians in their first year at medical school often brought up physicians' pay. Students and interns agreed that doctors' pay was scandalously low: *peanuts*, to use the word many favored. Poor salaries added insult to the injuries of heavy workload and limited clinical resources.

Brian Msukwa had initially wanted to go into medicine "to help the nation." At the time I interviewed him, halfway through his internship, he was embittered, tired, and angry.

> One thing that I would say is that in Malawi, now that I am in the system, the government doesn't care what we need here. You present your problems, they do nothing about it. It's like really *slavery*, the work. It's no wonder most of the doctors just leave the government. . . . You may have that heart in you to work—but, I mean, you need *some* money to support yourself!

Brian planned to use some American connections to arrange for postgraduate training there and expressed doubt about whether he would ever return to Malawi to work.[8]

Whether the financial situation for these doctors was really that bad depended on one's vantage point. New doctors in Malawi earned much more than the average citizen—eighteen times as much, in fact. But students rarely compared themselves to ordinary Malawians, who were among the poorest people in the world: "too poor to buy soap," as the students often put it.[9] They compared themselves to college classmates who went on to become lawyers or accountants (each requiring fewer years of training than medicine), or to the politicians who determined their pay. They compared themselves to peers who owned cars, lived in houses with plumbing, and sent their children to school without worrying about the cost. They also

TABLE 6.2. Pay scales

	Annual pay in 2003 US$ (PPP-adjusted)[a]	
	Malawi	United States
Putting wages in perspective		
Per capita GNP	160 (570)	35,277 (34,320)
Population living on less than $1 per day (%)	41.7	<1
Typical starting salaries		
Secondary school teacher	696 (2,479)	27,989 (27,229)
Intern	2,148 (7,652)	38,000 (36,969)
General practitioner	2,904 (10,346)	130,000 (126,473)
Accountant	6,312 (22,487)	39,397 (38,328)

Sources: General economic data are from UNDP 2003. Malawi salaries were taken from my field notes, where I recorded civil service wage scales for 2003; they include housing and other special allowances, which could be quite a high proportion of salary, and have been converted to US dollars using the average 2002–3 exchange rate of MK95/US$. United States figures (except intern salaries) are from the *Occupational Outlook Handbook*, 2002–3 edition, published by the Bureau of Labor Statistics (bulletin 2540). United States intern salaries were averages found in a 2003 online search of positions advertised.

Note: The *Occupational Outlook Handbook* did not distinguish between primary and secondary teachers. It also did not give starting salaries for physicians; figures for United States primary care doctors are averages.

[a]See footnotes to table 2.1 for a brief explanation of purchasing power parity (PPP). To be consistent with the other calculations here, I have used PPP adjustments from UNDP 2003.

compared themselves to the trainee doctors who came from abroad, showed up intermittently on the wards for a few weeks, then disappeared on safari or to the expensive lakeside resorts. In these comparisons, Malawian doctors' salaries fell scandalously short (see table 6.2).

In fact, the salary figures presented here may be too optimistic. Salary packages were supposed to include housing near the hospital, but few places were available, and most interns had to seek their own rentals. Their housing allowance was not enough to rent even a fairly basic place to live; minibus transport back and forth to the hospital further ate into their take-home pay.[10] Salaries also all too often went unpaid for months at a stretch. The nurses and interns working at Queens Hospital got no paychecks in November or December of 2002 due to "computer problems" at the Ministry of Health. At the end of January, they began receiving monthly paychecks again but six months later were still waiting for their back pay.[11] Similar "computer problems" kept some interns working for months without pay in 2007.

Doctors' feeling of being underpaid was exacerbated by several perceived injustices. First, most were aware that pay scales for other public-sector employees had been upgraded in recent years. Junior lawyers earned considerably more, for instance, despite being civil servants at the same level as junior doctors; the government had found improvements in pay essential to ensure an impartial judiciary. In contrast, the possibility of upgrading pay scales for doctors had been "under study" for some years, but the only change that had actually occurred was to make the housing subsidy taxable starting in 2002, representing a real decrease in total income of about 18 percent.

A second injustice was more specific to the College of Medicine: the Ministry of Education, through which faculty salaries were paid, used different pay scales for expatriates and Malawians. Faculty from outside Malawi not only took home substantially larger paychecks but were allocated better-quality housing and had their children's school fees paid, unlike their Malawian counterparts.[12] Junior faculty, some of them College of Medicine graduates, felt the dual salary structure doomed any efforts to "Malawianize" the College of Medicine. Dr. Arthur Gumbo, one of the first Malawian faculty members I interviewed, responded with a dismissive wave of the hand when I asked him how he thought things would change as the teaching staff became more heavily Malawian:

> This college is not going to be Malawian. That is a theory, but it will never happen. . . . Why would Malawians want to come here? The more Malawians we train, the more will just go outside, to the UK or other places. The salary is too low. You go outside, you see what else is available. Or you stay here and you see that expatriates are paid much more than Malawians. . . . If I get the opportunity, I will go, sure. So I don't see this place being Malawianized.

When I challenged him, saying that faculty I had spoken with predicted otherwise, his retort was brusque. "Who are the others? If they are Malawians, they are afraid. They are being political. And the other ones—well, it's in their interest to say that they are going to Malawianize the school. It is a nice theory." The dual wage structure meant that expatriates could keep their well-paid jobs, he held, even while imagining themselves as agents of African development and deploring the insufficient patriotism of Malawians who emigrated.

Whether the expatriate faculty were speaking cynically or simply underestimating the effects of pay discrimination on their Malawian colleagues, Dr. Gumbo was right. Only expatriates predicted the Malawianization of the school. The College of Medicine, championed by Dr. John Chiphangwi, started as a Malawian project, but it risked becoming an expatriate one.

Many students initially talked about wanting to teach "even here at this college," but plans to teach in Malawi diminished with years in training, and by internship, several doctors specifically mentioned the pay disparity as a factor in their loss of enthusiasm. It is difficult to overestimate how embittered young physicians felt about unequal pay for equal work, and how much it contributed to a desire to emigrate among those who had wanted to teach. As a registrar who had recently found out about the differing pay scales said, "I won't stay in that world. I wanted to stay here, but now I am preparing for my exam. I have to get out of here unless the conditions are to change."

New Malawian doctors perceived the sharpest injustices in the public excesses of national politicians. Discrepancies between politicians' and doctors' lives, in terms of workload, responsibilities, pay, and perks, came up in conversation and interviews more than any other comparison. Politicians would line their own pockets at the expense of the public in any way they could, even treating hospital budgets as sources of personal revenue, students and interns complained. Although no one I spoke with espoused the return of dictatorship, many linked increasing rapacity among the political class to democracy.[13] "Ever since we have had democracy," one young graduate explained, "it has been a matter of get rich any way you can."

Lawyers, politicians, foreign teachers, doctors traveling in from other countries, all could live luxuriously while they exhorted their Malawian medical colleagues to greater sacrifice for the sake of national development. The new graduates wanted to help their country, but they did not want to be fools or pawns. Few graduates saw any reason they as doctors should be the only ones expected to give up a decent living for Malawi.

Family Obligations

The attractions and disincentives of work in Malawi were not just financial ones. The new doctors sometimes felt compelled to stay by their extended families and at other times felt pushed to flee. Large kin-based networks of mutual obligation and support have historically been, and remain today, the major mechanisms for both social security and social regulation in this region. Among other duties, a doctor in Malawi was expected to facilitate health care access for family members, something students had occasionally anticipated as a benefit of their positions in medicine. But what was seen in theory as a privilege sometimes became a time-consuming burden in practice. It was not a matter of telephoning a receptionist and using one's title as doctor to get a relative a prompt medical appointment, as it might be elsewhere. Accessing the Malawian health care system for family (or anyone else, as Enelesi Nyirenda's story illustrated) involved shepherding the patient bodily through the maze of the hospital, buttonholing clinicians and laboratory technologists and nurses in person, using all one's connections until something got done, and likely paying for prescriptions or bandages or sutures at the end of it. It could easily take a day or more, and one was obliged to do it for even the most distant connections.

> We are taught—like in our culture—that your mom's aunt or somebody like that, my cousins, they are all part of us. We all belong together. So we have to respect it. If somebody comes to the hospital I've never seen before and says, "I need some help, I'm your—your daddy is my so-and-so," I still have to help. . . . Otherwise, I would be considered—like I have taken another foreign culture, if I don't help my relatives. (Catherine Gunya, clinical student)

Family expectations went well beyond medical access. Any employed person was obligated to take responsibility for extended family members, responsibility that could include anything from paying for school fees, weddings, or funerals to taking in orphaned children. As poverty, unemployment, and illness worsened in Malawi, these responsibilities became heavier. If students already had wealthy parents, aunts, or uncles, members of the extended kin network could go to those people for assistance. In contrast, students from humbler backgrounds were often already serving as "senior" persons in the family, and some were sole providers. Families in desperate need might pressure students to quit their long training in order to earn a living, or ask them to divert their scholarship funds to support relatives. Several interns were supporting kin out of their $179 monthly wage and benefit packages.

> You know here in our, in our setting, it's like—the children work to support the parents, to support the elders. Unlike the situation in other countries—for example, in European countries—where the parents are the ones who expect to do something like educate their children. So you find that you have just qualified, and yet you have this *stream* of people to look after. This stream of relatives. So you cannot look away, which makes life—which makes life tough. (Crispin Kamwendo, intern)

Conflicts between students' ideals about medical practice and their obligations to family were common. First-year student Saul Kaleso, who was already paying his sisters' school fees from his book money, mused aloud about work possibilities: "I need to serve the people at low cost, in order to help them and not just to be getting their money. But on the other hand, I have my sisters to help. . . . It's tough. I don't know how it will work out." The conflicts tended to worsen during internship, when family members who had been waiting during the long period of training assumed doctors' pay finally matched their status. "As Malawians, we are so *obligated*," fifth-year student Itai Chilenga lamented, pounding a fist into his other hand as he spoke of his imminent graduation. "Your family knows where you are working, so you, like, you take responsibility." In the face of these heavy obligations, it could be tempting to seek work some distance from the extended family, where it would be more difficult for relatives with financial demands and time-consuming health problems to track one down. Interns sometimes requested postings in districts far from their homes for this reason.

Working the System

The picture was not wholly bleak for the new doctors, however, even as the financial injustices rankled and family pressures worried them. Their status could make up for their poor salaries in some ways. In addition, there were opportunities to extract resources from the medical system through research, private practice, and workshops.

Doctors were important figures in their communities, and they could accrue social capital much more quickly than actual money.[14] A clinical officer who had worked in a rural area explained that one's reputation could make a difference to one's financial situation in ways not reflected in the actual salary.

> Well, Malawians—if a person comes to you and gets better, when he goes to the community, he says, "Such and such a person is a good person." And maybe the person he is talking to in the community has some facilities. Like, let's say maybe they have a shop. You go there, you can take things on credit easier. Maybe you need something, maybe he has that certain thing. Or maybe he works for a certain company and they have that thing. It will be easier for you to, to get access to that thing. Because people know you. (Phillip Tembenu)

In the commercial world of southern Africa, deals and purchases and financial matters were very often managed through social webs of mutual obligation, people who "know you." People might offer small gifts or services in gratitude for good medical care freely given (as happened to me), or to ensure that they could access care in the event it was needed. Social capital could go very far toward making up for limitations in economic capital. It was also morally blurry. The line between gifts in exchange for care and informal payments, or bribes, was far from sharply drawn.

One could make a good living as a doctor in Malawi with social capital and also with creative resourcing. Just as staff in the public hospitals routinely patched together supplies from several sources, and department heads became experts at wheedling donated goods out of foreign contacts or NGOs, many Malawian doctors in the public sector added up various financial resources into good incomes. Mission hospitals were more restrictive. They paid somewhat better than the public sector, while still providing the opportunity to treat poor patients, and many College of Medicine graduates sought mission employment. The disadvantage, as experienced nurses and doctors explained, was that mission contracts sharply limited opportunities for private work on the side, for additional training, or for research—all of which could add substantially to one's income.

Few graduates had the necessary experience or capital stake to open a solo private practice, and by 2007, none was doing so full-time. Opening a *chipatala* for paying patients required a considerable up-front capital investment: it was something for "old people who have got money," a student said. (It may be that the COM graduates who hoped to enter private practice had simply not yet accumulated adequate funds and that this situation will change over the next decade or two.) Several graduates supplemented full-time government positions with part-time private work, however.[15] Money was the big incentive, but private practice had other benefits, as one graduate with both government and private jobs explained. "There, I have antibiotics. I want to use a cephalosporin, I want to use a quinolone [two categories of antibiotic not available in the public hospitals], I have them. I want to get a urinalysis done, I can have it done."

Research contracts with nongovernmental organizations were also potentially lucrative. Trainees tended to see research work as unpredictable, sometimes morally suspect, and desirable.[16] Students in one focus group explained:

ALICE MATEBULE: A research job, you just hear *research*, and you know it's money. And that's what everyone wants, too.
MUKONDWA NDIUZANI: Yeah, they don't think "research for—for what?"

ALICE: It's just money.

MUKONDWA: And what do I have to do to get it!

Although all the students in this focus group hoped to participate in such projects, they also expressed desires to push the system toward research that would be more relevant for Malawians: "Maybe we need to own these things. Maybe we should feel they are *ours*. It's for *our* benefit, and not— right now we just think it's for *them*. Our benefit is just the money. And that's where it ends for us; we don't care." Everyone who had spent time in the hospitals had seen many an NGO-funded and foreigner-designed health-research project come and go. The Malawians who inevitably did the ground-level work of surveys or blood draws felt little commitment or con- nection to such research, students said; some claimed they knew research- ers who simply made up data to get the pay, and all agreed data quality was generally poor. These projects often produced clinical recommendations impossible to execute for lack of resources—or feasible recommendations that never got back to anyone with the power to implement them.

Several medical students spoke admiringly of those doctors and nurses they knew who had stayed in their government posts and resisted recruit- ment by the large research laboratories or other NGOs. But they also ad- vised others to make the connections they would need to open doors.

> Work hard and get to know people. Like *real big, big* people! Because if you have to do something big, or after training—what happens is if you know some big people, some consultants or other people who works in these research labs like Wellcome or Johns Hopkins, sometimes when they know you're talented, you get more opportunities in terms of funding and scholarships. Because otherwise, if you—if you don't find a scholarship, you are stuck. You end up doing things which you never wanted to do. (Catherine Gunya, clinical student)

Catherine spoke from experience. A bright, quiet student from a modest family background, she had wanted to do infectious disease research. Lack- ing connections to pursue additional training, she anticipated working as a primary care doctor in a rural setting instead—and four years later when I followed up, she was doing exactly that.

If students felt both desire and distaste for research work, they had similarly complex feelings about administrative work. Most of them ex- pected to become district health officers, and the DHO's job allowed some flexibility in the proportion of time spent on administrative duties. All

DHOs had to manage health personnel and budgets, oversee the supply chain, monitor and respond to shifting patterns of disease, and represent the district's health needs to its political overseers. Especially in larger (or sicker) districts, these tasks could consume considerable time. Many of the DHOs, however, also continued doing a great deal of patient care: surgeries, complicated obstetrical cases, hospital rounds on the sickest patients. Others dropped their clinical practices entirely. Students early in training were likely to speak contemptuously of those who relinquished clinical work for administrative oversight as "not fruitful," "not real doctors." As they progressed in their training, however, they grew more likely to view administrative work positively.[17] Some may have seen it as less dangerous or distressing than clinical work; many came to think of administration as the way they could have the greatest impact on the community's health.

Administrative work had other attractions, among them opportunities for workshops and meetings. Readers may recall that the DHO who was to supervise Evelyn Kazembe during a district hospital attachment was away at workshops and meetings for seven of the eight weeks she was there (a fact she mentioned casually when speaking warmly of her experience learning from clinical officers there). Another student, one with considerable previous hospital experience, spoke with admiration of a doctor he knew who sometimes chose *not* to attend meetings: "You know how it is with district health officers. They normally go for workshops and that. But sometimes he skips the workshops! He doesn't normally go there. Because he's too dedicated, he is much involved in the clinical part of things." Clinicians presented the desire to attend trainings and workshops as part of what many called a "natural urge to upgrade" one's skills, to learn something new rather than stagnate under the burden of the same old patient care obligations. But trainings and workshops were not just ways to learn or to avoid clinical work: they were also money-making opportunities. The international NGOs that ran workshops often offered generous fixed per diem payments to cover hotel fees and meals at conferences but did not require receipts. If a doctor stayed at a dollar-a-night rest house, or with a relative, she could pocket the difference.[18] As a Malawian administrator said dryly, "The workshops are why you will still see some doctors who are working for the government who are also driving Mercedes."

Clinical Impunity

Evidence from interviews, from informal conversations, from observations, and from my work at the hospital suggests that students and interns were exposed to a nearly dichotomous set of role models, some of the best and the worst doctors to be found anywhere.[19] Students describing good doctors they had worked with referred to qualities that to me sounded saintlike: humility, selflessness, love, patience, gentleness, tirelessness. In describing bad doctors, they told stories of clinicians who shouted at patients, handled them roughly, or refused to show up when needed or scheduled. I saw both sets of behaviors among the senior doctors at Queens.

The conditions that made such a dichotomy possible were complex. Malawi offered very low pay, risky work, endless numbers of needy patients, and a lack of material and human resources; there was not much of a "carrot" for doctors. In 2003, there was also virtually no "stick": little disciplinary action or surveillance of physicians, and no medical malpractice litigation. The Malawi Medical Council, a small and poorly staffed body, handled licensing and the occasional complaints it received, but few nonclinicians even knew the council existed. Patients in general were uninformed about their rights. Most did not know that they had the right to refuse surgical operations (such as tubal sterilizations), for instance, or the right to explanations of their diagnoses and treatments.

Clinical impunity—doctors' freedom from sanction for carelessness or error—must therefore be included in any discussion of the real situation of work. Iatrogenic injuries and deaths, of which I saw many, disappeared into a background of very high morbidity and mortality. Typically, no one was held responsible. This impunity, too, shaped the possibilities for doctors. It was possible to take a government job and simply not show up. If a patient died on your watch due to your negligence, your incompetence, your drunkenness, or your absence, you were unlikely to have to defend yourself even to your peers, not to mention to a lawyer.[20] Common justifications for inaction included the absence of blood in the blood bank or the assumption that a patient was "chronically ill" (one of the most popular euphemisms for HIV/AIDS) and would soon have died anyway. There was little push to better care. "This is Queens Hospital," one consultant said, dismissing an idea I had about improving perioperative antibiotic delivery. "We fix this problem, a hundred others take its place. There is no point." Clinical impunity did not create this sort of fatalism, but the absence of sanctions allowed fatalism to turn into inaction. What was the point in showing up to work, after all?

Most trainees were probably unaware of how little regulatory surveillance they worked under, compared to other settings. Clinicians with experience outside Malawi, both nurses and physicians, had a sharper sense of the implications of impunity. In 2003, one faculty member with experience in the United States anticipated (correctly) the imminent arrival of mal-practice law, as Malawi's schools continued to turn out lawyers in numbers far exceeding available civil service vacancies. Malpractice litigation would drive even more people away from practice, he believed, but this dark cloud had a silver lining: "At least the medical profession is going to be forced to upgrade. Because currently the system is such that *nobody* is forced that much to be on their toes, as far as health issues are concerned."

A Malawian nurse discussed at some length her disappointment with the way public-sector doctors treated patients, and particularly with the way doctors rarely explained a problem or discussed treatment options.

> They take advantage of Malawians' ignorance of what to do when that happens. People here do not know that they have rights—that patients have rights! If they come in to a clinic and they are examined by a doc-tor, or by a nurse, and nothing is explained to them, nothing is said, they think, "Ah, but the doctor has seen me, so it must be all right." Because professionals hold a very high place in this society, so people think what they do, it must be right.

She went on to describe the "wonderful, thorough" doctors she had worked with during training in the United Kingdom: gentle with patients, good at giving explanations, punctual. I knew this nurse well and had often heard her speak glowingly of medicine in the United Kingdom. When I asked her why the doctors there were different, I expected her to say something about their characters or their training. Instead, after a pause, she said she be-lieved that if they didn't have to be "cautious," if they were working with patients who didn't know their rights, over time they would behave just as badly as some doctors at Queens. As evidence to support her belief, she de-scribed her early experience with an expatriate physician now well known for his negligence:

> He was a *wonderful* doctor. Wonderful. Spent time with patients, al-ways here, always teaching. And he is a *very* smart man, you know. Just an excellent doctor. But when I came back [after several years abroad], everything was different. Now he is never here, he doesn't care. He is one of the worst.

The relative absence of external pressures to keep behavior in line, cou-pled with lack of external incentives to perform well, allowed for practice patterns at both ends of a range of commitment and effort. If anything, it was difficult to find a middle ground, to do a decently competent job for eight or ten hours and then go home. There really were a hundred problems to solve when one had been fixed, always more patients to see, always more inadequacies of staff or equipment to work around. There was always someone knocking on the door at midnight with a dire emergency. Many senior doctors seemed to escape into cynical fatalism, neglecting their patients to make a few kwacha in other ways wherever possible.[21] Others seemed to draw on—or perhaps to invent—alternative models of what it meant to be a doctor, models that allowed them to trade sacrifice for engagement and to make peace with the suffering they could not alleviate without becoming blind to it.

Responding to Crisis

Studies of medical training have often characterized the impossible workload as responsible for a sort of remaking. The student begins medical school as one sort of person, is crushed, and then is rebuilt into a new sort of person—a doctor. Memoirists and social scientists alike describe the process as a "boot camp": violent, painful, and humiliating.[22]

The transitions Malawian students made also involved rebuilding. Their processes exhibited interesting parallels with the changes described among Northern students during the same years and even more interesting divergences. Moving into the clinical milieu, whether in Malawi or in wealthier countries, commonly led to feelings of being demoralized, of eroded idealism, of being buried under endless and impossible work, of failure. Dreams of logical and scientific curative work ran up against a reality in which clinical failure was highly likely. (After all, everyone does die ultimately.) Students became cynical and angry, typically exhibiting an "us versus them" mentality. But who constituted the "us" and who the "them"? Malawian students and Northern students directed their hostilities toward strikingly different targets.

For North American and European students and doctors, the boundlessness, hopelessness, and potential for failure of their work tend to become embodied in *the patient*. First-person narratives and sociological studies consistently describe a cynical hostility toward patients, particularly patients (alcoholics, hypochondriacs, chronic pain sufferers, the morbidly obese) likely to inspire or exacerbate feelings of clinical failure. Patients have impossible expectations; patients are noncompliant. You can never be certain you've done "enough" for a patient. Patients will disavow their own responsibilities and the doctor's authority, and then turn around and sue you. Chris Feudtner and Dimitri and Nicholas Christakis (1994) coined the term *ethical erosion* as a way of capturing what happens when medical students become immersed in a cynical hospital culture in which patients become "whales" or "dirtballs."[23] There is also a subtler way in which failure is embodied in the self: your own knowledge will never be enough; you must pretend a greater knowledge and a greater confidence than you feel, and that makes you an impostor.

Malawian students also experienced a failure of the medical project, but I never heard them attribute this failure to their patients, and only very rarely to the deficits of their knowledge. Most did not perceive their knowledge as inadequate; it was just irrelevant. None described their patients as impossibly noncompliant; they were just impossibly poor and sick. Although cynical talk about patients is among the most consistent findings in medical socialization research, noted in every study I have read, it was absent here. In many a set of trying circumstances and in well over a year at the hospital, I never once heard a student or an intern speak cynically or in a derogatory fashion about patients—not in interviews, not in meetings, not on the wards or in the clinics. I have no reason to believe that this difference was a matter of some intrinsic culture of kindness. Nurses and doctors could handle patients roughly at times, apparently indifferent to pain or distress. Students were usually gentle, but they, too, could act indifferent: not all bothered to explain what they were doing during a physical examination, for instance, and occasionally some spoke about patients as if they were not in the room. But the antagonistic hostility toward patients consistently found in Northern settings seemed simply to be absent.

In Malawi, the gaping inadequacies of the health sector were so apparent that students' anger was directed instead toward a political system—and, to a lesser extent, a medical profession—that allowed such devastation. Medical students faced with clinical failure had an obvious nemesis. Clinical failure, embodied in neither the doctor's self nor the patient's self, was laid at other feet. The shortfalls of the *system* made it impossible for them to succeed clinically, and the *system*—not the patient—came in for their anger and cynicism.[24] As a fifth-year student put it, "The government pretends to care for the people as if doing something, yet it has no concern for the poor masses." Malawian medical students in their clinical years did not seem to feel a need for distance in an antagonistic relationship with their patients. Instead, they were already beginning to sense an alignment with patients as fellow victims of a government seen as brutal and uncaring—an alliance that they developed further as they moved out of the world of school and into the world of practice.

Reimagining the Doctor

As Malawi's medical students slowly became doctors, many reflected self-consciously on what made their work distinctive. In these reflections, the unique benefits of medical work in Malawi were not separate from its unique pains. The young doctors sometimes felt that the very suffering of their patients and the burdens of their work gained them a hard-won wisdom that enabled them to transcend some of the more problematic aspects of medicine. As intern Zaithwa Mthindi explained to me, the peril of working as a doctor in Malawi was that "you become so absorbed in the trauma that you miss the gift." Their reflections on the gifts of work amid the trauma clustered around four themes: resourcefulness, teamwork, empathy, and activism.

Technology Revisited: Working Resourcefully

In a medical world where "routine" medical technologies were rarely available, good doctors had to use flexibility and creativity to make do with inadequate resources. Students watched their supervisory faculty refurbishing used equipment, arranging for donations by sending heartfelt pleas and pictures of dying children to wealthy contacts, improvising from the tools at hand. They quickly learned to do the same. Resourcefulness—the capacity to secure any available tools, equipment, social networks, and funds—was essential to successful practice in Malawi. It was perhaps even more crucial for rural sites than for the urban hospital settings primarily discussed in this book. Two interns who had a weekend off the surgical schedule "organized" some donated medicines and bandages from a religious charity and spent a rare off-duty weekend in a rural village running an impromptu free clinic, treating anything for which they had the supplies. These two women came back shocked, red-eyed with fatigue but galvanized, having seen over six hundred patients in two days. Many of the people who came to be seen, they reported, were too poor to afford the thirty-kwacha (then about twenty-five cents) trip to the district hospital and had been living with ailments and surgical problems that had reached advanced states.

The line between the "resourcing" of funds and supplies (by diverting them to uses or to people for which they had not been intended) that the students I interviewed admired, and the corruption they spoke strongly against, was less than perfectly clear. But resourcing was a necessity.

> If you want to do things the standard way, the ideal way that people do it maybe in the book, with our resources you wouldn't achieve much here. So you have to be creative. Creative in terms of using our own resources. And also in terms of sourcing funds, where you can as much as possible source funds and try to help the people here. (Dumbisyani Zinyemba, fifth-year student)

A flexible creative sense could even transform the lack of equipment from problem into opportunity. Clinical student Kamwachale Mandala planned a career involving research and design of inexpensive technologies to aid diagnosis and treatment of locally important health problems.[25] "It really gets *into* you," he said of watching a patient die for lack of equipment, but quickly added: "To me, it doesn't put me off. To me, it doesn't put me off. It gives me the sense of—seek more knowledge, and in the very end, you'll be able to do *something*, however basic it might be."

Flexibility and creativity were realms in which Malawi's medical trainees came away from their encounters with medical tourists feeling that their *own* style of medical diagnosis and practice was the real thing. Several commented that their foreign colleagues, used to relying on radiologic and laboratory examinations, were not very good at physical diagnosis. Medical students from abroad did not know how to measure an enlarged liver with their hands, diagnose twins without an ultrasound, or confirm a ruptured tubal pregnancy without a pregnancy test. Two interns who thought "flexibility" was the most important hallmark of a good doctor found that doctors from outside were just too rigid. Outsiders thought, as one said:

> OK, this person has pain in the neck, I *have* to order a CT, I *have* to do this and that. . . . But here—well, in our situation you can't *get* a CT! You tailor it down to basics. You see what you can do based on the physical exam, based on the history, maybe an X-ray. But some people just are not able to do this: they have one way that everything should be done, only one way. (Diana Kondowe)

Technology could be helpful for the practice of medicine, to be sure. But in its absence, these trainees saw their own and their patients' resourcefulness as essential to a better kind of medical work for Malawi.

Months before she interviewed with me, clinical student Tuntufye Chihana had been caring for a patient with a worsening medical complication at thirty-one weeks of pregnancy. Anticipating that a baby with lungs too premature for survival would soon be born, she and I tried to get the mother a few doses of a steroid that improves newborn survival, but the hospital pharmacy had none. Tuntufye explained the situation to the patient's husband, who borrowed money from his family and went to every pharmacy in town until he found not the best drug but something not too different. We gave the injections in time, and the infant born a few days later survived and eventually went home, to everyone's great delight. "Here you really have to work with, make the most out of minimal resources," Tuntufye said later. "And people do improve! And you can help people, *even with* the minimal resources that we have."

Status Revisited: Trading Authority for Teamwork

Students also learned to be more flexible about authority as time passed. Several studies have shown increases in authoritarianism and need for power among medical students as they progress through their curricula. (Important exceptions exist, and I will discuss one of them below.) Not only did my research fail to demonstrate an increase in authoritarianism, it suggested the opposite. On questionnaires, the belief that doctors should share leadership with other members of the health care team correlated positively with increasing years in training. In interviews, clinically experienced students and interns often listed poor teamwork among the qualities of a bad doctor. Failing to seek consultation from other "subordinate" members of the health care team, such as nurses or clinical officers, was censured by students as often as failing to listen to patients.

In practice, some of these alliances could be matters of necessity. Evelyn Kazembe learned appreciatively from clinical officers in part because her supervisory doctor was absent. One morning a weary and baggy-eyed intern, Bridget Nyasulu, spoke warmly of the theater nurse who had walked her through surgery for an ectopic pregnancy the night before, showing her what clamps to use and where to tie: "It was my hands, but it was her brain." It was Bridget's first case of ectopic pregnancy, her second surgical operation ever, and her consultant had refused to come in.[26] Doctors learned from nurses and clinical officers in part because they had to.

For these medical trainees, cooperative effort with other members of a health care team could be not only a clinical obligation or a practical necessity but also a social benefit of medical work. Several clinical students and interns mentioned the opportunity to work side by side with people from varying social strata as one of the most appealing aspects of medical practice. Malawian society could be quite hierarchical, they told me, but medical work allowed one to interact with people from different gender, racial, ethnic, and educational backgrounds in pursuit of a common goal. If you become a doctor, as intern Crispin Kamwendo explained,

> you are not just mature in knowledge, but you are also becoming mature in the business of humanity. . . . [We] tend to meet people with different cultures, with different backgrounds. Just like you. We are working with people who have trained in other countries, people of different races will come together—we all work together as one to overcome difficulty.

It would be well to remember that the starting point for these students was a rigid medical hierarchy and an unquestioned high level of authority among physicians. A nurse would get up from the one chair in a room if a physician came in, even if the nurse was very experienced and the doctor was an intern. In practice, a few interns acted as if asking advice from a midwife was beneath them and asking for help from a consultant was an impertinence. Because students appeared to become more egalitarian did not mean that they had an unusually high degree of respect for teamwork. I cannot demonstrate, nor do I believe from interacting with them at work, that Malawi's medical students were less authoritarian than European or American ones; I contend only that they became less so in the course of their training.

The high status of medical students and doctors in Malawi may actually allow them to feel more secure about sharing authority. The socialization research that demonstrates increasing authoritarianism among North American students also shows that psychological needs for authority increase during times when trainees feel particularly powerless: internship and the clinical years of medical school. Trainees in these years often feel they are the lowest of the low[27] and struggle to create positions of power for themselves within the medical hierarchy. Some medical students and junior doctors have their needs for power assuaged in interactions with patients, but not all do. Female and ethnic minority students, both groups less likely to be called "doctor" on the wards, show greater needs for power when compared to white males (Beagan 1998; Kressin 1996). Nancy Kressin, a psycholinguist who coded transcripts of American medical student interviews for power-related imagery, concluded that white students' need for authority *diminished* over time, in a process parallel to that found in my research. The minority students she interviewed, who were often taken for hospital cleaners or orderlies, did not demonstrate such a decrease (Kressin 1996).

Malawians in medical training generally experienced a world in which their status was secure or even increased when they entered the wards. Unlike their Northern counterparts, these students could write orders on patients' medical files and often took charge of certain patients or even entire wards. Unlike American students, they were treated as doctors by the nurses. (When I mentioned to a student that nurses in the United States were well known for harassing third-year medical students, he was shocked: "That's something that would never happen here.") Their authority was not threatened, and perhaps this security allowed them to feel more generous about teamwork. One suggestive piece of evidence supports this explanation: the realm of authority was one of the very few areas in my research in which a gender difference was significant. Male students were much more likely to view sharing leadership with nonphysicians positively when they reached their clinical years. Female students were not. In interviews and focus groups, several women spoke resignedly about being taken for nurses, or about patients who asked them for "a real doctor, a *man* doctor." Women on the wards in Malawi may not have felt especially powerful, and their authority may have been too insecure to be shared safely.[28]

Mission Revisited: Transcending Helplessness with Heart

Resourcefulness and teamwork were a good start, but to be a good doctor, and to survive the emotional turbulence of the hospital, one had to have something students called "heart." Readers may have noticed already that in Malawi, interns and students throughout their training used this and similar metaphors commonly. The good doctor had "a heart for patients," "a heart for the work." "You have to put your patients at the heart." Many spoke of "love for patients." Over two-thirds of all the trainees I spoke with used the terms *love, heart, passion,* or *spirit* in describing medical work. *Heart,* as these young doctors used it, translated best as a sort of responsible empathy, or empathetic responsibility, and medical trainees saw it as the sine qua non of a good doctor. The concept is particularly interesting because it seems to lie in opposition to the quality of emotional detachment scholars of medical socialization have found so consistently among Northern students at this point in training.[29]

When Malawian medical students scored qualities of the good physician (from a questionnaire list of over twenty qualities that had come up in interviews), in the early years of training, they ranked love for patients as second only to thoroughness, and by the fifth year, love was first. In all years, love for patients ranked far above objectivity or technical skill. Clinical students often claimed that heart was more important than technical capacity or intellectual brilliance. After working with a physician who was cold and discouraging to patients, fifth-year student Itai Chilenga said he realized, "It would be better if I'm just an average doctor, a doctor who has enough information, and can *assist* people—rather than being a genius." Assisting people, for Itai, meant developing warm working relationships. Without that, "you're not a good clinician." Another fifth-year student put it more strongly:

> Medical profession is different from all other professions. Like when somebody is doing finance and the like, somebody has just got to do the job. Do it right. And it doesn't involve the emotions. But then in a medical profession, you are supposed to deal with people and their concerns. You are supposed to have the emotional feeling of what the patients, what the *people* are feeling. And then, if that is lacking, eh, I don't think that would be enough. (Alex Mkweu)

In the United States, I have often heard students, residents, and practicing physicians say of a colleague, "He may be an asshole, but he's a really good doc." (In years past, I have said it myself.) I never heard anything similar in Malawi and have come to believe that it would be heard as nonsensical there. The work itself, for these students, required heart.

Why, at a juncture when many Northern students come to prize objectivity and detachment over empathy, would these students move in the other direction? Malawians themselves gave several explanations. Some friends and colleagues whom I asked to reflect on this puzzle connected it with the emotional experience of life in an extended family. Africans learned to love many people from an early age, they argued, and therefore found it relatively easy to extend that love to an even wider circle.

Others made a religious argument for the centrality of heart to a Malawian doctor's self-image. The language was reminiscent of evangelical Christianity, and occasionally an interviewee would explicitly link religious beliefs and heart. Other interviewees, including some who identified as very religious, made a distinction:

> It's not just Christian. I mean, there can be a Christian doctor who will pray with you, who will carry around a Bible, who will do his best in terms of medicine and preaching, but you don't feel a *part* of them, you

don't feel *loved*. You have to have a real passion for understanding, for understanding who other people really are. . . . The heart of a doctor should be: what if it was me? (Thokozani Sokela, preclinical student)

Most commonly, however, Malawians connected "heart" neither with family nor with religion, but with the circumstances of clinical work. In interviews and in the hospital, most discussions of heart, love, or spirit came embedded within discussions about the actual working conditions for clinicians in impoverished Malawi. One needed a "spirit to treat," or a heart for one's patients, to continue doing good work in a setting of intractable patient problems, inadequate equipment and medication, and little external pressure to do good work.

In my clinical practice in the United States, even in an underfunded clinic among very poor patients, there was always some medication to give, some test to order, some surgical procedure to try, some referral to make. This was simply not true in Malawi. In response, the new doctors *expanded* the definition of what they could give that was important, and empathy and love took pride of place.

Malawi is a poor country. Poverty is the issue. . . . If you can give them *hope*, they know at least that there is somebody who cares, and there is somebody who can help them. There is somebody who understands their situation and can sympathize with them. I think that helps quite a lot. (Crispin Kamwendo, intern)

We are a nation that would *like* to love one another. We want to be loving, and we want to feel loved. We know the nature of the work that medical doctors do, we know they work in sometimes very nasty conditions. So when they are seeing patients, even if they do not have the medication to give, if they have the love, if that patient feels loved, then it can really help them. (Dr. Daniel Njobvu, faculty)

With the problems that the Malawi nation is facing, especially of the patients, I think there is more need for somebody who can *really help* the people. Like the HIV situation, and the poverty that is taking the people. We need somebody who has got a heart for the people. (Alex Mkweu, fifth-year student)

In contrast to the emotional detachment and objectivity Northern students value as central pieces of the doctor identity, these Malawians saw attachment and love as key to doing good work in a situation of suffering. A saying in Chichewa (and in many other Bantu languages) has it that "a person is a person through persons." One's very identity is based on connection and relation; community is as much a part of the self as body or spirit. This collective sense of humanness is known as *uMunthu*, and although no student I interviewed referenced it directly, it is not hard to read *uMunthu* in the importance of heart.[30]

Experience on the wards deepened the conviction that technical ability without a loving spirit could not make a good doctor. When students naïve to the clinical world discussed having a heart for patients, it usually meant sacrificing one's own well-being for the sake of others. They described doctors who lived in poverty, were persecuted politically, or even died of AIDS, accepting these hardships as consequent to the mission of medicine. Among experienced students and interns, the sense of heart seemed to shift. Many still spoke of selflessness and suffering. For experienced students and interns, however, the term tended to be used less in the context of accepting a difficult lot and more in terms that suggested imaginative empathy, participation, a sense of shared humanity. On the wards, said Andrew Kanyenda, he got "that feeling that at least I am contributing to my fellow poor people." Or as Evelyn Kazembe said, "I might have a heart for the people and all that, but I think I am learning more." A sense of purpose had led her to mature on the wards, she said: "I am beginning to understand more the realities of *what happens in life*. I am becoming more clear than before. . . . Every day being in the hospital? Now the ward is part of my life." Becoming a part of life (and death) in the hospital led some students to feel a strong connection to their fellow Malawians, and that, in turn, obligated them to advocacy, as we will see below.

At least one medical socialization researcher has concluded that the central tenet of American biomedical training is that "a doctor is not a patient." Howard Stein (1990) concluded that medical enculturation serves to protect the practitioner against recognizing his or her common human condition with the patient: vulnerable, fragile, sexual, passive, infirm, mortal. For some Malawian physicians, clinical experience pushed them to the opposite conclusion. Not insulated from suffering by technology or equipment, or private patient rooms with walls and curtains, or high staffing levels that allowed nurses to do all the dirty work, or vaccines or postexposure prophylaxis that limited their risks of contracting killer diseases when they stuck themselves with bloody needles, these student doctors were made constantly aware that they were, as Zaithwa Mthindi said, "as human as everybody else."

Feeling the needs of the people and then acting on them became central for some students as they struggled with the overwhelming burdens of hospital work. They reinvented the purpose of the doctor in a way that allowed them to fulfill that purpose. "A good doctor," as Zebron Ching'amba said, was "somebody who feels the needs of the people." But what could feeling the needs of the people really mean when one had a hundred or more patients to see each day, with little time to make a connection and not much curative medicine to offer them?

Nationalism Revisited: Holding the State to Account

One answer to this conundrum lay in politics, for their location as witnesses of suffering and injustice gave the new doctors a way to revisit their earlier sense of nationalism. Malawi's medical students did not show the declines in political commitment, the trend toward "neutrality" found among students in North America. Clinical students actually showed a small *increase* in the belief that doctors had a responsibility to be politically active when compared to preclinical students.

The transformation of trainees' nationalist impulses bore many similarities to the transformation of their concept of medicine as heart. Both tended to move from a vision of rather abstract sacrifice—to offer oneself up for the nation or the people—to one of greater engagement, a feeling of shared identity or political purpose. Itai Chilenga was one of the students who had initially wanted to enter medicine in order to improve Malawi's doctor-patient ratio. When he spoke with me later, as his internship approached, he reported a growing interest in health policy-making and political activism. It was the best way, he felt, that he and his colleagues could "uplift the life status of the people."

> It will be encouraging, it will be more rewarding to the country because particular illnesses in Malawi, there will be more people who will *actually know* about the common type of illnesses the people are suffering from, and they will get much more interested in finding out the best way to help those sick people.

Sometimes an engaged nationalism might become confrontational, as students discussed provoking their government into backing up its ostensible commitment to the people's health with resources.[31] If Malawi's grim clinical situation was a fixed reality, one's choices were to flee or to sacrifice oneself to the benefit of others. In either case, the context remained static. In

contrast, an engaged nationalism rejected fixity, and rejected also sacrifice
that was perceived as unnecessary and conditioned upon the perpetuation of
unjust—and alterable—circumstances. Instead, uplifting the nation might
mean vigorous engagement in a struggle to revise those circumstances.

By the late colonial period, hospital buildings and training programs
had been used as testaments to the beneficence of government, but without
the necessary long-term follow-through. Students saw this same strategy
used in the postcolonial state at the turn of the millennium. A member of
Parliament might agitate to get a hospital in his district to boost his prestige, but then leave it unstaffed and unsupplied. The buildings were there,
the doors were open, but it was often hard to see what went on inside as
medicine. Complicated births were unattended, or attended by the hospital cleaner. Urgent surgeries were postponed indefinitely for lack of suture.
Critically ill patients were warehoused without treatment and often without diagnosis until they died, or until their families took them home in
despair. Nutritional rehabilitation units had no food. Hospitals and clinics could not count on long-term allocation of the most basic resources,
including human resources. Students held the government responsible for
the failure of that allocation; with increased clinical experience, most came
to see their national economy as pathogenic and the government as pathological: "not normal."

In 2007, resources were a little less straitened, and the electricity was
on so regularly that the interns had begun to use PowerPoint to present
cases of maternal death at our biweekly mortality review. (The screen saver
showed a lurid painting of three gowned, masked, and gloved figures clustered around an anesthetized patient. Two were visibly white; the third—
and the patient—in dark shadows. Behind them all stood a robed Jesus,
emanating light, sadly beatific, hands on the surgeons' shoulders.) Phillip
Nkhandwe presented the complicated history of a woman referred from
a mission hospital to a district hospital, and from the district to Queens.
She was two days out from Cesarean on arrival with a very badly infected
wound. Her surgical care at Queens, where she had needed three operations
to clean out pus and remove an ever-growing number of infected organs,
was impeccable. But at every step, management decisions had to be made
without basic diagnostic information, monitoring was slim to nonexistent
because the postnatal ward was desperately understaffed, drugs were chosen on the basis of what we had rather than what she needed. Her room, in
which the window screen was broken, Phillip described as smelling "offen-
sive, with flies plus plus." In her final two days of life, she was on inappropriate antibiotics because "unfortunately, we do not have metronidazole at

the moment," she got no intravenous fluid because the obstetrics unit ran out, and the sole nurse on duty did not record any vital signs: pulse, blood pressure, even temperature.

The interns were encouraged, according to the standard curriculum, to look for avoidable causes of death at "personal, medical, and administrative" levels. One faculty member who never lost a chance to lecture on excessive fertility ("personal") contended that the patient should have been urged earlier to get a sterilization, as this was her sixth pregnancy. Because she only had two living children, however, Phillip did not think she would have been likely to accept this idea. Someone questioned whether it was an administrative mistake to transfer her, but no one really thought it was the transport itself that killed the patient. It was difficult to identify medical errors in this case but painfully easy to identify what was missing. A young faculty member finally summed things up: "Should postnatal nurses be able to record [vital signs]? Yes, but they don't. Should we be able to get pus swabs [wound cultures]? Sometimes we become used to things that are *not* normal. You can't get antibiotics. You can't get pus swabs. You can't find fluids." The interns must remember, he said, fixing Phillip with a stare: this was not normal.

Students and interns recognized that becoming involved in issues of resource allocation could be politically dangerous, but felt they were obliged to take the risk for the sake of their patients. Patricia Zembere, whose family had suffered greatly under the Banda regime, found herself torn between wanting simply to do clinical work and feeling that she might have to be active in higher-level health-sector planning to allow her to do that work effectively. "I fear politics," she said bluntly, yet "sometimes I really think, given the chance, I know I can do this better."

Davies Msiska had a close relative who was a DHO. "Medicine is tough," his relative had warned him. "It needs someone who will love the job." Part of the toughness was politics, Davies explained.

> The DHO writes a budget, and it is funded for 10 percent of what the district should have—this they must not accept, not work with. They should say, "We cannot work under these conditions," and close the hospital doors, make political pressure. . . . I think if all the DHOs together did this, the government could not ignore. This is what must happen to change the health care system in Malawi.

The situation would only worsen, Davies said, if doctors accepted their lot, if "they tolerate this thing which they should not tolerate." He was far

from the only student to advocate collective action, a proposal that clinically experienced students often made.

Everyone was aware that recent attempts to exert collective political
pressure in the health sector had been harshly repressed. In 2002, a hospital-
wide strike at Queens in response to the government's failure to implement
promised pay raises was negotiated to a close (without the raises). Immediately after the strike ended, the twelve hospital negotiators—presumed
to be strike leaders—were arrested despite earlier government promises
they would not be penalized. Just before these interviews began, the courts
had determined that all twelve were to be censured and dismissed from the
Ministry of Health *retroactively*: that is, not only would they lose their jobs,
they would also not be paid for the fourteen months of work they had put
in between their arrests and the judgment.[32] Medical trainees feared such
repressive measures, but many remained convinced that widespread collective action was their only hope of holding their government to account
for the health and health care of Malawi's citizens. Several specifically suggested that educating patients about exactly *why* there were no drugs or
resources available could lead to collective action of doctors, nurses and allied health professionals, and the wider community. If a patient knew that
the only pain medicine for her fractured hip was aspirin because a politi-
cian was diverting medicines, she might be angered enough to help agitate
for change. If guardians knew they had to buy their sick relatives food (at
the higher prices charged by vendors who worked near hospitals) because
the budget for the health sector had been slashed again, they might join
doctors and nurses in protest.

A few students, particularly but not exclusively previously trained clinicians, had entered their medical training with activist agendas. Ernest
Dzongolo, for instance, had begun his first year with the long-term goal of
working in the arena of health and human rights. His experience as a clinical officer had convinced him that he needed a doctor's clout to be really effective. Even those who did not enter school with such an agenda, however,
sometimes developed one on the wards. (Zaithwa Mthindi, whose story follows this chapter, was one such trainee.)

This was another arena in which students often made a distinction
between Malawians and the foreign doctors who visited the country. In
pointed contrast to "experts" or short-term medical tourists, they said,
those trained in Malawi simply could *not* remain blind to the ultimate
causes of health problems: poverty, poor governance, inequality, and the
ways these problems interacted. Therapy for this deeper pathology would

require collective action, grassroots work, and public education. If they had earlier learned to see deeply into the body and see through false explanations for disease, as they believed, now their medical vision enabled them to see beyond simplistic models of disease causation and superficial solutions to health problems. Despite a curriculum not all that different from that in most Northern schools, it appeared that biomedical training—and especially clinical exposure in these poor African hospitals—could be politically galvanizing.

✧

The realities of practice in Malawi placed significant constraints on the new doctors. Their salaries, while far above the income of most Malawians, were still low enough that they could be difficult to live on, at least in the style to which the new doctors and their families felt their social rank entitled them. Their extended family networks imposed extensive, sometimes crushing, obligations on them. Their district hospital settings offered very scarce resources, which meant these doctors often had little or nothing to give their patients, save love and witness. They saw the political and economic system in which they were embedded as one that both limited what doctors could do and perpetuated injustice. In light of these constraints, many sought to leave the country, or at least to leave the public sector in search of less frustrating and more lucrative work. Many also came to new understandings of what was essential to medical work. Evidence from this study supports an increased emphasis on resourcefulness, teamwork, the importance of bearing witness to suffering, and collective political action as students completed their clinical training and became interns.

Malawi's new doctors appropriated and reworked material resources to new ends, converting intravenous drip containers to catheter bags and fishing line to suture. They also appropriated and reworked cultural resources to new ends. Social networks got used to mobilize jobs and goods. A culturally important value of uMunthu—one that already linked body, spirit, community, and work—got mobilized to become the "heart for the people" a doctor needed.

The paths these students followed presented striking contrasts to the findings of much previous medical socialization research. Certain paths were blocked—it was perhaps difficult for students to be the representatives of disembodied knowledge when they felt their bodies at risk, difficult to be technocrats without many technologies—while others were less enticing than they might have been elsewhere: clinical impunity, for instance, meant error was less likely to drive one to detachment; unquestionably high status probably meant a less urgent need for authoritarianism. In the final chapter, I will explore some theoretical considerations their journeys raised.

⚜

Someone Else in This World
Duncan Kasinja

Duncan had set up an interview at the end of a thirty-hour stretch on call. I met him on the ward on his way back from the hospital director's office. He and his fellow intern on the service had just delivered an ultimatum, he said. "It's so hard. It's unbelievable. It is just the two of us. . . . We are taking call every other [night], most of the time, we are working very hard, we have no help. We said either find us some help or we stop working." They didn't know how this challenge would work out, Duncan said, but they felt they had no choice but to try.

Over chicken, stewed pumpkin leaves, and *nsima* at a small local café, Duncan's indignation settled and he told me about his route to medicine. His parents had lived separately since he was small, but they shared ambitions for him, he said. Both were educated themselves; his mother was a secretary, and his father worked in a law office. They were not wealthy enough to put him through the expensive private schools, but they found other ways to keep him moving upward through Malawi's educational system. After primary school, "I sat the exams, and I did fairly well but not all that well, and I was not selected for government secondary school. So, in fact, I went on to a mission school, that was in the North." He did well in classes there, particularly the sciences, but once again fared poorly on the exams. "And I was not selected to go to college." Duncan was not bothered, but his father was. Eventually, a friend of his parents talked him into repeating the exams, and he was finally admitted to college. The college was closed for "water problems" for a year, but Duncan ultimately made it through two years of study and was admitted to the medical school.

Why medicine, I asked? "In truth, here in Malawi there are not that many choices," Duncan explained. If you study the sciences, "you will be just a mere teacher when you are finished." A few people may get scholarships to do further studies, it's true:

> But you have to look at what there is for them back here when they return. If you look at the salaries of lecturers, they are not that attractive. And besides being a lecturer, there is not much to do with that advanced training, so it is not much of a choice. So I was working hard in college, I got good grades. Chemistry, bio, math especially. So I said, what are my choices? The problem here in Malawi is with BSc you will just be a teacher. You get further training, you come back, and again you are a teacher. So I said, ah, maybe I should just do medicine. . . . At the end of the year, I saw the list in the paper, and I saw that I was selected. I've been at the College of Medicine five years now, but now my life is more tough. Anyway, I don't regret it that much.

Duncan had five younger siblings, and I asked him whether he would recommend medicine to any of them. He was quiet for a moment, his bearded face still as he looked toward the hospital.

> If it were my brother or my sister, I wouldn't discourage. I would give the pros and the cons. I wouldn't discourage very much, but I would just be very honest, tell them what the situation is like, what the environment is like. But for my own son or daughter, I would say no. I wouldn't want to see this for someone of my blood, you know? It's too frustrating, it's too hectic, you go through all that suffering. So, for a son or daughter, I would say no. I would emphasize strongly the disadvantages.

Medical work in Malawi was not solely a matter of suffering, he noted. Admittedly, there were advantages, too.

> The recognition you get from society is very good at the end of the day. Like your parents are happy, they say, "We have a doctor in the family," your relatives are happy. When you go home, everyone is asking your advices and things. . . . The respect we get as doctors is very great in this society, and that does make a difference, even though the money is poor. Girls, girls are always after us! When they find out you are a doctor—ho! Like now I have friends, we were in college together, and they maybe did accountancy or civil engineering or what, and they are driving a *car*,

and they are living in a *house*, and we go out to some drinking spot and they are buying *drinks*, but I can't buy drinks since I have no money. But then, as soon as they say, "But he is a doctor," girls start coming around and they are very interested in you! . . . And then you feel very much encouraged, compared to your accountant friends.

Overall, however, Duncan thought the status (and the girls) were just not enough to compensate for the difficulties of being a Malawian doctor. He intended to leave the country as soon as he could.

I think—I think this is a hard time to be a doctor here in Malawi. Because I think really things are getting worse and worse. In the older times, when there were also very few doctors in Malawi, eventually they became very prominent. Not at first—maybe at first they struggled, but then later on they were very prominent, and very rich. But in their young and tender days, it was definitely tough. But now you can't really say it will be better later. The environment is just not that good. The hospital doesn't make doctors welcome. Housing is a problem—it's hard to find housing if you are an intern. You go to the director, but they say, "We have no room for you." There is no common room. There is no place you can sit and study, or even relax with other interns, or leave your books. And then on the wards—there are no nurses. There is no equipment. There are no syringes. You come in to work, you leave patients suffering because there is nothing you can use to help them. I have to say I think things are getting worse. The government seems like its priorities are upside down, they are really draining the health sector, and the future doesn't look good. All my friends are saying, "I have to move on in my life, given another choice." And I am, too—I want to finish my internship, then go to the UK, study, and pass my exams there, maybe specialize there once I have passed the exams. I don't want to end up here. I want to be someone else in this world. That's why even now when I go home, I study late. I am so tired, it is so hard because the environment is not too conducive, but I try to do at least a little studying at night to prepare so I can take exams outside Malawi.

Once again, Duncan's studies—along with some connections in the United Kingdom—paid off. I lost touch with him not long after he finished his internship. One of his classmates later confirmed that he had made it to London. As of this writing, he had passed his examinations and was in specialty training, well on his way to being someone else in this world.

꙳

As Human as Everybody Else
Zaithwa Mthindi

When I first met Zaithwa, he was an intern. He spent many long days in the outpatient department (OPD), where hundreds of patients waited in line to be seen by only one or two clinicians. Other days he was primarily in the operating theater. We met for a long lunch one afternoon, after his "surgical list" (of operative cases for the day) was finished, and before he needed to go back to see his patients for evening rounds.

Zaithwa was the last child born into a large family. Raised in a rural area, he moved to a nearby city to attend secondary school and, later, to a more distant city for college. Four of his siblings were still alive, as were his parents, a social worker and a primary school teacher. No one in the family had worked in medicine. Zaithwa himself had for many years intended to join the army and described himself as choosing a medical career almost by chance, and at the last minute, during his first year of college.

> For me, it's different because I didn't grow up in town. I grew up in the village, so the only medical personnel I came in contact with were nurses and medical assistants. Not even clinical officers: medical assistants. So there was no exposure to medicine, law, engineering—you know? I just went to a rural primary school, and I had very little knowledge about the outside world. So mostly that whole first year, when people were talking of medicine, I wasn't thinking of medicine at all. And then, towards the end of first year, you can either apply for law—so others were applying for law, but I wasn't interested in that. But I think maybe something like a week or so before closing the applications for medicine, well—ha, why don't I do medicine? Eh? It wouldn't be a bad idea to do something like that! Ha! . . . So I submitted an application just casual like that. [*laughs*] And then when I got into medicine, they just couldn't believe it!

Early in his medical training, Zaithwa most enjoyed the intellectual variety. There was always something new to learn, and although he found the amount of material to be mastered overwhelming, the range of it was compelling. When I asked him to reflect on the rewards and challenges of internship, he initially returned to similar themes.

For those who work with papers, it's mostly routine work: you compile, you type things, you copy memos. I wouldn't be very comfortable in a job that you lock yourself in a room, and you're working with paperwork and machines and everything. I wouldn't enjoy that kind of work. I like the work where you deal with people. The challenge is, you have to be humane, to show your humanity. You can ignore some machines for some time. "Ah, I will work on them tomorrow. I am too tired, I will just leave them for some time. You can bang them!" [*makes whacking motion with his fist*] But that you can't do with people, OK? You come, you have had a bad night at home, you are not quite fit for the work, but you can't import your own problems and bring them to your working place. Yeah, so I think it really tests your abilities, which is an enjoyable part of it. And also many times your work—your work—makes a critical difference in people's lives. Sometimes it defines life or death.

When the queue in OPD seemed miles and miles long, however, it tested his abilities in a way that was not so enjoyable.

It's always a challenge. Many times the demand is more than you can cope with. So you deal with one patient, and you know that "really, I am doing less than I am supposed to do—or less than I would wish to do for this patient." Or the examination is not as thorough. I think that's one of the—the distressing things. When you know that this patient, I would wish to do a more thorough examination, yet you know that you cannot do that because of the queue. So you just sort of give subminimal attention. Subminimal examination. Like, cheap attention to the multitudes. Which is—it's not very good. Many times you feel bad. "Oh, I really wish I could offer what I am capable of offering." Yeah, but then you cannot do that.

Toward the end of a two-hour interview, I asked Zaithwa how he thought he had changed since his medical training began. He laughed, then paused for over a minute. Flies circled the remnants of our meal as I watched him, waiting. On the tape recording, only the hoarse croaking of Malawi's ubiquitous pied crows filled the quiet until he finally spoke.

Ah, well, working in the hospital for me is not just working with sick people as a healer, to heal them. But many times I—it's as if I'm participating in their suffering. Now this may be a bit theological, or spiritual. But many times I think that when you've got an economic base, when you've made it up, you've got a job, things are going your way—it's as if you are cushioned from problems that your fellow humans are struggling with. And so you can hear about it over the radio, or read it in the newspaper as well perhaps, but by and large you are insulated. I think working as a doctor means I find that I have—I participate. I am not insulated. I am fully aware, and many times I think I get to a point where I feel the suffering in our society. So that I think it has, ah . . . changed the way I look, especially at the disadvantaged part of the society. When you are staying in good areas, good environments, everybody seems well nourished, happy, well clothed. But always I am constantly reminded of the disadvantaged and the sick, the suffering.

"But," I asked him, less perhaps an anthropologist at this point and more a fellow clinician, "how do you deal with that as a human, without becoming enormously depressed?" He paused again.

Mmm, I would say that it's not—the way I look at it, it's not something which has to be defeated or has to be overcome. Ah, what will I say? I will use this illustration. Many times when I am talking to friends, they will say, "Eeee, your job is difficult. Eeee, your job is demanding. Eeee, I couldn't afford being a doctor. Eeee, you do this or you do that." OK? But my point is that even though a job may be very dirty if you think about it in that way, even though a job may be dirty, still it has to be done and it has to be done by somebody. So I think, well, it may be a difficult thing, but somebody has to do it. It may be a cross—but somebody has to carry the cross. Maybe that is me. So that's—many times I think about it in that way. So I don't necessarily look at it as something which has to be fought against. I think on one hand I would say it helps me be sober. Live a sober life. Not live a life of assumptions. Because sometimes I think we have too romantic ideas about life. You can't fall sick. You can't lose a leg. Yeah? You can't be confined to a wheelchair. But when you look at all those people who are sick, it's not that you are more clever in one way or another than them, or that you are more educated—I think some people have that notion; they don't necessarily put it in words, but their attitude towards life seems like somehow these things can't affect them. So it sobers me.

Learning to be a doctor in Malawi, Zaithwa said, one could not forget, "You are still as human as everybody else." Plenty of other lessons could be learned, too.

I have never had any training abroad, so I think I cannot compare my training with any other place. But what I have learned—many times at the hospital we deal with problems that are not clinical, so to say. Some of our problems are not diseases that are caused by microorganisms or any body pathology, necessarily. Somebody talked of medicine as an end stage of social pathology. What he said is, many of the problems that are in society, their end stage will be in the hospital.[33] They will manifest as disease. Some of them are poor governance, some of them are financial mismanagement. Some are illiteracy. Inability to handle social pressures or personal problems. Inability to handle stress. Things like that, they will all end up in hospital. And if you don't know your field of play, you will think that answers are only drugs. And maybe health education very specifically confined to medical issues—disease and pain and things like that. I think many times when you are able to do your training here, you are able to know the interlinking of issues. The interlinking of problems. Which I think is a good starting point! It's OK to go abroad, do some five-year or four-year training and then come back. But you already have that initial foundation, you are able to know that.

The interlinked problems that ended up in the hospital had much to do with distorted government priorities, he believed, and perhaps even a misplaced faith in curative medicine.

The government priorities are really a problem. Really a problem. It's not just the salaries—in fact, I think that's a small thing, really. Sometimes I think the Ministry of Health should be renamed the Ministry of Illness. Or even the Ministry of Death! There is no attention paid to the real causes of suffering and death here. Our country has the highest mortality rate from road accidents in the world, and the ministry comes to the hospitals and says, "You must do better with this, you must handle trauma better." But it is foolish to call road accidents a hospital problem! You can improve trauma care all you want. But when there is a road accident, how are those patients to get to hospital? What about ambulances? Or how about preventing the accidents in the first place? What about better roadblocks? What about police actually enforcing the laws about overloading in minibuses and *matolas*? Making the COF ["certificate of fitness," indicating a vehicle has passed a safety inspection] really mean something, and really enforced? So there is that sort of problem. These politicians don't really care about the causes of death or illness, only about appearances.

This priority of appearances over realities was also evident inside the hospital walls, Zaithwa said. "MPs want to know that a hospital is open in their district, but as long as the doors are open, they don't really care what is happening inside. If it has any drugs, any equipment, if you can really say it's 'running,' doesn't matter in the end." The only hope for change was collective action.

> Cooperative collective action—health workers and patients. Nearby there is a district that was given 10 percent of its requested budget last year, and the hospital chooses to function. There is a septic tank leaking directly outside the main ward. It has been leaking for over a year, but repairing it is a "luxury." So in the main ward, there is always a stench. The entire hospital has one ambulance that works. Patients do get one meal a day, but the guardians bring in the rest, anything they can find. This is in a region where there has been a big problem with famine! But the guardians just don't know any better. They think this is how things must be, and the DHO does not close the doors of the hospital. He knows he would just lose his job, and the hospital would stay open with a different DHO. But if we acted *together*, this might change. What would happen if all the districts closed their doors? Right now, patients and guardians have no voice. We must be the voice for them, and we should choose to be this voice and to help them find their own voices. We must inform the patients. Right now, patients in Malawi don't know that things can be different. That things should be different! And we don't tell them, and we should. I will give an example, eh? You do a lumbar puncture, but the hospital has no lignocaine [a local anesthetic], so you do it without lignocaine. And the patient doesn't know it shouldn't feel like this. In this case, we should tell the patient! We should say, "In other countries, you will have some medicine that numbs the skin so that this LP is not so painful. But here, because the hospital has not received necessary funds from the Ministry of Health, we must do this test without the lignocaine." Thus, if health systems in Malawi are inadequate, we must blame ourselves because we are the ones who know the conditions—and we are the ones who know what they should be.

Zaithwa and I have stayed in touch on and off over the years. Soon after this interview, he was selected for advanced training in a country famous for high-quality and high-technology medical care. The stipend was excellent, the living and working conditions strikingly different from those in

Malawi. During his years abroad, more than one of his former Malawian colleagues suggested to me that he would never come home; he would be a fool to do so, said one. But he did. He continues to work in a large Malawian public hospital and does research with a university-sponsored group. He's an active teacher and by several accounts a superb mentor to medical students.

CHAPTER SEVEN

Doctors for the People:
Theory and Practice

Turning Practice into Theory

"Disembodied" knowledge is never really disembodied, as I argued in the first chapter of this book, and "value-free" science reifies social values all the more effectively precisely because its practitioners and beneficiaries understand it as neutral, value-transcendent—that is, because its values are so deeply embedded as to be invisible. Scientists, including practitioners of medical science, typically understand their knowledge to be culture-free; social scientists and historians have convincingly demonstrated that the separation between facts and values is *itself* an artifact of reductionist science.

The imbrication of fact with value is perhaps more apparent in medicine than in any other science. It is especially difficult to sustain a belief in knowledge as disembodied in medicine, precisely because the universal body clinicians use to think with, medicine's subject and object, is always and everywhere encountered in the real bodies of actual people. It takes an act of significant cognitive violence to strip these medical subjects of their individual vagaries, their lived realities, to "expose" (or rather, to create) the pure medical phenomena beneath. Central to the demonstration of medical competence among North American doctors in training, it is also an act that has functioned to legitimate the power of the state and the dominance of the elite, and to naturalize oppressive hierarchies of gender and race.

In one sense, then, my central research finding—that as these Malawian students acquire a body of medical knowledge, they also take on a distinctive set of medical values, a sort of practical ethics—is nothing new. What *is* new and significant here is that the moral values at the heart of medical science turn out to be not at all the same as they have been shown to be elsewhere, and as they have sometimes been assumed to be everywhere. Malawi's new doctors did not reject the biomedical knowledge that claims to understand the workings and pathologies of a universal human body. Instead, while embracing that knowledge, they challenged the radical reductionism, technological focus, and individualizing (and therefore depoliticizing) strategies that have been theorized as its inevitable consequences. They changed the social relations around biomedical knowledge, the ends to which that knowledge was put, and the moral purpose of the doctor as agent of medical science. A biomedical epistemology of the body remained; the values with which it has been identified did not.

The values from which medical facts cannot be separated turn out to be no durable moral *order*: they constitute rather a moral *economy*, constantly re-created and renegotiated in specific historical, material, and political milieus—whether those milieus are physically located in Blantyre, Manchester, or Madison. In this final chapter, I move from students' accounts of their experiences to a theoretical analysis of how this postcolonial breach in the canonical narratives of medical science happens, and from that analysis on to some of its implications.

Moral Economies and Medical Science

What I mean by *moral economy* here bridges two somewhat different senses in which the term has previously been used. Historian of science Lorraine Daston understands a moral economy as a "web of affect-saturated values that stand and function in well-defined relationship" (Daston 1995:4).[1] The sense of the term more familiar to most anthropologists is the one used by E. P. Thompson, James Scott, and others, to indicate the legitimating ideas, emotions, and practices that characterize the relations between dominant and subordinated groups (Scott 1976; Thompson 1971). Thompson studied eighteenth-century food riots in England, Scott twentieth-century peasant insurrections in Burma and Vietnam. In both cases, peasants understood uprisings as legitimate responses to violations of accepted economic relations, the norms and obligations that determined which claims on their labor were justified or what prices for bread constituted exploitation. By combining Daston's use of *moral economy* and that of Thompson and Scott, we can think of a moral economy as something malleable on two levels: not only a set of emotionally charged values used to negotiate changing economic and social relations between dominant and dominated groups, but also as values that *are themselves* open to negotiation and change.[2] The moral economy of medicine, in this sense, is both process and product: it is the shifting set of values developed and used to legitimate, evaluate, and potentially alter the relations between those seeking medical care, those providing it, and those paying for it or profiting from it. This sense of a moral economy benefits from the dual meaning of the word *value* as used both to indicate an ideal good and to signify worth negotiated through exchange and subject to ideas of fairness.

Among Malawian medical students, the affect-saturated values of heart, of resourcefulness, and of activism were clearly bound up with understandings of responsibility, economic justice, and exploitation. They allowed some new doctors to make sense of their work, and allowed medicine to remain for them a tenable intellectual and moral project. In this moral economy, value was not simply assigned, but created and exchanged; value was dynamic although not completely flexible, shifting while not completely fluid. When novice doctors *could not* perform one kind of value, they sought out another—political action, for instance, became more central to the purpose of the doctor when the wielding of technology was unavailable. The new doctors creatively forged a practical ethics in which there was always something to give: drugs or surgery or bandages, if they could be resourced; love or heart, whether resources were available or not; political activism and a public health focus that drew on a larger regional history in which healing in general was always already social, national, and transnational. This is nothing so stable as an order. We can see these values worked out in practice, tried on and abandoned and then tried on again, reformulated (as when, for instance, "heart" seen as sacrifice is modified to a form that does not compel complicity with an unjust status quo), circulated, exchanged. What may look in a snapshot view—stilled momentarily—like an "order," unchallenged and unchanging because it is unseen, appears in lived experience to be a challenged and changing economy, one in which the technologies and epistemologies of a Northern biomedicine are only one set (if a powerful set) of component parts.

Abstract Presences and Material Absences

Anthropologists of science and medicine know that new technologies can reshape the medical imagination, producing new values and making "moral pioneers" of clinicians and patients alike (see, for example, Casper 1998; Rapp 1999). Such effects have typically been examined where the technologies are materially present. The ethnographic fieldwork presented here suggests that biomedical technologies may also shape values even where they are absent: that is, they alter the medical imaginary, and in so doing, they alter its economy.

Here in this materially impoverished place, the newest diagnostic and therapeutic technologies were present in various more or less abstract forms: in the textbooks from which students learned; in formal lectures from visiting faculty and informal conversations with visiting medical students from the wealthy parts of the world. Sometimes they were present physically, in enclaves at once geographically near and pragmatically inaccessible. Viral loads and CD-4 counts could be measured in the transnationally funded research facilities surrounding the public teaching hospital. Coronary stents could be placed for ischemic heart disease, or in vitro fertilization used to treat infertility, in the South African clinics to which elites flew for care. In the actual clinics and wards where Malawi's student doctors encountered their patients, however, an abyss gaped between clinical reality and medical possibility. The student doctors could see the other side, they could see the countless lives lost in that deadly gap, but they were powerless to bridge it.

This tension between the abstract presence and material absence of new technologies like gene assays or magnetic resonance angiography (or considerably older technologies like radiation therapy, mechanical ventilation for newborns, or dialysis) might have been expected to foreclose a Malawian biomedicine, to imply that real medicine was something that happened elsewhere. For some medical trainees, and at some points, it did. For others, or at other times, the disjuncture between regimes of technoscientific knowledge and realities of everyday practice was a major impetus forcing them to reimagine the work, and renegotiate the moral economy, of medicine.

I emphasize the *new* here to refute any suggestion that Malawians simply learn and practice a medicine of the past. Such a characterization can be tempting, especially from the perspective that sees modernization as a set of stages through which all societies progress sequentially. This model of linear development remains influential outside academia.[3] It also appeared in the language of the Malawian students who wanted to help bring their country to an "advanced," "mature" level.

Some of the ways in which Malawians responded to learning medicine do echo historical analyses of medicine in the North. Reiser (1978, 1993) connects alienation between clinician and patient with the increasing use of diagnostic technologies, both in the profession as a whole over many decades of medical history and among medical students as they progress through training. In his analysis, even as proficiency with such technologies grants physicians greater access to the interior of a patient's body, the patient herself becomes more and more a distraction from the task at hand and the "art" of medicine is abandoned in favor of its "science."[4] Sharon Kaufman (1993) argues that social good was better articulated and individualism less predominant in American biomedicine before the post–World War II knowledge explosion. As medicine's therapeutic powers increased, medical focus narrowed to the individual and "curing began to supersede caring in importance and emphasis" (Kaufman 1993:294). The empathetic and social aspects of medicine that these authors describe dying over the course of medical history in the North appear to be alive in Malawi's present.

In addition, Northern physicians who write about global health often frame African medicine in terms of the past. A geographical trajectory becomes a temporal one: in Africa, students are encouraged to learn from "a nineteenth-century spectrum of advanced disease" ("The Overseas Elective: Purpose or Picnic?" 1993:753). Sometimes geographical and temporal journeys can also be moral ones. Northern physicians may believe that when they spend time in poor countries, they move the world to a better future by recapturing a better personal and professional past: "The obvious challenges of global health provide Western physicians with the opportunity not only to work towards a critically important goal, but also to regain our center and our focus, and in the process remind ourselves of the fundamental values that define our profession" (Shaywitz and Ausiello 2002:355). The language of regaining and reminding calls for a return to an imagined past when medicine had more meaning, and perhaps more status, than it does today: at the very least, medicine reclaims abroad a patina of heroism it has lost at home. These authors conclude that by working in poor countries, "not only can we improve the health of people throughout the world, but we may also revitalize ourselves while renewing the dignity of our calling" (357). Just as Malawi's elite urbanites might become true Malawians by a stint in "the village," constructed simultaneously as geographical Other and temporal past, so elite physicians of the North can become true physicians by a stint in Africa, constructed similarly as geographical Other and temporal past.

Malawi's medical trainees did give less evidence of alienation from patients, and many did articulate social good as crucial to effective and appropriate medical care. They themselves often used the language of modernization. We can see this in two of the ways they spoke of healing the nation: by doing the *work* of medicine, they became agents of modernity for Malawi, and simply by *being* doctors, they were evidence of that healing modernity.

Their reconfigurations of medical work did seem to draw upon historical precedents—albeit precedents of the region and the regional diaspora. These reconfigurations, however, had everything to do with the disjunctures between their twenty-first-century medical knowledge and a twenty-first-century Malawian clinical reality that might have evoked a simpler (or sicker) past to outsiders, but felt like an unjustly deprived—not past but "not normal"—present to those who could not remain insulated from social suffering on the wards. In the medical future they envisioned, their scientific capacities could be put to good clinical, political, and social use.

A model of modernization that fixes Malawi's new doctors as followers, stuck at a past stage of medical development, allows us only to see them as catching up to a Northern present (whether that present is seen as advanced and mature or as alienated and devitalized)—or as failing to do so. It does not allow us to see their genuine creativity. Rather than theorizing their transitions as a matter of returning to or moving out of the past, then, we should understand them as the innovations in the present they are: epistemological innovations in which these doctors-to-be enlarged what constituted scientifically relevant evidence for medical practitioners, and practical innovations with which—as a necessary result—they enlarged what constituted medically relevant practice for biomedical scientists. In this process of enlargement, the new doctors came to experience their work as the basis of a new sense of communal identity, which, in turn, gave them a new purpose for their work. Being doctors made the trainees I knew feel they had access to the lived realities of ordinary (poor) Malawians. That personal and vicarious experience on the wards authorized *and even commanded* their activism. Scientific medicine, rather than enforcing through the need for "neutrality" a separation from the state and the people, gave students both the authority and the duty to make claims on the state in the name of the people. It was their lived experience of the contradictions between the medical imaginary in which they had been schooled and the practice realities they encountered daily on the wards that catalyzed those innovations.

Contradictory Consciousness

I am not the first writer to describe how realities encountered at the worksite can uproot hegemonic concepts that previously seemed no more than common sense while bringing to the fore counterhegemonic narratives. That distinction belongs to the Marxist theorist and political activist Antonio Gramsci, who long ago described a similar disruption. Gramsci's concept of contradictory consciousness proves to be a very helpful way to think about the transition Malawi's doctors made as they encountered clinical realities.

The export of a medical curriculum to a poor place did bring with it hegemonic concepts of the normal and pathological body, and of technical intervention as the goal of medical knowledge, concepts that challenged and partially replaced other ways of viewing the body and health. Other ways were not wholly lost, however; they remained available for reworking when the theoretical knowledge of biomedicine was itself challenged by a more experiential knowledge. Students were unable to maintain biomedical assumptions about the individual locus of pathology once confronted daily, hourly, by the human suffering that results when severe poverty is met with state and supranational neglect. Nascent beliefs in technology as the ultimate means of healing were frustrated by technology's absence (as in antiretroviral drugs that could prolong and improve lives), its irrelevance (as in donated high-tech equipment that broke down promptly after its arrival in Malawi), or its paradoxical harmfulness (as in injections given with unsterile needles because no sterile ones were available). The perceptual dispositions and inclinations to action, the habitus of the doctor-scientist that students began to learn and enact through their medical curriculum, confronted a working-world reality in which scientific technomedicine was both scarce on the ground and ambiguous in its effects.

Gramsci, who articulated the concept of hegemony later used by many critical medical anthropologists to analyze biomedicine, also discussed what happens when hegemonic consciousness confronts a working world too disparate from it.

> The active man-in-the-mass has a practical activity, but has no clear theoretical consciousness of his practical activity, which nonetheless is an understanding of the world in so far as it transforms it. His theoretical consciousness can indeed be historically in opposition to his activity. One might almost say that he has two theoretical consciousnesses (or one contradictory consciousness): one which is implicit in his activity and which in reality unites him with all his fellow-workers in the practical transformation of the real world; and one, superficially explicit or verbal, which he has inherited from the past and uncritically absorbed. (Gramsci 1988:333 [from *The Prison Notebooks*, 1929–1935])

This "contradictory consciousness," if it remained inchoate, could result in a feeling of alienation and produce a state of "moral and intellectual passivity," Gramsci went on to write. This state of alienated passivity is perhaps something akin to the fatalism I saw in a few expatriate doctors in Malawi. But if, instead of remaining inchoate, this consciousness were articulated, it could be enacted as ideological struggle and ultimately as revolutionary change.

In Gramsci's formulation, if Marxist intellectuals could be clear about how their philosophy ratified the *real working experience*, the practical activity of the "man-in-the-mass," counterhegemonic consciousness could make possible meaningful political change. Malawi's new doctors were obviously neither the Marxist intellectuals nor the Italian proletariat Gramsci had in mind, yet the concept of contradictory consciousness describes their experience too well to dismiss.[5] Critical medical anthropologists' concept of biomedical hegemony, in this case a hegemony exported through a medical curriculum brought from the North, fits reasonably well with the doctor-scientist identities students began to take on early in training, and that indeed some of them struggled to maintain. It does not explain the radicalization that others experienced through their medical work, or their reconfigurations of the doctor as one charged with the complex task of healing the nation: diagnosing pathologies beyond the level of corporeal bodies and calling on networks of political and social resources to treat them.

Doctors for the Body Politic

The language of science is often mobilized to make political claims, and social scientists and historians have found the concept of citizenship fruitful for analysis of such practices (see, for example, Heath, Rapp, and Taussig 2004; Rose and Novas 2005). People who share (for instance) a biological condition like diabetes, or a genetic vulnerability like cystic fibrosis carrier status, forge social ties; those alliances can then be used to seek access to forms of social welfare or therapeutic technologies. Two ethnographic examples are particularly apt for this discussion. In post-Chernobyl Ukraine, as Adriana Petryna (2002) has shown, radiation-induced illness became the *only* basis upon which to make valid claims on the state. Ukrainians suffering in a devastated economy and a nightmarish bureaucracy mobilized various kinds of evidence and social networks to demonstrate ties to harmful Chernobyl-related radiation exposure, and thus to stake their claims to "biological citizenship." In an example closer to the Malawian experience, Vinh-Kim Nguyen (2005) described new forms of social identity related to HIV-seropositivity in Burkina Faso. When a few HIV-support-group members began antiretroviral therapy, then still unavailable to the general infected Burkinabe public, these newly formed and still-fragile groups became politicized, mobilizing transnational networks, invoking their human right to be treated, and enacting what Nguyen calls "therapeutic citizenship." Those with access to treatment were expected to advocate on behalf of those who did not yet have it. Nguyen's version of citizenship was one that went *beyond* the level of the state, "whereby claims are made on a global order on the basis of one's biomedical condition, and responsibilities worked out in the context of local moral economies" (Nguyen 2005:142). In post-HIV Burkina Faso, as in post-Chernobyl Ukraine, national or transnational citizenship became the basis for articulating injustices and seeking redress using the authoritative (if sometimes ambiguous) language of medical science. These new forms of citizenship arose from experiences of suffering in situations of widespread poverty, where state systems of health care and social welfare had collapsed.

In the ruins of such systems, it is not only the sick person seeking help who suffers; those who are charged with alleviating illness and providing curative care may also feel distress, anger, a sense of injustice. If we understand the notion of biological citizenship as, to some extent, an instance of the traditional "patient" role writ large (that is, a collective patient identity, based in shared biological vulnerability or pathology, and entitled to make therapeutic claims on the state), then we might also conceive a parallel reconfiguration of the traditional doctor role on the national or transnational stage. Here the doctor's responsibilities for diagnosis and treatment are exercised in relation not (solely) to the individual patient's body but rather in relation to the collective patient, the body politic. Where biological citizenship describes a strategic political use of the patient identity, mobilized as a collective to make collective claims upon the state, there is evidence that Malawian medical trainees made a parallel move on behalf of physicians in their articulations of being "doctors for the people."

When these doctors-to-be talked about their work, they used *spirit* (or *love* or *heart*) for the work interchangeably with *spirit* (or *love* or *heart*) for the people: "the people" were Malawians, and the people *were* the work. Making the people's/nation's health better, then, was the responsibility of a doctor, whether that work was actually done through collective or individual political action, through hands-on encounters in the clinics and wards and operating theaters of Malawi's hospitals, or through epidemic mapping and creative resourcing of staff and drugs in a district health office.

The knowledge of scientific medicine was a necessary but not sufficient basis of their moral authority as doctors of the body politic. Early in their training, they had learned to see deeply into the body and to see through the explanations of nonmedical practitioners. Later, they understood themselves as having learned to see deeply into the pathologies of society, and to see through the superficial and apolitical explanations of disease and suffering proffered by outside experts. They also drew upon the acts of imagination we call empathy, experiencing the ward as part of their lives (as Evelyn Kazembe put it) or feeling the suffering of their society (as Zaithwa Mthindi did). The heart of a doctor, said Thokozani Sokela, must be "What if it was me?" Imaginative empathy, hearts for the people, was critical to the moral authority they needed to critique the state. Their own emotional responses to the wards, like the suffering of their patients, were not extraneous distractions to be suppressed for the effective performance of scientific medicine. They formed the basis of a solidarity between patient and doctor that allowed the latter to act as advocates on the national stage. They gave access to the heart of the work.[6]

Doctors for the people, in the articulation given by many Malawian trainees, were entitled and obligated to make claims on the state on behalf of the people. They were entitled and obligated to reject notions of saintly self-sacrifice that left abuses of power and systemic injustices unchallenged. They were entitled and obligated to make their fellow-Malawian patients aware of the medical deprivation they met with: this spinal tap would hurt less with anesthetic, but we have none because the government has not made health care a budget priority; your child's pneumonia should be treated with antibiotics, but we have none because the MP has been diverting them to the black market; a nurse should change your dressing, but the nurses' salaries are so low that many have left to work as secretaries.

This last strategy—making patients aware of the structural components of their suffering—engages Malawian physicians in the political mobilization of their patients. Coming from the mouth of a physician in the context of treatment, such analyses may be understood to be tantamount to diagnosis; they describe to the patient the etiologies of his suffering, and they suggest remedy. In this case, both are located outside of the body and are positioned squarely in national and global structures. Such diagnosis performs several kinds of work. It aligns doctors and patients together in solidarity against the systems of global exploitation and inequity—or national failure and corruption—that give rise to suffering. It may also begin to engender in the patients so diagnosed a sense of their own collective suffering as patients, and so may begin to create a new biological citizenship in response. In this process, we can see how just as the traditional roles of doctor and patient are mutually constitutive in the biomedical clinical encounter, so, too, the strategic, politicized collective identities of the biological citizen and the citizen clinician are generated and mobilized in mutual relationship.

Collective citizenship and the imaginative empathy that made it possible had limits, and the conception of the "doctor for the people" role is not unambivalent.[7] These students had aimed for "the top" of a social hierarchy of professions; conversion of their experiential knowledge to authority put them again at the top, bolstering their status as elites in many respects. They tended to characterize "the people" as poor, deprived, suffering—generic. The body politic as worksite, while it did not allow a completely reductionist medical science, also did not necessarily require greater attention to the individual *subjectivities* of those seeking clinical help than would the body corporeal.

In addition, if their status as doctors gave them responsibilities as Malawians, it also engendered entitlements—to status, compensation, political power—and authorized other collective identities. Even as they positioned themselves as doctors for the nation, these students often also understood themselves to be "international doctors." Like the activists Nguyen studied, they forged alliances not only with fellow nationals but with outsiders who might be (or have access to) useful resources. "People who have trained in other countries, people of different races," said Crispin Kamwendo, could "come together as one" to overcome Malawi's difficulties. One could make claims on transnational networks of people and resources, too, and given the poverty of the Malawian state, it was crucial to maintain a position from which those claims were possible. And when self-sacrifice was too unfairly demanded, the experience of injustice too sharply felt, the risks too great, when one needed to become "someone else in this world," as Duncan Kasinja did, the doctor's status as international citizen could make emigration feel "only human."

Journeys and Stories

The concepts of moral economy, contradictory consciousness, and doctoring the body politic are helpful ways to think about what happened as Malawi's young doctors learned their profession. What none of them captures quite satisfactorily is the sense of direction that appeared repeatedly in students' own narratives of their experiences. Their stories did not consistently feature either stasis or struggle, although both were evident from time to time. More often, they referenced paths, routes, journeys. Students reflected on the past and projected themselves into the future, or positioned themselves in Malawi and imagined themselves moving elsewhere.

In these journeys, the doctors' own actions were parts of broader trajectories, often trajectories of development or decline. Duncan Kasinja needed to leave because things were only getting worse. Joe Phoya hoped that if enough doctors stayed in the country, Malawi's medical system, which was "just still developing," would "become mature." It was stasis, or directionlessness, that was most feared. Medson Namanja felt he had been plunged into the "deep end" of medicine in Malawi. Catherine Gunya lamented being "stuck" as a general practitioner, and Patricia Zembere hoped not "to be glued here." Several asked aloud, of themselves or of their profession, "How shall we know the way forward?" These journeys were moral, because they were saturated with judgments of value.[8] The lines between temporal and spatial points marked trajectories in which Malawi was understood as getting better or getting worse, or in which some places (inside or outside Malawi) were better or worse than other places, or in which the new doctor was developing more of a heart for the people, or the student who had once thought himself brilliant sadly discovered that he was not what he had thought he could be.

The stories they told of their own journeys also referenced available narratives of medical work. African learners are sometimes treated as if they were blank slates (Matos 2000), but of course they never are. Malawians arrived at the College of Medicine steeped in a regional history that made the equation of medical work with moral cleansing, healing individuals with uplifting society, curing with mission, feel natural. They were products of a nation in which the highest-status doctors, like the highest-status traditional healers, brought the wisdom of other places to Malawi. In their country, hospital work had been entwined with Christian mission for nearly a century and a half, and doctors had been preachers, revolutionaries, politicians, heroes, prisoners, a dictator. Their history prepared them to understand the status of healer, including that of physician, as one that entails the potential both for great power and for serious endangerment: physical, political, and moral peril.

Plenty of these students had family stories that recapitulated these histories. Relatives who had worked in Malawi's hospitals had fled the country under the Banda regime, suffered threats, were ordered to undesirable locations. Even for those students not personally touched by this history, it was recent and palpable. Everyone knew that a College of Medicine graduate had been relegated to internal exile in a godforsaken district for speaking truth to a corrupt power over the diversion of drugs for profit. Their own first principal had risked his position, and perhaps his life, by standing up to a powerful dictator who was also a doctor—another story everyone knew. The dangers did not end with the dictatorship. Most students and doctors had watched plenty of doctors, nurses, and clinical officers around them sicken and die, some from infections acquired on the job. To be a doctor was highly prestigious, but it was also far too risky to undertake simply as a means to power.

The vagaries of culture and history, the particulars of legal, financial, and other structural issues affecting medical practice, made certain social identities readily available to the new doctors even as they foreclosed others. The available narratives were different in Malawi than in the North. There were almost none of the fabulously wealthy doctor-entrepreneurs seen in the United States. (Malawian students and faculty sometimes spoke of one rich private practitioner, but it was always the same one.) There were few if any of the doctor-employees for whom medicine is a nine-to-five job, conscientiously performed and then left behind at the office; I certainly never heard students, interns, or practicing physicians speak of such an archetype or such a person, nor did I ever encounter one. Instead, there were doctor-politicians, using their credentials as stepping-stones to power, for good or bad or ambiguous purposes. There were doctor-experts working for transnational research projects, doing more or less relevant work for good pay. There were doctor-émigrés, prominent in the mythology of the medical school, working abroad and sending money home, both scorned and envied. There were self-sacrificing doctor-missionaries, offering their hearts to their patients and putting themselves at risk: some of these perhaps *only* sacrificed, accepting fatalistically the conditions of their work, while others also acted to change the larger structures of inequity. And there were doctor-fatalists, stuck and static, doing desultory and angry work among the poor patients and not trying very hard to help anyone, because ultimately there seemed not to be much point.[9]

Turning Theory into Practice; or, So What?

The research presented here, and the theoretical explanations I have offered for these findings, have implications for policy, for future research, and for medical pedagogy. It is not at all clear how generalizable the processes described here might be to other places, whether culturally African or materially deprived or both. It is not even clear that these processes will persist in Malawi itself. What is clear is that stories of training told and retold (and the processes of training studied and restudied) in the North are *not* generalizable.

The universality of science is a powerful narrative: the laws of physics behave the same way around the globe (and beyond it); the physical body, if not everywhere the same, is predictable enough that medical practitioners can perform some of their functions—if perhaps not very well—without thinking much about its variability.[10] Practitioners believe in the universality of science, and from there it is a short step to understanding our own experiences of medicine as also universal. However "global" medical science may (or may not) in theory be, though, in practice it is always and everywhere learned and implemented in a particular place, among people in particular social relations, with particular cultural and material resources available to them. Scientific knowledge is developed, and its applications delivered, in actual communities and through social and political processes specific to those communities.

Remembering this inevitable particularity puts African biomedicine back into its proper analytical place alongside all the other healing practices and theories of the continent. Splitting African healing practices into a reductionist and individualizing Western biomedicine and a social and public indigenous tradition has long been recognized as a distortion (Vaughan 1994). Although such a depiction is still fairly common in more popular approaches, it rarely appears in the scholarly literature now, and then only accompanied by numerous caveats and apologies (see, for example, van der Geest 1997). Biomedicine has been recognized for years to be one of many epistemological and practical resources upon which ailing Africans draw. Yet African practitioners of biomedicine keep slipping into the conceptual cracks. Few social scientists have found them of interest, although some historians have (see, for example, Hunt 1999; Iliffe 1998; Marks 1994). Hardly any anthropological research has been done in biomedical institutions in Africa (the work of Stacey Langwick is an exception), even while African traditional, neotraditional, syncretic, and religious healers continue to fascinate anthropologists. This omission has hurt our understanding of biomedicine as a form of African healing.[11]

People who study African healing empirically and ethnographically have for a long time shown the instability of any category we could think of as "traditional," and the resourcefulness of healers outside the formal sector in drawing from different theories and techniques—including those of biomedicine. Where this book is unique is in showing a similar resourcefulness at the heart of institutionalized medicine, within the very process by which students become doctors. During one of those rare times when everyone is consciously and explicitly focused on the production of identity, the new doctors themselves challenge values that have been assumed to be central to medical science. What is more, this challenge takes a shape that is distinctly reminiscent of other healing practices in the region: public, political, aimed at healing the nation and repairing the ruptures of the social world.

This research also puts the existing studies of medical socialization into a new perspective. The story (or stories) of learning medicine in Malawi I have told here are strikingly different in many respects from those that have been reported in the extensive literature on medical socialization in the North. If the analysis stops at "difference"—if what happens in the North is taken as normative and what happens in Malawi is taken as Other, for cultural or material reasons—then it has failed. I am arguing that these very differences challenge us to reconsider what has been thought of as normal, archetypal. If medical science in Malawi has a moral economy, negotiated and contested, contingent on material realities, available narratives, social networks, then surely so does medicine in the North. If these stories of medical students at Queens Hospital (like the histories of their patients) do not make sense without understanding their historical, economic, and social positions, then surely the stories of medical students at Harvard Medical School or University College London (or the histories of their patients) require similarly careful contextualization.

Economies are living, fluctuating, relational negotiations that can *appear* to be fixed when viewed consistently through the same lens or from the same vantage point. Thus, the North American location of previous work on the subject can give rise to the *illusion* that the moral economy is in fact a moral order, and that medicine as an institution has certain inevitable consequences for those who train within it and those who seek help there. Relocation to Malawi makes the fluidity of the process more *evident*, makes it obvious that the imbrications of medical knowledge and values are not static or acultural, but contingent and shifting. This relocation, in turn, allows us to look back at the North and see the dynamism there.

Implications for Malawi

While conducting and writing up this research, I was often asked—but never by a Malawian—whether I thought a medical school was a good idea for such a poor country. Perhaps Malawians had the reasonable belief that this was a topic on which their opinions should have more weight than mine. The Malawians who disclosed their thoughts on the issue all thought the country should have a medical school. Several, however, worried that not enough of the new doctors would stay. I am inclined to agree with them on both counts, although it is not easy to foresee what the ultimate effect of domestic medical training will be for Malawi and its health sector.

The University of Malawi's College of Medicine, as an intervention intended to improve the health of Malawi's people, is a giant, expensive, long-range gamble. At worst, it may suck up scarce national resources to produce an elite that will leave the country at the earliest opportunity, or stay and benefit only a few wealthy clients. At best, it may *also* produce at least a small, and perhaps a sizable, cadre of physicians dedicated to the poor of their nation. Such a cadre will have the power to make beneficial long-term changes through political activism, through research, through public health–oriented innovation, and through day-to-day clinical activity—activity that perhaps cannot be detected on any macro level in the ocean of medical need that the African continent sometimes seems to be but that nonetheless can be truly meaningful (to practitioners and patients), even lifesaving.

I believe that this research offers reason to hope for that best outcome. There are students and interns who demonstrate a passion that may sustain them as they struggle for larger changes. Their lack of cynicism about patients is surprising and encouraging. Five years on from the initial research project, most of these young Malawi-trained doctors were hard at work in the district hospitals, in the Ministry of Health, in research organizations trying to work out cost-effective interventions for the diseases that injure and kill too many Malawians. I do not know what will happen to them in the long run: whether they will burn out soon, become fatalists, or gradually slide over the none-too-clear border between resourcing and outright graft—or whether they will be the visionary leaders Malawi's health sector so desperately needs. I also believe it would be a mistake to count out those who have left the country, although it is easy from a policy perspective to see brain drain as the worst possible outcome of medical training in Malawi. Malawi's history is one in which healers have long come and gone across national borders, bringing knowledge and techniques and social networks with them, and in which diasporic figures have had powerful symbolic and material impacts on their nation—whether they returned to the country in the long term, the short term, or not at all.

The less tangible, more symbolic outcomes of the medical school are also important. Those who oppose medical schools in poor countries as "white elephants," inappropriate technologies, must be aware of the subtler implications of their opposition. Yes, medical schools are expensive. Yes, midlevel cadres such as clinical officers can perform the basic work of curative medicine as well as doctors can, and at a fraction of the cost, in many (probably most) settings. But donors and other critics who push for *only* such midlevel training must be aware of the racist legacy of some such strategies, in which two-tiered medical training was a deliberate way to keep black Africans in a subordinate position. They must also think seriously about whether promoting a medical hierarchy that stops at the level of clinical officer perpetuates an exploitative system in which poorly paid Malawian workers are inevitably managed and supervised by high-salaried expatriate "experts." Like it or not, and there are many reasons not to like it, physicians internationally exercise considerable power in health affairs. Producing more Malawian physicians should ultimately put the health sector in Malawian control. The high status accorded to Malawian physicians may be problematic in many ways, but it may also be a lever with which they can effect beneficial change, and a source of national pride and hope.

Africa is bursting with human capability. In addition to the corrupt politicians, child soldiers, and starving babies that figure so prominently in the international news, the continent is packed with motivated workers, bright and hopeful students, resourceful innovators, people with great ideas and the energy to run with them, doctors and nurses and clinical officers who long to help their people thrive. In my own opinion, countries like Malawi need fewer outside experts to inform, educate, "empower," or otherwise tell people how to do things. Rather, they need adequate resources to nurture, train, and retain home-grown talent. Northerners—clinicians and others—who feel a fierce need to reach across borders and help would do well to identify who is already doing good work and then humbly ask how we can be of service. We can also pressure our own leaders to dismantle the transnational structures of oppression that hobble African capacity to respond vigorously to poverty and sickness—that actively mitigate against healing the nations.

Implications for the Critical Anthropology of Medicine

Medical anthropologists struggle over the role of medicine in society. At opposite poles of the debate, curative biomedicine can be a moral obligation, a salvific required by the call to social justice (Farmer 1999), or it can be a tool of exploitation, systematically masking social injustice and serving the needs of a powerful elite (Taussig 1980).[12] African understandings of healing practices from many places on the continent may provide a helpful precedent in moving away from this kind of polarized understanding. In many accounts from Africa, healing power is understood as inherently dualistic: because healing involves accessing an invisible realm in which harm and help may both be worked, the power to heal *is* the power to harm (see, for example, Ashforth 2005; Davis-Roberts 1992; Geschiere 1997; West 2005). In Malawi, the word *muti* reflects this duality: *muti* is medicine, and it is also poison.

Emily Martin (2006) recently explored a similar dualism in the context of Western psychopharmaceuticals. Observing that the Greek word *pharmakon* also connotes both remedy and toxin (as others have also noted), she discussed the way pills are symbolically split into good and bad parts. Rather than recognizing that the helpful and harmful are intrinsically connected, she suggests, Northerners displace the bad parts: by calling them "side" effects, by setting off warnings in confining black boxes, by conducting clinical trials far away, and by other mechanisms.

In my own experience, the paradox Martin begins to explore goes far beyond tranquilizers and antidepressants, deep into the heart of biomedicine itself—and perhaps, as the ambiguity of words for medicine in widely divergent language groups hints, of any healing tradition. For biomedicine, almost any example will serve. Cesarean section can save a mother and newborn from death due to obstructed labor, and it can condemn a woman to die slowly, painfully, and unnecessarily from septic shock following an infection and a burst abdomen, without saving her infant. Cardiopulmonary resuscitation can restart a heart and save a person's life, and it can ensure that an elderly person's last living moments are spent naked and sprawled, ribs cracking and needles jabbing, for the dual purposes of teaching the medical students how to "run a code" and reassuring the family that "we did everything that could be done." Smart, careful, hardworking clinicians can make difficult diagnoses and deliver lifesaving therapies, and can make terrible mistakes that cost their patients injury or even death. High-quality, high-technology biomedicine—and not just in the global South—can give people the chance to survive HIV, multidrug-resistant TB, trauma, or childbirth. It can also engender ecosystem-wide antibiotic resistance, taint tap water with estrogens and antidepressants, and function as an incredibly expensive distraction from other serious causes of inequality, injustice, suffering, and death—and not just in the global North.

To desire rain is to desire mud, as a Malawian proverb goes: *Walira mvula walira matope.* The bad comes with the good. A theoretical commitment to skepticism about either-or assessments of biomedicine (or any other healing practice), following rather an African model in which healing and harming are instead presumed to be integral, would allow critical medical anthropologists a subtler take on the effects of medicine on individuals and populations in poor *and* wealthy, culturally Western *and* culturally Other, places. The findings presented here suggest that medicine in practice may have such ambiguous effects, neither perhaps as useful as its defenders hope nor perhaps as imperialist as its critics charge. In addition, they help to disentangle critical analyses of medicine and health from a related policy problem.

Two types of errors commonly afflict health policy in poor countries, as Barbara Jackson and Antonio Ugalde (1987) pointed out long ago. The first error, one promoted by international economic regimes for decades, is to believe that economic development alone will suffice to improve a nation's health.[13] To those who take this position, providing doctors, nurses, hospitals, and drugs is *not* the responsibility of the state: curative medicine is at best a distraction from the economic reforms that will solve health problems and at worst a diversion of essential funds. Those who criticize biomedicine as neocolonialist hegemony must be aware that their arguments can be used to support policies like the neoliberal "health-sector reforms" that essentially force poor states to gut the civil sector of nurses and doctors, drugs, and even basic primary care in the name of improving the GNP.

The second error is to conflate biomedical technologies with health: more doctors, more nurses, more hospitals, and more drugs mean better health. Critical medical anthropologists commonly charge this error to doctors and health policymakers (many of them doctors as well), especially in the global South. A policy focus on health *care*—as opposed to health—minimizes the role of the economy and the state in the production of health and illness.[14] In the eyes of some critics, medicine's individualist, curative focus will *inevitably* lead medical practitioners and like-minded policymakers to depoliticize health problems in poor countries.

It should be clear from the material presented here that Malawian students and graduates in general rejected an exclusive focus on health care technologies even as they refused to consider abandoning health care as a national priority. Ambulances—although desperately needed—were not the solution to Malawi's terrible road-traffic-accident-related mortality, any more than drugs were the solution to the malnutrition that landed hundreds of children in Queens every hungry season. Nearly all of the new doctors had highly politicized takes on Malawi's health. The impact of state-level decisions and of systemic poverty were all too clear to them as they struggled in the country's devastated public hospitals. Their critiques had some limits. At the time I worked among them, when few had long-term clinical experience, they did not challenge the central *ethical* primacy of the state: they held Malawi's government to be critically responsible for the welfare of its citizens, even as its actual ability to provide for that welfare was undermined by the transnational forces of globalization.[15] It is also true that much of their concern was directed at the lack of resources flowing to the public health sector, a focus clearly linked with worries about their own salaries and the support of their own extended families. But they did not typically conflate biomedical technologies and health: in fact, some believed it was impossible to do so if one was paying attention during clinical training in Malawi. Their concerns extended well beyond the health sector, to wider problems of corruption, poor education, mismanagement, inattention to issues of public safety and well-being. Both the significant emphasis on public and community health in their didactic medical training and their practical activity on the wards in the clinical years reinforced the messages of preventive care and social responsibility.

In this case, the ways that students negotiated a moral economy of medicine mean that biomedicine in Malawi cannot comfortably be thought of either as culturally neutral technology or as inherently neocolonialist project. The contradictory consciousness students and interns developed in their everyday working experience led them to articulate counterhegemonic ideas about health in this poor place. I am not suggesting their ideas or practices will produce revolutionary changes in Malawi's health sector or beyond; I have no evidence to support such a claim. However, they are sufficiently different from mainstream Northern concepts of medicine as technoscience that they provide some hope for practical, if incremental, change.

Anthropologists have been accused of "missing the revolution," to use Orin Starn's (1992) term—relishing cultural difference so much that they ignore political and economic upheaval around them. It may be that our theoretical perspective leads critical medical anthropologists to an opposite error: watching for the revolution while missing the real possibility, and real effects, of small and incremental changes made every day in the practical interactions of doctors and nurses, patients and bureaucrats. Both errors can allow us to see stasis where there is dynamism. J. K. Gibson-Graham (1996) argued that academic Marxists, demoralized by the oppressive practices and subsequent implosion of the Eastern bloc, failed to recognize and encourage the everyday forms of resistance to capitalism that in fact surrounded them. Critical scholars of health can sometimes do the same, lamenting the devastating health effects of large-scale political economic processes while failing to examine seriously the small ways that people everywhere may resist the processes that exacerbate their suffering (see, for example, Paley 2001) or commodify their succor (see, for example, Pfeiffer 2006).

Implications for Medical Socialization

These findings also have theoretical implications for those who study medical socialization in the North. If, as I argue, biomedicine's "moral order" is actually a fluid, negotiated moral economy, then the separation of subjectivity from rational science and social responsibility from medical activity must be seen as cultural moves, and fresh explanations for the persistence of medicine's values must be sought in the North. I suggest two areas for potentially fruitful exploration: the impact of history and culture as demonstrated in existing medical narratives; and the material circumstances of medical practice.

Narratives have tremendous power. In Malawi, stories of sacrificial missionary doctors, medical-school graduates bravely exposing corruption, and medically trained émigrés sending money home from the wealthier parts of the world circulated among students and new doctors. These stories drew upon the historical and cultural locations of medicine in Malawi. The stories then performed work as students considered who they were becoming. Reading the literature on medical socialization in the global North, I have been struck by the frequency with which students and interviewees there also referenced stories about doctors—often fictional. The importance of stories as touchstones for doctors-in-training can be seen in the work of Terry Mizrahi (1986), a sociologist who studied internal-medicine training in the American South in the 1980s. Interns and residents she spoke with there often suggested that she need not interview them to understand their experiences; she could simply read *The House of God* (Shem 1978) instead. Kit Boyes (2007) describes similar comments—thirty years after the book (set in Boston) was published, and halfway around the globe in New Zealand. It is not uncommon for American students to refer to characters from television shows or movies. Perhaps it is time to pay more attention to the circulation of the stories told about medicine, or written, or shown on the big or small screen. What sorts of narratives are available to students? What cultural resources do they draw upon when the going gets rough?[16]

If historical and cultural narratives are important to the construction of doctors' working identities, then so are the material conditions of medical work with which these narratives are entangled. The findings presented here suggest that a half century of research on medical education has overstated the importance of student and curricular factors on identity, and understated the impact of the actual conditions of work—conditions including infrastructure, bureaucracy, financing, social arrangements, tools and technologies. Northern research on professional identity, like the personal (and even the fictional) narratives about medical training, has generally been situated in elite, resource-rich, *materially* virtually interchangeable sites. My research shows that poverty and resource limitation matter profoundly to medical training in at least one country in the South. A reasonable hypothesis, then, would be that the material conditions of work, largely ignored in most research on medical training, should have similarly profound effects in the North.

This hypothesis suggests new avenues for research. Economic and social conditions of practice have changed substantially since the days of the classic American studies. (Most recent ethnographic studies of physician training have been conducted in countries with national health plans, in the United Kingdom or Canada.) American medical schools since the 1980s have increasingly relied for their financial survival on the funds brought in by research grants, by highly paid specialty care, and by the rapid throughput of primary care patients. Pharmaceutical and medical-device manufacturers now fund about 70 percent of all clinical research trials and over half of all continuing medical education (Schafer 2004), contributing to the entrenchment of a highly technologically focused and for-profit model of medicine in medical schools and teaching hospitals. Kenneth Ludmerer (1999) has argued that the shift is so substantial that academic medical centers no longer function meaningfully either as integral parts of the university or as public trusts; rather, they have become extensions of corporate power. He sees the rushed environment of medical practice in the managed-care era as particularly problematic for doctors' training.

> Habits of thoroughness, attentiveness to detail, questioning, listening, thinking, and caring were difficult if not impossible to instill when both patient care and teaching were conducted in an eight- or ten-minute office visit. Few learners were likely to conclude that these sacrosanct qualities were important when they failed to observe them in their teachers and role models. (Ludmerer 1999:361)

What Ludmerer understands as a change in the context of training and practice, other observers commonly assume to be a generational divide. Medical educators and a senior generation of doctors often grumble about what they describe as the "Gen-X" mores of today's medical students, residents, and junior faculty. This generation gets characterized as *culturally different*: unwilling to work as hard as their predecessors, less thorough or careful, less committed to medicine, more likely to seek "balance" between work and other pursuits, inadequately deferential (Bickel and Brown

2005). Such characterizations probably reflect a fundamental error of attribution: the common human tendency to attribute other people's behaviors to individual or group characteristics, and to underestimate situational factors. Training doctor-scientists and then setting them to work in situations of tremendous poverty alters how they behave and think and feel. It seems likely that setting them to work amid abundant technology, which they are to wield as quickly as possible in the service of an enormous profit-making machine, has similarly profound effects. New research on American medical training in the corporate era—or, better yet, comparative research across materially and culturally different settings of training—could explore more deeply the ways that medicine's moral economy gets negotiated under various conditions of practice.[17]

Medical educators often contend that the primary goal of a medical school should be to produce humanistic, socially responsible doctors.[18] No doubt some believe it—even though the attempts to make it happen are typically so underresearched, so underfunded, and so often (if unofficially) derided as "soft" medicine that it would be difficult to think of a more effective way to produce the appearance of change without the discomfort of actual change.[19] Meanwhile, much critique of professional education in the North characterizes it as dehumanizing, a process that enables technical expertise while disabling the capacity to make human connection, the capacity to care. Arthur Kleinman (2009) has recently gone so far as to characterize medical education as a process of moral impoverishment. Whatever they are taught formally, students learn through medicine's "hidden curriculum" that the lived experiences of their patients and the social and economic structures in which they fall ill are irrelevant to medical work and that students' own affective responses to that work are unacceptable and must be buried.

If empathetic, humanistic, socially responsible doctors really are the goal, medical educators might find the research presented here worth pondering, particularly in connection with some research from the North. In a study of American medical students who volunteered at a clinic for the homeless, Beverly Ann Davenport found that students learned to "witness" patients' lives rather than treating them with an objectifying reductionism (Davenport 2000). Witnessing meant two things to these students: paying respectful attention to the stories and experiences of their patients, and advocating on their behalf in city and state politics. The study was small and far from definitive, but the results are provocatively similar to some that I have presented here. If educators truly want students to believe that a human connection with patients is crucial to being a good doctor, one option they might test would be to have students spend time in locations where they sometimes have only that connection to offer.[20]

Imagining Communities

People move in and out of Malawi following routes pioneered by others: between Livingstonia and Meharry, Lansing and Blantyre, Lilongwe and Manchester, Zomba and Uppsala by way of Durban or Accra. Medical ideas, practices, photographs, textbooks, lab coats, CT scanners, microscope slides, drugs, stethoscopes, and stories also travel between the representatives of one locale, marked as "African," and representatives of another, sometimes marked as "Dutch" or "American" but sometimes as "international."[21] These journeys can have complex effects in more than one direction.

Encounters between Malawi's doctors-in-training and the medical-student tourists and volunteers who visit from the wealthy world were one important force that pushed the Malawians to reflect on what it meant to be doctors. They relished what they saw as a chance to transcend the borders of nationality, race, and class. They described a real feeling of community with those Northern students and doctors they met on the wards. Yet these encounters also troubled them, enhancing their awareness of the contradiction between their high status, product of a globalized idea of the doctor, and the realities of their day-to-day work, firmly lodged in the poverty-stricken postcolonial South. New Malawian doctors, like their Northern peers, were unquestionably among the elites of their country. Their status was high, their income *by Malawian standards* was high, their education was unmatched among their age-mates. Yet they earned much less than the graduate student who came to interview them, and even adjusted for purchasing power, their incomes were lower than those of Americans working fast-food counters at minimum wage. They took serious risks at the hospital, as they faced long lines and crowded wards of the desperate and destitute. Their working conditions were such that a thoughtful doctor could talk about medicine, without irony, as a dirty job that someone had to do.

Benedict Anderson (1983) described the way in which nationalism created "imagined communities" that could bind different people together in service to a common ideology and identity. It may be that occupational identities in the era of globalized, service-based economies also form "imagined communities." "Global" medicine, like global science or economics, is always and everywhere practiced locally (W. Anderson 2002). There is no real physical space called the global, as many analysts of globalization have pointed out, but there is an imagined social space—in this case, an imagined community of clinicians—with effects in many physical localities. The Malawians felt themselves to be members of such a community, built up as medical people and medical goods and medical stories moved from place to place; they used the social networks within this community, when they could, to material and symbolic ends that they considered important to the work of medicine.

Do Northern doctors and medical students also imagine the Malawians as members of our shared occupational community? If so, how does that change how we think about our work? If not, how might it?

Arthur Kleinman (1999), who has written extensively about the uses of narrative in theorizing about illness, contends that ethnographic research can give us invaluable information about the local worlds of moral experience within which decisions are actually made, negotiated, reworked. In this case, close attention to the narratives students and interns use to explain their experiences allows us to see how economic and political circumstances shape subjectivities that, in turn, shape the moral values of medical work: how contradictory consciousness happens in practice. Close attention also allows us to see their stories *as stories*: as constructions in which what may have seemed random is revealed (or made) to be coherent; in which they relive their experiences and reflect upon them simultaneously; by which they justify their decisions, make sense of the past, and project themselves into the future.

"Clinicians are often impatient with stories, but stories are what keep us going in the face of our inevitable mortality," Laurence Kirmayer has said. "More, they are the agents of individual and collective memory, and it is precisely through them that we can begin to appreciate the ways in which choices can be enlarged and value found in places beyond those sanctioned by the purveyors of desire" (Kirmayer, in Farmer 2004:321–22). How do the stories of these Malawian doctors and doctors-to-be affect those of us who are members of their imagined professional community? If their encounters with us trouble them and give them hope, do their struggles implicate us? Are their griefs and joys resonant? Do we think, What if it was me? If we identify with them as members of an imagined community, do we become conscious of the stories *we* tell about ourselves and about the world? When we move from believing our own ideas as truths to examining them as stories, we open up new possibilities.[22] What kinds of decisions, political, economic, educational, make our stories end the way they do now, and what kinds of decisions might lead in different directions? The expansion of our own imagined community, through narratives like the ones recounted here, introduces instantiations of medical practice that differ from the one with which we are most familiar, the one in which reductionist rationality, individualism, politically "neutral" authority, and love of technology are the inevitable accompaniments of science.

∽

Malawi's new doctors are frustratingly ambiguous figures. They really are, as they perceive themselves to be, both elites in some respects and an underclass in others, both subaltern and powerful. They critique the government, even while they are employed by and representatives of the government. Their resourcefulness can slide easily into corruption, their status into impunity, their bent for political action into a way to avoid painful clinical encounters. Their own depiction of themselves as agents of modernity (in a nation imagined as insufficiently modern) can lead us to overlook how innovative their understandings of medical science sometimes are. Their social class, education, and status divide them deeply from most of "the people" with whom they nonetheless feel (perhaps unilaterally) a strong bond, and to whom many profess a fierce commitment. Their hopes for healing the nation and "uplifting Malawi" depend upon both the specificity of their experiences, on the wards of Queens and in the dusty hamlets outside Mangochi, and on a quite nonspecific understanding of themselves as members of a global profession. Their dream of community solidarity and collective action against the depredations of national (and perhaps international) structures of power seems badly out of step with a neoliberal moment of privatized salvation in which health, like the economic and spiritual well-being with which it is bound up, is assumed to be a private matter: just between the individual and the free market. The power of this moment—which was, after all, once thought to signal the end of history—is such that to an outsider, their vision can appear naïvely utopian, unrealistically romantic, even doomed. And yet it can also seem, just possibly, cause for hope.

These doctors complicate theoretical narratives, too. Just as Malawi's medical trainees drew upon a range of resources to make their work feasible and meaningful, I have "resourced" a heterogeneous set of theoretical tools, from postcolonial history to science studies, from Marx and Gramsci to Bourdieu and Kleinman, to make sense of their sense-making processes. Their science is neither an easily portable set of universal truths and techniques nor a moral order inextricably bound to the West: probably no science is. Their responses to learning and applying it cannot readily be seen only as resistance or as accommodation, unless we are to ignore large parts of what they do and say. If we consider them to be doctors of modern bio-medicine, as we must, our theories of medicine and medical socialization must change substantially to accommodate them. If we call them African healers, as we also must, we lose a theoretical dichotomy that—however problematic—has been very useful to maintain, for both the medically and the anthropologically trained. The experiences these students recounted should be sobering for anyone who imagines the global spread of biomedi-cal technologies as a secular salvation, a triumphal advance of scientific modernity. Yet their responses to those experiences also unsettle dystopian visions of a hegemonic biomedicine that functions above all to extend the power of the state and the corporation without anyone noticing.

I have heard it said that Clifford Geertz once claimed that the true pur-pose of anthropology was to increase the number of stories in the world (an attribution I have never been able to verify). It seems a worthy purpose. The story of Malawi's medical citizens and would-be émigrés, its doctors for the people and its dirty workers, allows us to map the dead ends and unexpected pathways that open out of one particular space where material and medical need, historical and cultural patterns of meaning-making, and the forces of globalization meet. The recognition of this (and other) alterna-tive workings-out of the moral economy of medical science can not only enrich and expand our sense of what *is*, but by reanimating the theoretical base of our observations, expand also our sense of what *is possible*.

EPILOGUE

Departure

L ila Abu-Lughod, in her famous essay "Writing against Culture," proposed that anthropologists write "ethnographies of the particular" to
make others less homogenously, mysteriously, timelessly Other:

> The special value of this strategy is that it brings out similarities in all
> our lives. To say that we all live in the particular is not to say that for
> any of us the particulars are the same. It could well be that even in
> looking at the everyday we might discover fundamental differences. . . .
> The particulars suggest that others live as we perceive ourselves living,
> not as robots programmed with "cultural" rules, but as people going
> through life agonizing over decisions, making mistakes, trying to make
> themselves look good, enduring tragedies and personal losses, enjoying
> others, and finding moments of happiness. (Abu-Lughod 1991:158–59)

As my plane bumped off the runway, circled up past the crowded slums
that climb the sides of Mount Ndirande, and rose into the clouds, I found
myself thinking about Malawi and about the people I had come to know
there. It seemed likely that to them I was one more in the parade of *azungu*:
the medical tourists, eager volunteers, and foreign experts who come and
go, most of us leaving behind not much of importance. But I could not
shake them from my mind.

The memory of a recent dream came to me so vividly that it blotted out
for a moment the sound of the plane's engines and the sight of the moun-
tains that guard Blantyre. In the dream, I was reading a surgery textbook
when the page I was on began to bleed. Compressing the bleeding point—as
any doctor knows to do in a hemorrhage—did nothing to stem the flow. In
desperation, I closed the book and pressed its covers together hard. But the

blood kept seeping out from between the pages, covering the book and my hands. I was marked, stained. Imbrued.

I shook my head to chase the images away and looked back down to the earth. You couldn't quite see the hospital from here, but I knew it was there. I could still smell it on my own skin. The sounds of its wards and hallways still rang in my ears: the eerie call-and-response songs of grief as families escorted a body to the morgue, the slapping of bare feet and cheap plastic shoes on the concrete floors as guardians brought *nsima* and *ndiwo* to sick family members, the shouts as one nurse called out for another: "A-*sist*-ah!" There in the crowded wards, tragedies and personal losses were happening right now. Someone was being born, almost certainly, and someone else was dying, unquestionably. Probably the interns were agonizing over a decision: it was to be Bridget Nyasulu and Arthur Kamkwamba on call together today, a good team. Some of the medical students were no doubt making mistakes; some were trying to make themselves look good. Some were likely wishing that they could fulfill the Western medical imperative, "You must always do everything," while others were beginning to make their own: "You can always do something if you have love." They, too, were haunted by dreams and propelled by imaginings of a better world, even if their dreams and imaginings were not mine. In the everyday realities of their work, they were finding bottomless frustration and moments of happiness.

I looked down toward the city, thought of the students working and the patients living and dying and being born down in the sprawling maze of Queen Elizabeth Central Hospital, and sent them a silent salutation, human to human. And then the plane moved up into the clouds, and I could see Malawi no longer.

TECHNICAL APPENDIX

Research Methods

This appendix provides detail on research design, data collection, and methods of data analysis. Strategic concerns, related both to gaining approval to do this work and to communicating the work effectively to different audiences, shaped the final research protocol significantly. Evidence of this kind of shaping rarely appears in published materials, and I discuss it here in case it may be useful to others planning anthropological work in the professions. In addition, I discuss the major methodological and ethical difficulties encountered throughout the research process.

Research Philosophy and Goals

This book drew upon informal conversations, clinical work, and day-to-day life in Malawi as recorded in field notes from 2001, 2002–3, and 2007, with occasional reflections back to a 1990 journal from my first Malawi journey. The primary data sources, however, were semistructured interviews and focus groups, and to a lesser extent written questionnaires.

Much excellent interview- and questionnaire-based research, most conducted by sociologists, describes the transition from student to doctor in the North. I used the results of some of these studies in the preceding chapters as a background against which to examine the experiences of Malawian student physicians. Had I actually adopted the protocols used in one of the North American projects, I could have essentially had a ready-made comparison group. The choice not to do so therefore requires justification. Because the range of questions dictates the range of possible answers, I was concerned that this approach would impose categories and issues that were not relevant in Malawi and miss others that *were* relevant. The research findings bear this concern out. For instance, had I used questionnaire protocols derived from North American studies, rather than basing questions on issues that arose in interviews, I would likely have introduced concepts like "balance" between work and home life, an issue of central concern for trainees in many North American studies and one that almost never arose among Malawians. I might also have concentrated inappropriately on specialty "choice," a socially and emotionally freighted but otherwise largely unconstrained decision for many Northern trainees and an extremely pragmatic and very limited one for most Malawians. More important, I would not have known to explore with students concerns such as how to support their extended families, or the significance of having love for patients.

I chose instead to use a more classically anthropological approach, trying to immerse myself as much as possible in students' worlds, working to understand how they came to think about their own experience, and gradually crafting more targeted research questions to test my tentative insights. Many anthropological field studies use such a strategy, combining different methods (for instance, participant observation and interviews) over a substantial period of time in order to uncover local ways of thinking and acting. The major weakness of this approach is that, because the primary tool of research is the researcher herself, such studies can seem subjective to the point of irreproducibility. Long-term multimethod immersion approaches also have powerful methodological advantages, however: researchers can come to near-native understandings of complex situations; they leave open the possibility of uncovering findings and exploring questions they had not initially anticipated; and they can appreciate both normative trends and patterns of variation among those with whom they work. These three advantages cannot be readily attained with other research strategies.

To learn about the moral economy of Malawian medicine and how students assumed, negotiated, and understood it, I needed a research protocol that was sensitive, flexible, rigorous, and open to unanticipated findings. Two strategies were important in developing the final protocol: a collaborative approach in which a Malawian colleague and I worked together closely to design the study; and a research method designed to elicit broad areas of interest at first, and gradually to narrow the range of concerns to be investigated, moving from open-ended inquiry to narrower, more specific questions as the study progressed.

Collaboration as a Research Method

The initial research project was designed in collaboration with Dr. Chiwoza Bandawe, who was at the time Malawi's only clinical psychologist and head of the Department of Community Health at the College of Medicine. Working collaboratively was important for several reasons, both philosophical and practical. Malawians are no strangers to the long and ongoing tradition of exploitative "safari research," as some outside-sponsored biomedical studies in Africa have been characterized. In order to discourage this extract-your-data-and-then-leave approach to research, the College of Medicine's Research and Ethics Committee, which must give approval to any project conducted within the college or its teaching hospital, has made collaboration a requirement for approval of any externally funded work. Thus, a collaborative approach was a strategic necessity. At times, such mandated teamwork can be very fruitful, a whole greater than the sum of its parts. At other times, it is more theoretical than actual—visible on the paper of the research proposal but not on the ground. Dr. Bandawe and I hoped that a real collaboration could be useful to the College of Medicine as it struggled to improve the health status of Malawians. "Expert knowledge" on Malawi, we both felt, should not just benefit outsiders. It should also be produced and applied as much as possible within the country.

Collaboration necessitated some difficult decision making related to the political economy of intellectual production. Social psychology, Dr. Bandawe's disciplinary home, and anthropology, mine, differed in many respects: from the academic customs of authorship to assumptions about what constituted argument and evidence. Multiple authorship was accepted in his discipline and looked down upon in mine. Quantitative data amenable to statistical analysis were essential for his work, marginal to mine. "Thick description" was an important goal of my work that would have been questionable at best in the mainstream of his field. We had to think carefully and speak openly about potentially touchy issues of authorship, ownership, funding, credit, and evidence at an early stage when we barely knew each other. That we managed to do so is a testament to his flexibility and generosity. Dr. Bandawe and I were aware that both the dissertation produced from the original data and the book that followed would need to be my "products," as my funders, graduate program, and academic career prospects all dictated. We agreed that I would need to do all the data collection, nearly all the analysis, and all the writing to make this degree of ownership legitimate. The collaborative work would be concentrated in research design, to ensure that the study would be relevant to Malawians' concerns about the role and impact of biomedical training, and in coauthored work directed to a medical—and Malawian—audience. We made plans to publish jointly a pair of articles based on the major findings of the initial research study. Those articles would be written for doctors and other clinical personnel: in other words, they would include much quantitative analysis and exclude most descriptive material. We planned to write these collaboratively, my initial draft fleshed out and corrected with Dr. Bandawe's comments, and place them in a journal to which Malawi's medical students, interns, and faculty members had ready access. We have since done so.

In addition to its complications, collaboration offered benefits to both of us. Dr. Bandawe, who was named dean of students for the College of Medicine just before my first phase of data collection began in 2002, had a pressing interest in the process of student development but lacked both the time to research it intensively and the relative anonymity of a position outside the college administration that might allow the students to feel safe talking. In me, he gained a colleague who had both. I expected my position as a white expatriate physician in a former British colony to be potentially problematic. Talking over these concerns honestly with a thoughtful Malawian colleague could not make issues of power and status disappear, but I believe Dr. Bandawe's insights did mitigate their effects. I also gained the input of a coinvestigator immersed in the challenges of medical education, accustomed to the bureaucracy, and attuned to the concerns and aspirations of powerful actors within the college. He helped me to avoid several political pitfalls and, most important, helped to ensure the practical utility of this project.

We worked out the details of our collaboration and drafted a research proposal during a preliminary field visit I made to Malawi in August 2001; that research proposal was approved by the College of Medicine Research and Ethics Committee two months later. Dr. Bandawe was closely consulted in the project design and served as a resource throughout the data-collection phase; we coded the first three focus-group transcripts together, and he also assisted me in thinking through interpretation of my initial findings. Although he was not involved with my 2007 research (he was in South Africa for most of that time), I was still guided by some of his insights from the earlier phases of this project. All of the data collection, interview and questionnaire coding and analysis, and writing were my own.

Data Collection

To begin to understand the forces working upon these students as they negotiated their training, I had to speak with trainees from each year in the medical curriculum and with graduates in internship and beyond. In many respects, the ideal way to examine the shaping of doctors' ideas about their work would have been to do a longitudinal study. Pragmatic concerns—I had only one year's funding for fieldwork—did not allow a longitudinal project, and the original research was cross-sectional in design. I have been able to add limited longitudinal follow-up since that time. (Most other studies looking at change over time during medical socialization [for example, Becker et al. 1961; Sinclair 1997] are also cross-sectional, probably for similar pragmatic reasons. For a rare genuinely longitudinal ethnographic approach to medical education, see Konner 1987.)

Cross-sectional studies have disadvantages. Particularly in a place like the College of Medicine with a small student body, random variations between classes may explain some of the differences found. At the same time, a cross-sectional study does have the advantage of studying several groups of students at the same time, creating a snapshotlike image of professional socialization. Like many other Third World countries, Malawi is undergoing rapid political, economic, cultural, and ecological change. A longitudinal study following the same students for five or six years would likely find them in a very different setting at the end of their training than at the beginning. (The change in available HIV diagnosis and care from 2002 to 2007, for instance, has already had a notable impact on some of the working conditions students found most troubling. I have discussed this and other changes above.)

The core of the study was accomplished in three phases. Investigation began with broad, open-ended questions posed to focus groups of students at several stages in their training. In the second phase, individual interviews combined open-ended and more specifically targeted questions, based on themes that had arisen in the focus-group discussions. The third and final phase was a questionnaire administered to all current medical students, in which we explored quantitatively aspects of physician identity and experience found to be important in the interview stage. Of the 144 students enrolled in the College of Medicine, 23 (16 percent) participated in focus groups, 31 (22 percent) gave individual interviews, and 121 (84 percent) completed and returned the questionnaire. Focus groups, interviews, and questionnaires were in English, the language used for postprimary education in Malawi and all instruction at the college, and the only language in which all students and faculty were fluent.

The overall strategy of data collection, in which responses elicited by observation and open-ended discussion were then used to design more specific questions, comes from grounded theory (Glaser and Strauss 1967; Strauss and Corbin 1998). Dr. Bandawe and I both believed that this strategy would work well to uncover unanticipated issues in students' trajectories rather than simply replicating earlier research. While incorporating some of the methods of grounded theory, however, we rejected the theoretical assumption that data would generate theory. Theoretical concerns were explicitly interwoven at every level of data collection and analysis. The simple central hypothesis behind each level of questioning and observation was that the cultural and material (meaning both political and economic) circumstances in which medical education takes place would alter the process of becoming doctors.

Focus Groups

I had planned to begin the research process by recruiting focus groups of six to eight students in each of the five years of the medical training program and asking each group several open-ended questions. Focus-group discussion is relatively uncommon in anthropological research, but it can be useful early in a project when little is known about a subject or population, and therefore investigators want the broadest possible latitude for response (Bernard 1995; Schensul et al. 1999). Data can be enriched and the range of variation among informants explored by disagreements, debates, and discussions that arise in focus groups. Dr. Bandawe and I developed focus-group questions together, with the intent of eliciting students' understandings of what it meant to be physicians and of beginning to compare students' experiences to those of their Northern counterparts. Three questions asked students why they believed people chose medicine as a career, how their own thoughts about medicine had changed, and what they believed patients wanted from doctors. These questions were intended to allow us to sketch out a preliminary picture of physician roles in Malawi. Presocialization to the profession (socialization that began before medical training proper but after students had decided to become doctors), we believed, should be reflected in differences between students' ideas about popular expectations of doctors and their own ideas when entering medical school. Socialization would be reflected in differences between ideas on entering school and at the time of questioning. Additional questions, which centered on students' experiences of medical school and their expectations about medical work, were intended to allow early identification of important professional values and norms, and how these shifted over the course of training. Findings from the focus groups were to aid us in designing an interview protocol for the second phase of research.

That was the theory. In practice, the focus-group phase of the study was the most difficult to conduct and complete. I began by presenting an overview of the study to each year of medical students at times they were collected in classrooms, handing out to each student a written abstract and invitation to take part in the study, and asking them to write on a short form whether they were interested in participating in a focus group, an interview, both, or neither. When these forms had been returned, I set about making contact with students who had expressed interest in focus groups. Two unanticipated problems arose immediately.

First, despite a preliminary field visit, I had failed to register a recent change in the university's academic calendar. I arrived in September 2002, assuming it to be the beginning of the academic year, only to find that in Malawi the academic year now ran from January to November (thus allowing a break during the December planting season), not September to June as it does at most Northern institutions—and as it had at the College of Medicine until 2002. Complicating matters further, although I had thought all necessary hurdles had been cleared to allow the research to begin, I was wrong. In addition to clearance from my home institution and from the ethics committee at the College of Medicine, both of which I had in hand, I was informed on my arrival that I needed approval from the college registrar before I could speak to any medical students. This clearance was not especially difficult to obtain, but it took several weeks. Just when I finally secured permission to proceed, the students were heading into their year-end exams. Their schedules were fully booked with make-up lectures and review sessions, and by the time I had met with every class to explain the study to them, another month had passed. As a result, I completed only three of the anticipated five focus groups—those with first-year, third-year, and fifth-year students—before time pressures forced me to begin the interview phase of the research project. (The second-year student focus group met within the first month of interviews. The fourth-year class was a small one known to have difficult interpersonal dynamics, and one with which I had made a serious blunder [see chapter 5, note 15] early on. Only three students from the class expressed interest in a focus group, and those three never agreed on a time to meet at all.)

Second, lack of institutional and national infrastructure made contacting students to set up focus groups—and later, interviews—unexpectedly difficult. Cellular phone service was fairly new in those days. Few students had cell phones, and the network seemed to be down or overloaded more often than it was working anyway. (It functioned much better for most of my 2007 fieldwork, although a catastrophic fire took down one of the two major networks for a month.) Almost none had land lines; the waiting period for a land line in Malawi at that time averaged ten years. All students technically had Internet access, but the excruciating slowness and frequent breakdowns of the College of Medicine server and the very small number of working computers available to students made this a less than reliable way to contact them. The students also did not have mailboxes. Letters sent to them were put in a pile on a table in the cafeteria to be picked up (with a little luck, by the addressee) when someone saw them. I ultimately used all three methods—snail mail, e-mail, and cell phone—to reach students to arrange interviews and focus groups.

All focus groups were tape-recorded, with the permission of the students involved, and the recordings transcribed. After I had altered any potentially identifying data on the transcripts, Dr. Bandawe and I together analyzed the first three focus-group transcripts to brainstorm a working set of codes and to develop a protocol for semistructured interviews.

Our intent had been to write all of the interview questions based on the major themes that appeared to influence students' experiences of becoming doctors. Two limitations of the focus-group data made us reconsider this plan. First, I had only been able to complete three focus groups before proceeding to interviews, and those groups averaged only five or six students. Although the completed focus groups incorporated the beginning, end, and middle years of the medical program, neither of us could be sure the data were as robustly representative of the student body as we had hoped. Second, the first three focus groups were entirely composed of male students. A fourth group, which met after interviews had begun, was entirely female. Women form a minority of the school's enrollment, particularly in the upper-level classes. Later, both male and female students volunteered that women often felt uncomfortable speaking up in a group of men and would not elect to do so.

In the end, we chose to reuse for the interview protocol the broadly open-ended focus-group questions that explored students' experiences of medical training and their expectations about medical practice, making only minor wording changes where it appeared that the original questions had been confusing. These questions had demonstrated their worth by eliciting intense discussions of economic, political, and social factors affecting the process of education and the practice of medicine. (The set of three focus-group questions specifically addressing professional identity as seen by students or by community members had turned out not to be especially enlightening, and we did not reuse them.) Other interview questions were derived from findings in the focus-group phase as planned. Two groups' spontaneous discussions of particular "good" or "bad" doctors offered interesting insights into the ways students categorized, identified with, or rejected various medical roles. We therefore included in the interview protocol two questions asking students to discuss—without naming them—actual doctors they thought of as particularly good or bad. Focus-group participants also often volunteered discussion about changes they had noticed in themselves and others, and about what it took to feel like a "real doctor." Discussions around these two themes often uncovered the "of course" comments about doctors that can be clues to hegemonic ideas, and we included questions on both.

Finally, as part of a commitment to making this research practically relevant, I had asked students what information I could gather that would be useful to them. The ethics committee prohibited offering incentives at any part of the study, so this question was also an attempt to give back in some way to those who generously volunteered their time and ideas. Students involved in the focus groups felt that the opportunity to deliver anonymous feedback to the school's administration would be valuable, so at their request, we included a question asking about changes students would like to see in their training. I agreed to write up the answers to this question as a report for the principal of the College of Medicine and discuss that report with him, and did so in 2003 before leaving Malawi.

Interviews

Interviews typically lasted forty-five minutes to an hour, but ranged from thirty minutes to over two hours. The interviews were semistructured: occasionally, if a student had particularly limited time, I would drop one or two of the questions; in most cases, I asked additional questions, pursuing topics that students brought up or seemed to feel strongly about. After the first few interviews, whenever time allowed, I added a question asking students in what sorts of situations they imagined themselves working in ten years.

Before beginning their interviews, all students read and signed consent forms giving permission to proceed. In addition to obtaining this written consent, I verbally reiterated to students that all data collected would be anonymous and that they could also choose whether to have their interviews taped or not. No student or intern waived the right to anonymity. (A few have since said they would prefer to have their real names used, but the approved study protocol does not allow me to do so.) Most agreed to be taped; some declined taping. In each of the untaped interviews, I took particularly copious notes and typed up the reconstructed interview as soon as possible. Inevitably, some material was lost in the untaped interviews: interviews reconstructed from notes were about 25 percent shorter by word count than interviews of comparable duration that I transcribed from tapes.

I planned to recruit a minimum interview sample of 23 students distributed among the five school classes, a sample size that would have represented 25 percent of the student body at the time recruitment began. At the beginning of 2003, enrollment increased rapidly to 144 students, and the 31 student interviews I did represented 22 percent of the student body (see table A.1).

Difficulties in actually contacting students persisted during the interview process but were less troublesome than they had been in the first phase of research. Partly, as the students got to know me, face-to-face contact took on a larger role in scheduling interviews. Students would drop by my office to see when I'd be in, or would find me in the school or hospital hallways and set up an appointment. The importance of face-to-face contact probably explains the particularly high interview rates among third-year students and among interns, as these were the two groups with whom I had consistent contact in the hospital. This improvement was probably also a matter of my own acclimation, of coming to expect five or ten failed attempts for each successful one and being pleasantly surprised when the ratio was lower. Initially, I had been wary of badgering students by making too many attempts to contact them, imagining that if they hadn't come in after one or two e-mails, phone messages, or letters, they had changed their minds about participating. Dr. Bandawe disabused me of this notion: "Just keep asking them. They'll tell you if they don't want to come in—you aren't bothering them. Have you listened to our music? We *like* repeti-

TABLE A.1. Student and intern interview sample by year in training

Year in medical school	Students interviewed (% of all student interviews)	Total students in each class (% of 2003 students)	Percentage of class interviewed
Year 1	11 (35)	66 (46)	17
Year 2	5 (16)	28 (19)	18
Year 3	6 (19)	14 (10)	43
Year 4	4 (13)	17 (12)	24
Year 5	5 (16)	19 (13)	26
Interns	7	13	54

Source: Total class sizes from College of Medicine records.

TABLE A.2. Medical student interview sample demographics

Demographic factors	Students interviewed	Total student body
Males (%)	22 (71)	96 (67)
Females (%)	9 (29)	44 (33)
Father's education: mode / mean[a]	5 / 4.39	5 / 4.25
Mother's education: mode / mean[a]	4 / 3.48	5 / 3.61

Sources: Gender distribution for the student body as a whole is from College of Medicine records. Gender of four students was not included in these records, so the total adds up to 140 instead of 144 students. Parental educational status for the student body as a whole is from the questionnaire portion of this research; no student socioeconomic indicators are gathered by the college. Educational status indicates highest level begun, not necessarily completed.

[a] 1 = none, 2 = primary, 3 = junior secondary, 4 = secondary, 5 = college.

tion!" His guidance bore fruit: each attempt to contact students resulted in additional interviews.

I ultimately interviewed a higher proportion of the students in the third year than in other years (43 percent versus 19 percent, $p < .05$), and a higher proportion of interns than students (54 percent versus 22 percent, $p < .01$). Beyond that, it is not possible to be certain whether the students interviewed were generally representative of the student body as a whole, in part because the college has almost no demographic information on entering students. I found no significant differences between interviewed students and other students in gender or in parental educational status, used here as a social class marker (see table A.2).

It is also impossible to determine what sort of information students chose to conceal in interviews. This study, like all that rely heavily on interviews or questionnaires, presents primarily students' self-reports about their thoughts and behaviors. Students seemed vocal and forthcoming, even on topics I had imagined would be quite sensitive, such as dealing with corruption and political pressure in hospital practice, or with substance abuse and casual sex in medical school. Nonetheless, I have to assume both that students were the best source of evidence about their own process of becoming doctors and that some evidence was missing or misleading.

Questionnaire

In the final phase of this project, after all student interviews had been completed and half of them coded, I distributed a short, anonymous questionnaire to all students at the College of Medicine. (The complete question-

naire can be found in Wendland 2004, appendix E.) It included a limited
set of demographic questions—limited for time reasons, but also because
the focus-group and interview phases had made it clear that most students
were very concerned about anonymity. I also included an item asking students to identify whether they had interviewed with me or not to allow
comparison of interview responders and nonresponders.

The bulk of the questionnaire, which Dr. Bandawe and I wrote together,
concerned four major themes: motivations to enter medicine, aspects of
being a doctor, career objectives, and factors influencing those objectives.
Each of these themes had arisen as an important focus of discussion in the
interviews, and all individual questions grouped under these themes were
also derived from the interviews. We used Likert-type items throughout
the questionnaire, as Likert scaling was developed specifically for the measurement of attitudes (Likert 1932) and has been used extensively to elicit
values and norms (Bernard 1995). We had initially intended to use clusters of questions to construct scales measuring various professional values
but ultimately decided against scaling for two reasons. First, we had been
granted a limit of fifteen minutes (by the faculty members whose classes I
was interrupting) in which to administer the questionnaire, so that total
numbers of items had to be restricted. Second, multi-item scales have little
validity if they are not pretested. No comparable test group existed outside
the medical school, and we did not want to sacrifice any of our very small
pool of potential respondents to a pretest group.

I obtained permission from faculty members to take fifteen minutes of
class time for each group of students and handed out questionnaires in person. A portion of the fifth-year class was away at a rural health site, and
this group received mailed questionnaires. I explained to each class that the
questionnaire was the final phase of this research project, that it was completely anonymous, that the questions were derived from interviews with
them and their colleagues, that there was absolutely no obligation to fill it
out but that I hoped that they would find it interesting.

The response rate (84 percent, 121 of 144 students) was well above the
20 to 75 percent generally expected for a self-administered questionnaire
(Bernard 1995; Dillman 1983). Because the response rate was high, analysis of questionnaire responses, in addition to being a means of triangulat-
ing, allowed a reasonable comparison between students who interviewed
and those who did not. This phase of research also provided a much larger
sample size to evaluate shifts in professional identity and goals over the
course of training. The single-item responses used in the questionnaire
must be interpreted more cautiously than multi-item scales, and in this

book, I have tried always to present questionnaire results in light of the more in-depth qualitative data from interviews, focus groups, observations, and other sources.

In 2007, I was able to return to Malawi for a five-month period. Although I was there beginning work on a different research project, this relatively brief fieldwork visit afforded me the opportunity to follow up in person with a number of the students and interns I had interviewed years earlier. Some had stayed in touch in the intervening years with occasional e-mails. Many had graduated and moved on; a few had been "weeded" out of school; two more were in the United Kingdom. I had asked students at the time of their initial interviews if they would be willing to be contacted for follow-up later, and all had agreed. As I had not included follow-up interviews in the initial protocol submitted to the College of Medicine ethics committee, however, it seemed to me that asking these students and young doctors for formal taped interviews was not appropriate. Nonetheless, I did have the opportunity to chat informally with several of them about their experiences during the previous few years and where their work was taking them next. Those conversations inform the work presented in this book as well.

Other Research Activities

I supplemented student interviews with interviews of seven interns and four other recent graduates of the College of Medicine who were beyond internship, asking them to reflect upon their training experiences. In addition, I conducted nineteen semistructured interviews with College of Medicine faculty and administrative personnel selected because they were particularly closely involved with the students. These interviews helped me to understand the institutional priorities and constraints that shape recruitment and teaching of would-be doctors.

The Malawiana Archives at Chancellor College in Zomba and some uncataloged gray literature found on a manual search through the shelves at the College of Medicine library both provided archival materials that illuminated the historical development and institutional structure of the medical school.

I also sat in on classroom lectures and labs, although fewer with preclinical students than clinical students, and hung around in the campus library and computer lab. I had the sense that my attendance in classrooms was somewhat disruptive, and that in the basic science setting in particular, teachers felt that they were being evaluated by yet another foreign "expert" despite my reassurances to the contrary. These experiences gave me a feel for the places in which students worked but did not in general provide much additional data. After the first three months, I did not pursue additional basic science classroom experience. In the hospital, because I also had a work role there, I was much more readily able to blend into the background. Attendance at occasional teaching rounds and many didactic conferences in the clinical setting strengthened my picture of clinical training. I also spent a day at the community health training site in Mangochi, and was able both to tour the district hospital there and to sit in on a long debriefing session as students returned from their "Learning by Living" experience of community placement with rural families. Many informal conversations and observations recorded in field notes, from the medical school, the teaching hospital, and outlying medical settings, also were vital in understanding the paths students took as they became doctors.

Finally, during both my initial fieldwork in 2002 and 2003 and during the shorter five-month 2007 visit, I spent two days each week working as a volunteer obstetrician at Queen Elizabeth Central Hospital, the urban referral center that functions as a clinical training ground for the College of Medicine's students (as well as for nursing students, clinical officer students, and other allied health trainees). Although it was approved as part of my initial research proposal, I had been dubious about doing clinical work in the teaching hospital—the Obstetrics and Gynaecology department was at the time widely regarded from without as both clinically weak and politically a snake pit. (Both assessments were correct, although changes since 2003 have resulted in very significant improvement.) In addition, I was concerned about working as an instructor to the study cohort, fearing that it would impose unacceptable pressure on students I asked to participate in the study.

My colleague and research collaborator Dr. Bandawe ultimately prevailed on this point. He felt strongly that clinical experience in the public sector in Malawi would be crucial, giving me a much richer sense of the realities that medical students and new doctors there face, and he was unquestionably correct. The two days a week I worked at the hospital consistently proved exhausting and emotionally difficult. Supplies and equipment in "Chatinkha," the obstetrics and gynecology annex at Queens Hospital, were limited if not completely illusory: women gave birth on bare metal trolleys or uncovered vinyl mattresses; the operating theater frequently ran out of iodine, suture, gauze, soap, and running water. Even diagnostics I had considered "basic" were rare; for instance, in all the time I have worked at Queens, I have never been able to use a pregnancy test. I learned to treat infection with any antibiotics currently available, usually without benefit of any laboratory diagnostic testing—unless that particular patient was fortunate enough to be enrolled in some transnational study. I found the bureaucracy byzantine even by US standards, the patients sick, and the resources skeletal.

My hospital days were Tuesdays and Wednesdays. Monday night I never slept more than a few hours, dreading what was coming next, and Wednesday I inevitably came home depressed, exhausted, and angry. Hospital work was by no means a wholly negative experience, however. Difficult and painful, it was also rewarding, and although often I dreaded going to Queens, there were other times when I wanted to stop all my research and stay in Chatinkha's wards working as hard as I could as a doctor. My participation in clinical care—a handful of difficult deliveries for which I was consulted, seventy surgical cases, hundreds of ultrasounds, hundreds more clinical visits with high-risk antenatal patients in the clinics or on the wards—was nothing in the face of Malawi's overwhelming clinical needs. It is no false modesty to recognize that my time as a doctor there was meaningless from a public health perspective, but I believe it was not meaningless to my patients, and I know it was not meaningless to me.

Although the personal involvement of the researcher often introduces new levels of ethical, emotional, and methodological complexity (Stacey 1988; Visweswaran 1994), as it did for me, anthropological work has also benefited from such personal engagement (Behar 1996; Rapp 1999). Working clinically, for all the emotional upheaval involved, had its uses for this study. My worries about contaminating data by too much clinical contact with the study cohort did not materialize. Ultimately, it was fairly easy to lay low and to avoid teaching or evaluating the medical students. I had minimal informal clinical teaching contact with third-year students and interns, but gave no formal lectures until my return in 2007 and played no part in evaluating their performance at any level. (I had much more extensive teaching contact with nurse-midwifery and clinical-officer students, teaching that was one of the most rewarding parts of my clinical work experience.) Nonetheless, the fact that I was working clinically got around, as such things will in any small community, and seemed to give me a certain amount of "street credibility" with the interns, students, and other clinical staff. The hours in the hospital were also useful in terms of opportunities for informal interviews and in planting the seeds of a few real friendships.

Because I assiduously avoided spending much time with the students in the hospital setting, I cannot quite bring myself to call this clinical work "participant observation." It may be better characterized as what Loïc Wacquant (2003) and others call "observant participation." I have tried not to generalize from my own experience of this work to that of the Malawian trainees who learn in the hospital. However, my long days in the hospital unquestionably informed the project, providing another level of insight into the lived experiences of Malawi's physicians, its physicians-in-training, and its patients.

Data Management and Analysis

These research methods produced roughly two thousand pages of transcripts, field notes, maps and sketches, summaries of archival material, and questionnaire results to be coded and analyzed.

Coding

Dr. Bandawe and I developed an initial set of codes by reviewing the first three focus-group transcripts line by line and looking for recurrent themes. This "open coding" method is considered especially well suited to identify new themes (Glaser and Strauss 1967). We modified the line-by-line technique only to make it sentence-by-sentence, finding in practice that a single line was often too short to understand the speaker's point but allowing more than one code per sentence as needed.

After completing and transcribing the first three interviews in each class of students, I extended this initial set of codes, developing a branching system of themes in which general areas of interest were divided into more specific or focused codes. I tested these codes with the help of three research assistants, all educated Malawians but none involved in any way with the data collection or the medical school, who each recoded these first fifteen transcripts so that I could detect and correct areas of ambiguity.

Qualitative Analysis

I used this more focused code set to analyze the remaining interview, focus-group, and field-note data. The process of coding and analysis was facilitated by QSR N6, a text-management software package designed for anthropological research (Qualitative Solutions and Research International 2002).

Like the process of study design, the process of data analysis was also guided by theoretical concerns. Coding the focus groups together, Dr. Bandawe and I did not concentrate exclusively on areas in which students ex-

pressed consensus, as we were interested in variation as much as unifor-
mity. While we considered statements students introduced with "I believe"
or "I think" as possible reflections of students' values, we also paid close
attention to simple declarative statements, and to statements bracketed by
"of course," "as you know," or other similar markers, as offering insight
into the commonsense assumptions that signal hegemony. In subsequently
coding interviews, I attended to interviewees' choices of metaphors. I also
looked for the proximity of concepts to each other in the transcripts; if
discussion of one concept (for instance, love for patients) was consistently
embedded within discussions of another (for instance, Malawi's poverty), I
took this contextualization to be significant.

Quantitative Analysis

The quantitative measures reported here are quite minimal, but what is
presented builds upon an extensive statistical analysis of interviews and
questionnaires. I used the statistical software package STATA 7.0 (Stata
Corporation 2001) to analyze this material. Because interview topics
tended to be binomial (students either raised a particular issue or did not),
when statistical significance of a particular interview topic was in order,
I used two-tailed proportion testing (or Fisher's exact test for smaller cell
values, as appropriate) to assess differences between groups, and ordered
logit analysis for trends among more than two groups. For the questionnaire data, when assessing the impact of binomial categories (for example,
student gender or interview status) on Likert scores, I used t-testing. For
correlation between two linear variables—for instance, Likert score and
year in training, or Likert scores on two different items—I used simple linear regression. For ordinal but nonlinear categories (maternal and paternal
education, which students answered by category rather than by completed
years of education), I used ordered logit analysis. In the very rare cases in
which results of statistical analysis appear in the book, I have given results
in terms of p-values; for linear or logistic regression, I also noted correlation coefficients (Pearson's r or pseudo-r). Although correlation coefficients
are reported for both linear and ordered logit analyses, these coefficients are
calculated differently in the two models, as the term "pseudo-r" for logit
calculations suggests, and are therefore not directly comparable.

In the dissertation developed from my 2002–3 fieldwork, I used quantitative analysis fairly heavily. (Readers frustrated by the minimal statistical
evidence presented in this book are referred to Wendland 2004.) I have not
done so here, and I have not in fact conducted any quantitative analysis on

the 2007 data. Instead, I have chosen primarily to use semiquantitative language like *most, over half, several,* or *a few.* This choice is partly stylistic; an incessant parade of *p*-values disrupts the flow of the text. It also reflects my growing discomfort with using statistical analysis to buttress this kind of data, creating a sort of false certainty that is especially problematic when samples that may not be random are used. I do think statistics can be quite useful to consider the *limits* of certainty in qualitative analysis, especially in comparisons between groups. When I have reported group-to-group differences here (between men and women, for instance, or clinical and pre-clinical students), I have done so only after statistical analysis has given me a probability of over 90 percent ($p < .10$) that these differences really reflect what would be found in a larger sample of students. Another way of thinking about this, statistically speaking, is that one in ten of the intergroup differences in interview results I report does *not* reflect a real difference between groups, while I may have missed nearly one-third of actual differences. (Because of the larger sample size of the questionnaires, I used a limit of $p < .05$ when reporting intergroup differences for questionnaire results. At the $p < .05$ level, the questionnaires have a 5 percent chance of type I error [reporting a "difference" that is not real] and a 5 percent chance of type II error [missing a difference that *is* real] between two groups of roughly equal size. Using $p < .05$ for interviews would have created an unacceptably high rate of type II errors, so I used $p < .10$ and accepted the higher risk of type I error.) Again, combining the primarily qualitative data from interviews, focus groups, and field notes with the primarily quantitative data from questionnaires should provide a better picture of students' thoughts and experiences than any single data source alone could provide.

Issues in Representation

Much of the material in this book comes directly from interview or focus-group transcripts. I edited transcript excerpts minimally (deleting stammers, *um,* and *uh,* for instance) but tried to keep both the substance and the stylistic flavor of the conversations intact. The extended interview excerpts presented between chapters—in the stories of Joe Phoya, Mkume Lifa, Evelyn Kazembe, Duncan Kasinja, and Zaithwa Mthindi—were edited more heavily for flow and clarity.

Malawian English differs from American English and even British English. Some differences are lost in transcription. For instance, in the English of most Malawians, *nurse* rhymes with *face* and *learn* with *pain*; tonal shifts are pronounced and may sound musical to an ear attuned to American speech. Other distinctions show even on paper: nowhere outside Africa have I heard *whereby* or *whilst* used so readily in casual speech. I have not corrected or marked unusual locutions except to add explanatory notes in brackets where the meaning may not be obvious or when interviewees used Chichewa words. The interview excerpts contain many repetitions, which I have rarely edited out; readers should be aware that in Malawi, repetition signals emphasis.

Most students and some faculty members were extremely concerned with confidentiality. Protection of interviewees' identities was also mandated by the ethics committee. For that reason, I used pseudonyms throughout. (The same caveat applies to casual conversations recorded in field notes.) The pseudonyms are all authentic names, and matched by gender to the interviewee, but as most Malawian surnames indicate the families' geographic and ethnic origins, I did not attempt to match other characteristics lest students be too readily identifiable. In a few places, I did not provide any identifying information at all, for fear the speaker might be too readily identified. (This issue was especially difficult for women in the later years of training and after graduation, as there were very few in most classes and only one in one class. In most cases, I simply listed female students as "preclinical" or "clinical.") I also changed transcript words, such as birthplaces or locations of prior employment, that might identify students. Changes in transcripts are explained in notes; changes in the other texts—such as the patient narratives—are not. They are not fictions, however: everything I've written here really did happen, and every quotation is something an informant really told me.

I did not like all of my informants, nor do I believe they all liked me. Some of the students, graduates, faculty, and staff struck me as grandiose, manipulative, or self-centered. Others seemed to be among the finer humans I've encountered: loving, intelligent, thoughtful, and committed. Anthropologists know that transcripts can be chosen or edited to make informants look a certain way or to conform to certain theoretical models. As much as possible, I have tried to maintain the diversity of perspectives I was presented with, to represent interviewees accurately, and to do my best to move into the speakers' frames of reference when analyzing material. I have also tried to apply what has sometimes been called the principle of interpretive charity: the assumption that the people who told me their stories were truthfully relating their own perceptions and experiences. When other findings contradict or support these perceptions, I have reported those, too.

༒

NOTES

PROLOGUE

1. That was in 1990. In 2007, the same hospital had intermittent access to methotrexate, two donated working ultrasound machines, and an old and very slow but
functional CT scanner. An MRI was on its way, thanks to a multinational research project that needed it. There were still no newborn ventilators, and there was still no radiation therapy. Those were all relatively advanced (and, with the exception of methotrexate,
expensive) medical technologies. The hospital was also without far more basic things, as
chapter 5 will elaborate.

CHAPTER I

1. Throughout this book, I use *medicine* and *biomedicine*, recognizing that these
terms are contested. The term *biomedicine*, as Frankenberg (1988) has pointed out, con-
flates biological knowledge with medical practice in a way that overstates the scientific
basis of the latter. *Medicine* can be both too broad and too narrow. Many scholars would
like to use this term for nonbiomedical healing practices; at the same time, among
physicians, *medicine* also refers specifically to the work of internal medicine, as opposed
to surgery or other specialties. The other choices sometimes used by anthropologists,
however, seem even more misleading. Describing this form of medicine as "Western,"
"cosmopolitan," "allopathic," or "AMA" makes too narrow a geographic or theoretical
circumscription.

My use of *the global South* represents another, and even more difficult, problem of
nomenclature. Over the decades, fashions for naming the wealthiest countries in the
world and the poorest have shifted. The instability of the terminology reflects the shifting
inclusion criteria and untenable boundaries of such a distinction. Because biomedicine
as we now know it is very largely a product of Western Europe and North America,
imported and exported as an intellectual and technical commodity around the rest of the
world, some set of terms to describe "the West and the rest" is important for this work.
I generally use *North* and *South* here, as a reminder that Malawi's major intellectual,

economic, and migratory ties lie primarily on a north-to-south axis rather than an east-to-west one. (I am aware that the terminology is problematic, however. In some parts of the world, the polarity is actually reversed: for instance, Australian medical practitioners and resources are often at work in Papua New Guinea, where the ideological North is to the geographical south of the South.) I also sometimes use *First World* or *Third, West* or *non-West*. All are inadequate in their connotation of geographical determinism, and none really stands out as more acceptable than the others. By shifting among them, I am attempting to keep the idea of the world's poor countries as unstable as the reality. I have tried to avoid the evolutionary suggestion embodied in terms like *developed, developing,* and *underdeveloped* (or in current fashion, *least developed,* the category into which Malawi falls in the listings of international lenders and charities). It is worth noting, however, that the Malawians who talked to me about medical and health issues quite consistently used *developing* or *poor* and *developed* or *rich* to contrast their own country, and those in similar plights, with Europe and North America. They tended to oppose *Western* and *African* when talking about cultural issues such as music and the globalization of fashion or behavior.

2. Both Beagan and Taylor critique the understanding of medicine as acultural and the effects of that idea on medical training. Taylor, borrowing a phrase from Traweek's (1988) study of high-energy physicists, explains how students enculturated into medicine's "culture of no culture" develop deeply rooted understandings of the *real* and the *cultural* as opposites. Beagan considers the effects of the demand for neutrality on those medical students who fit the ideal least and who thereby expose just what "neutral" means: ethnic minority, female, gay and lesbian, or working-class students. The "view from nowhere" is Thomas Nagel's term (Nagel 1986); see also Haraway 1988.

3. The concept of medicine as culturally neutral technology, because it is still widely held by scientists, medical professionals, and the general public, cannot be dismissed as a straw man. Even though it is not well supported by scientific evidence, even though it has been increasingly dismissed by social scientists and historians since the 1970s, it remains a powerful narrative with real effects in the world.

4. Scholars from a number of disciplines, many initially trained in the natural sciences, have produced a rich body of literature on science as culture. Good places to start for science in general include the reader edited by Biagioli (1999) or Pickering's edited collection, *Science as Practice and Culture* (1992). For medicine in particular, see n. 5.

5. Rhodes (1996) offers a helpful overview of research on biomedicine as a cultural system, touching on many of these points. Important early collections were those by Wright and Treacher (1982), Lock and Gordon (1988), and Lindenbaum and Lock (1993). Feminist scholarship has been particularly important in exploring the cultural construction of biological and medical science, and the ways that science furthers gender inequality by naturalizing it; see, for instance, Haraway's *Primate Visions* (1989) or Martin's *The Woman in the Body* (1987), both considered classics in this field.

6. I do not mean to imply that there has been *no* resistance: antimedicine movements that rejected colonial and mission medicine were especially notable in Africa in the nineteenth and early twentieth centuries. The spread of prophetic healing and the persistence of rumors about the true aims of doctors and hospitals can be considered subtler forms of resistance to biomedicine on the continent today (Geissler 2005). For a geographically

broad literature on contestation of biomedicine, see the edited collection by Cunningham and Andrews (1997).

7. For example, Libya's Muammar Gaddafi signaled his commitment to pan-African solidarity by promising to build a new hospital in Malawi, a project promised at the time of my initial fieldwork and close to completion in 2007. In another example, a writer in the *Guardian Weekly* offered this upbeat assessment of health in central Africa: "There is, of course, the scourge of Aids [AIDS], which has swept through Africa, but the Malawi government has been dedicated in its attempts to counter the problem, building six new hospitals in the past five years" (Hill 2001:11). This statement is comparable to suggesting that the government's commitment to countering poverty is shown by the construction of six new banks. The illogical conflation of hospitals and health, however, is so commonplace that it went unchallenged.

8. Biomedical research has also increasingly crossed national boundaries; more and more clinical trials are being carried out in the poorer nations of the world, many by contract research organizations working for multinational industries. The implications of this particular form of medical globalization are beyond the scope of this book; interested readers are referred to Petryna 2009 for an in-depth analysis, including ethnographic material from Poland and Brazil, or to Shah 2006 for a journalist's look at transnational medical research (particularly but not solely in India).

9. Morsy (1988) reverses the direction of this argument in her discussion of Islamic clinics in Egypt: she sees a veneer of Islamic revivalism as locally acceptable cover for the import of the ideologies and practices of Western-style biomedicine.

10. An article by Bradley Lewis (2007) drew my attention to this fascinating policy paper from the RAND Corporation, which also advocates that the United States choose Pakistan as "the first patient." Readers interested in a critical take on the global health movement will find Lewis's paper a useful resource.

11. In this section, I am drawing primarily on the literature of political economic or critical medical anthropology. Morsy (1996) provides a helpful if now somewhat dated overview of this literature; another, longer overview can be found in the volume by Baer, Singer, and Susser (1997). In international research, a critical medical anthropology approach often entails the analysis of mechanisms of economic globalization (Schoepf, Schoepf, and Millen 2000), the exploration of biomedical hegemony (Alubo 1987), and the examination of the effects of both on the health of the poor (Kim et al. 2000; Scheper-Hughes 1992, especially chapter 5).

12. For those to whom it is not clear, in this context I am referring specifically to an old debate: do ideas produce the material world and changes in it, or do changes in the material world produce ideas? Karl Marx propounded the latter argument in an era of contestation over the underlying mechanisms of human history and of revolutionary change. The influential German philosopher Georg Hegel, with other scholars grounded in the Romantic emphasis on individual thought, had taken the collective knowledge, thought, and culture of humankind (Hegel's "world spirit") to be the driving force of human history, creating the world as we know it. In the mid-nineteenth century, Marx and others essentially turned this idealism upside down in materialist interpretations of history and the contemporary world. Philosophy, religion, thought itself: all were superstructures built upon the material, economic base of a society's mode of production,

and of the class relations enabling that productive mode (Marx and Engels 1970). The "world spirit," rather than driving history as Hegel claimed, was actually the ideological means by which the ruling class legitimized its control over the labor of others. Critics of biomedicine working from a Marxist tradition tend to see biomedicine as one part of this complex ideological superstructure.

13. Gramsci's writing on hegemony is famously difficult and open to multiple interpretations. Discussions with Nan Enstad have challenged me to think about the term in a more complex sense (see also Enstad 2009). Here I am drawing not only on Gramsci's original work but on the interpretations of it by Raymond Williams (1977) and by John and Jean Comaroff (1991). The Comaroffs include a useful elaboration of the Gramscian concept of hegemony in their historical anthropology of mission in South Africa, *Of Revelation and Revolution*. They contrast hegemony with ideology, in which an openly identifiable power coerces belief. Ideologies may be in obvious conflict; hegemonies are taken for granted.

14. Antonio Ugalde has described similar consequences for the professional dominance of physicians in public health policy-making in Latin America (Ugalde and Alubo 1994). Other scholars see a different trajectory for biomedicine in that region, including some much more politically radical perspectives that identify poverty and inequality as root causes of ill health (Morgan 1998; Waitzkin 1981). The physician and socialist leader Salvador Allende was one key exemplar of this approach, which goes back for more than a century in South American medicine.

15. Medicine's social authority has led one anthropologist to characterize the profession in the United States as an enforcer of national morality tales (Stein 1990). Stein links contemporary "wellness programs" with historical purges and ascetic movements that always involve the scapegoating of some impure other, from the racially inferior of the nineteenth century to the mentally defective and inebriate of the twentieth to the obese of the twenty-first. Petersen and Lupton (1996) make a parallel argument in a more transnational context for the "new public health" as a morality-judging exercise. As medical and public health attention shifts from infectious to chronic diseases, disease-linked life "choices"—sometimes so highly constrained that it requires significant mental contortion to construct them as choices at all—are viewed as moral failings. The fat person, the sedentary one, the smoker, are not only *ill* (through a neat conflation of risk factors with disease) but *unworthy*. Studies of medical students show that it is exactly these people who become targets of disparaging humor when they enter the clinical setting, and for exactly this reason: having brought on their own illnesses, they are perceived as deserving neither their clinicians' efforts nor their hospital's resources (Wear et al. 2006).

16. Leigh Turner (2005) provides a recent examination of the "culture" concept with specific reference to medicine and global health.

17. Different analysts describe different core values grounding the knowledge and practice of contemporary medicine. Robbie Davis-Floyd (1992), for instance, makes the argument that science, technology, patriarchy, and the institution are crucial to American obstetrics. Many others see the consolidation of social and economic power as central purposes of medicine as an institution (see, e.g., Baer 1989; Starr 1982). Howard Stein (1990) contends that individualism, activity, authority over nature, and orientation toward the future are core cultural values of American medicine. Medicine in export

has been understood as inevitably bringing with it individualism, reductionist empiricism, social authority, and a curative (rather than ameliorating or preventive) orientation (Cunningham and Andrews 1997). Other attempts at characterizing medicine's embedded values and unspoken assumptions include Kleinman 1993, Comaroff 1982, Gordon 1988, and Lupton 2003. No one of these interpretations agrees entirely with any other, and several would disagree with my schema on one point or another. (Kleinman, for instance, suggests that Western medicine is actually *anti*authoritarian, although I do not find him convincing on this count.) I am not arguing either that medicine is monolithic or that those who study it have characterized it as such: either suggestion would be grossly inaccurate. But certain basic values or orientations do appear again and again in this scholarship, and perhaps even more so in the writing of physicians about their own work (see, e.g., Gawande 2002; Groopman 2007). The four pillars of medicine's moral order I choose here, based on reading, observation, and my experience as a practitioner, represent my own attempt to think about contemporary medicine—but they are only one of many possible ways to characterize it.

18. The Cartesian mind-body dualism long associated with medicine is now, I believe, eroding, incrementally replaced by a neurobiological reductionism that sees "mind" as an artifact arising entirely from brain.

19. Medicine is thus rational in the sense of possessing a scientific logic. It is also rational in the bureaucratic sense. Disease, suffering, birth, and death are removed from the realm of the sacred to the rationalized routines of the hospital and other medical institutions. No longer holy mysteries, they are tasks to be performed, managed, documented, and audited by highly trained technical specialists.

20. This reliance on technologically produced (and quantifiable) evidence is what Daston (1995) has called "mechanical objectivity." Evidence produced through mechanical objectivity is often considered superior to all other types of evidence, and for some purposes—such as scientific publication or the formulation and justification of medical practice guidelines—it is the only type of evidence that may be seen as truly legitimate. The superiority of this kind of evidence is by no means uncontested in clinical practice, however.

21. Authority over nature is a very old theme in science, traceable back at least to Francis Bacon, the seventeenth-century polymath commonly considered to be the founder of the scientific method. Nandy (1988:14) writes that to Bacon, "nature was an enemy which needed to be defeated and tortured—the expression was his—so that its secrets or powers could be extracted for the benefit of the human race."

22. The commitment to individual patient autonomy and responsibility is matched by a strong focus on autonomy and responsibility for the physician, with implications for how error and negligence are managed. Professional responsibility is inherently individual, not communal (Bosk 1979). This concept of individual responsibility is so deeply rooted that attempts to follow the lead of the airline industry by treating medical errors as systems problems, rather than as failures of culpable individuals, have met with serious resistance (Institute of Medicine 2000; Leape and Berwick 2005).

23. For literature on obstetrics that explores this imbrication of technology and authority, see, for instance, Davis-Floyd 1992, Hahn 1987, Jordan 1993, or Wendland 2007. For perspectives on cosmetic surgery, see the histories by Gilman (1999) or Haiken (1997).

In decades past, among medical specialties psychiatry was an outlier in the orientation to technology: many psychopathologies required subjective assessments and difficult-to-measure interpersonal therapies. In an era of advanced neuroimaging and psychopharmaceuticals, with surgically placed neural implants under investigation for the most severe pathologies, psychiatry is less and less anomalous within medicine in this respect (Luhrmann 2001).

24. A few women and ethnic minority students did attend the schools discussed in these foundational studies (although the title *Boys in White* might suggest otherwise). The researchers, however, interested more in the school as a social organization than in transformation processes of individual student doctors, primarily interviewed and spent time with the white male subjects they saw as representative. The representation of minority students in the medical schools studied by the Columbia group in *The Student-Physician* was even more fleeting. Women students appeared exactly once in the volume, in a footnote that simply stated "over 90 per cent of the medical students observed are males" (Merton, Reader, and Kendall 1957:120), and other minorities never appeared at all.

25. The depth of medical curricular reforms is a matter of dispute. Kenneth Ludmerer, a historian of medicine, shows that even the most ambitious were both relatively short-lived and without demonstrable lasting impact (Ludmerer 1999: see especially 201, 304–6). Demographic shifts are more visible, yet their impact on medical socialization is much smaller than many analysts had expected or hoped. Women entering medical school, for instance, collectively rate higher than male students on measures of empathy and interpersonal skills. Some feminists had hoped that the increasing presence of women in medicine might help to humanize the profession. Yet even where female students have reached a "critical mass" for a decade or longer, emphasis on humanism and psychosocial skills drops markedly for both sexes during training (Dufort and Maheux 1995; Leserman 1981). Because the drop is more dramatic for women than men, some studies show that gender differences found at matriculation narrow or even disappear by graduation (Beagan 2000; Dufort and Maheux 1995). See the collection edited by Takakuwa, Rubashkin, and Herzig (2004) for first-person accounts of the often difficult experiences of medical training by some students marked as nonstandard Others.

26. The author of one of the most recent systematic studies of medical socialization comments on this continuity:

> What is perhaps most remarkable about these findings is how little has changed since the publication of *Boys in White* (Becker et al., 1961) and *Student Physician* (Merton et al., 1957), despite the passage of 40 years and the influx of a very different student population. The basic processes of socializing new members into the profession of medicine remain remarkably similar, as students encounter new social norms, a new language, new thought processes, and a new world view that will eventually enable them to become full-fledged members of "the team" taking the expected role in the medical hierarchy. (Beagan 2001:289)

27. See Becker et al. 1961, Good and Good 1993, and Sinclair 1997 for general discussions of depersonalization, a long-standing concern in studies of medical training.

Rothman (1991:142) notes that the implications of students' mechanistic concepts of the human body and their worrisome emotional detachment were discussed among ethicists by the 1960s. Conrad (1988) refers to lamentations about medical students' loss of humanism going back to the 1920s. Anspach (1988) provides an excellent example of the wide literature on the effects of medical language specifically. Fox (1979, 1989) has written extensively on the related topic of detachment, providing a more nuanced analysis of medical trainees' trajectory from attachment through detachment and eventually to what she calls "detached concern." The experience of human dissection features prominently in her analysis of this process. Hafferty (1988, 1991) has also examined at length the specific effects of cadaveric dissection on students' perceptions of death, the self, and the body. Like others, he has understood depersonalization to be in part a mechanism by which students control unwelcome and unacceptable emotions.

28. See *Boys in White* (Becker et al. 1961) for an early report on the valuation of technological and procedural intervention, and Good 1994 for a deeper theoretical elaboration.

29. Some of this language is idiosyncratic or institution-specific; some is much more widespread. *Gomer*, for instance, is a term used for elderly and debilitated patients, an acronym for "get out of my emergency room" that originated with the antiheroes of a popular fictional (or fictionalized) account of medical training, *The House of God* (Shem 1978), and has since spread widely.

30. Wear and colleagues (2006) provide both focus-group data from students at one medical school and an accessible overview of the literature on cynicism and ethical erosion in medical training. For earlier data on the development of cynicism and loss of idealism, see, for instance, Becker et al. 1961 or Bynum and Sheets 1985. Becker and colleagues were among the first observers to record the disregard for patients save as teaching material, the increasing emotional detachment in the face of death and suffering, and the callous language used to describe undesirable patients that many other researchers cite as evidence of cynicism. The authors of *Boys in White*, however, disputed that analysis and renamed student responses to training "pragmatic idealism." They also elicited from their informants a strong belief that the opportunity to do anything that entails the risk of harm to a patient is a measure of both personal worth and quality medical education; this belief they classified under the rubric "medical responsibility." They argued that the long-range ideals students brought to medical school—such as helping others—had simply been replaced by more appropriate profession-specific ideals, such as never undertaking treatment without a diagnosis. (This rather counterintuitive analytic strategy was no doubt influenced by the then-current sociological emphasis on functionalist explanations for behaviors perceived in the wider society as deviant.) Terry Mizrahi's book about residency training, *Getting Rid of Patients* (1986), explores the theme of cynicism at considerable length and analytical depth. Memoirs (e.g., Klass 1987; Konner 1987) and fictional depictions of medical training (Shem 1978) are also rich on this topic. Articles by Hafferty and Franks (1994) and Feudtner, Christakis, and Christakis (1994) are good places to begin looking at the hidden curriculum and effects of ethical double standards in medical training.

31. See, for instance, Beagan 1998 or Konner 1987.

32. On medical trainees' growing unwillingness to criticize the profession or its members, see especially Beagan 2001, Light 1980, and Sinclair 1997. On status and

authority, see, for instance, Beagan 1998; Becker et al. 1961; Fox 1957; Kressin 1996; and Shapiro 1987. Authoritarianism among medical students is complicated by effects of social class, gender, and racial or ethnic minority status, and I will discuss the topic in more detail in chapter 6.

33. The term *cloak of competence* comes from Haas and Shaffir 1977. Fox (1957) had already demonstrated the process two decades earlier, and many others have since described it as well.

34. Some research (e.g., Helkama et al. 2003; Self et al. 1991) shows that medical students not only demonstrate a narrowed range of response to moral and political questions, but also demonstrate arrested—or even reversed—moral development when compared to other professions or other college graduates (Feldman and Newcomb 1969; Perry 1968). This reversal has been called "ethical erosion" and seems to be most striking when students reach the stage in training that involves intensive work with patients in hospital and clinic settings. On homogenization and trends toward political conservatism, see Leserman 1981, Maheux and Beland 1987, and Shapiro 1987. Beagan (2000) provides a useful and thoughtful analysis of how this homogenous "neutrality" actually functions in the world of medicine to replicate hierarchies of gender, sexuality, class, and race.

35. I have tried to list here only those issues on which there appears to be a reasonable consensus among researchers of medical socialization, an inevitably somewhat subjective choice. This tactic runs the risk of making the literature look more cohesive than it is. In fact, many significant aspects of medical socialization remain contentious. Do the extraordinary stressors of medical training and work really cause increased rates of substance abuse, depression, anxiety, and suicide (Dyrbye, Thomas, and Shanafelt 2006; Sinclair 1997), and, if so, does the greater prevalence of psychological distress among women reflect differences in the general population or gender-specific effects of medical school (Newbury-Birch, Walshaw, and Kamali 2001; Stern, Sloan, and Komm 1993)? Does peer culture or faculty and institutional culture influence students' development more (Becker et al. 1961; Bloom 1989; Bloom 1973; Merton, Reader, and Kendall 1957)? Is the shift away from primary care and toward specialization as students progress through their training an effect of greater status and income potential in the subspecialties (Bynum and Sheets 1985; Schroeder 2002), the perception that one can only truly master a narrower set of skills (Becker et al. 1961), lifestyle or personality issues (Mutha and Takayama with O'Neil 1997), or institutional priorities (Campos-Outcalt et al. 1995)?

36. Describing the realm of medical socialization research as "the global North" would be too broad, and my frequent use of "Europe and North America" in this book conceals just how narrowly confined this research is. The vast majority of empirical research involving anything more than questionnaires comes from the United States and Canada, and then mostly from elite institutions. I have found almost no empirical work on professional socialization in Africa, Asia, Central America, or South America in searches of literature published in English, French, German, or Spanish (for exceptions, see De Craemer and Fox 1968; Gallagher 1988). Jefferys and Elston (1989) speculate that this narrow focus may result from disciplinary traditions. Outside the United States, social science research was seen as associated with leftist politics; social scientists thus had difficulty gaining a foothold in academic medical centers, where such research could be perceived as threatening to institutional interests.

Although literature on medical *training* outside the North is scanty, some excellent research on variations in the *practice* (and even the epistemologies) of medicine does exist (see, e.g., Finkler 1991; Lock 2002). In addition, some studies of colonial medicine have explored the transition from a colonial medicine provided exclusively by (and initially for) expatriates to that provided by the colonized. Most of this work is outside the scope of this book; some will be discussed tangentially below.

37. See, among others, Arnold (1993), who documents doctors' involvement in anticolonial movements in India, Adams (1998) on the more recent Nepal revolution, and Peard (1997) on a group of nineteenth-century Brazilian doctors who called themselves *tropicalistas* and took an explicitly political-economic approach to "tropical" disease. Lo (2002) provides a fascinating and nuanced analysis of changes in the medical profession in colonial Taiwan; Taiwanese doctors saw themselves as "doctors for the nation" at some points and as members of an international professional community at others, and their critiques of Japanese colonial power, always couched in terms of modernization, were limited by their need to maintain market position.

38. For rare exceptions—from outside anthropology—see De Craemer and Fox's (1968) work on Congolese *evolués* who trained as doctors in France, and Iliffe's (1998) history of doctors in East Africa. There is an important, if small, historical literature on biomedically trained African nurses and medical assistants: see, for instance, Marks 1994 or Hunt 1999. African clinicians do make appearances in economics and development literature, often in the process of using their medical credentials as a ticket to elsewhere.

39. Caveats, asides, and the obligatory defenses of contentious terminology choices are also primarily relegated to footnotes. So is explanatory material intended to make the book accessible to an interdisciplinary audience.

40. Geertz was here discussing the work of Jerome Bruner on narrative and cultural psychology (see, e.g., Bruner 1991).

41. Some of the history of science raises the concern that researchers' standpoints may *entirely* determine the results of scientific study. Certainly, we have ample evidence of research that justifies a social order with the scientist at the apex: scientific criminology (Horn 1995), most nineteenth- and early twentieth-century sexology (Terry 1999), scientific racism (Gould 1996), anatomical studies confirming the inferiority of women (Schiebinger 2000b). Research findings in *complete* concordance with the interests of the researcher (particularly but not exclusively those suggesting that one group of people is inherently inferior to others) should perhaps raise the suspicion of bad science. In all of the examples given above, research results were later found to be willfully or subconsciously misinterpreted, misrepresented, or flat-out spurious. Scientific research has also featured plenty of findings that surprised or baffled researchers, loose ends or anomalies that could not be fit into science's theoretical models until much later (Fujimura 2006). An understanding of social location as the sole predictor of findings cannot account for the possibility of surprise, and surprising or inexplicable results, I would argue, can sometimes be reassuring evidence of good science.

42. Even in that brutal program, there were a few people who made it through with a modicum of grace, although most of us did not. In fact, my experience of medical training makes me question some of the emphasis on homogeneity noted in studies of physician socialization. In the interests of fairness, however, I should also point out that nearly

every doctor with whom I've discussed it believes her own experience to be different in some important way from the classic research findings (although we all do seem to recognize the "doctor identity" in colleagues). It is possible that the research is seriously flawed. It is also possible, of course, that we cannot see what would make us look—or feel—bad.

43. In recognition of this evanescence, and in solidarity with the theorists who critique anthropologists' use of the "ethnographic present," I use the past tense for ethnographic material through the remainder of the book.

44. HSAs are community health workers, trained for educational and health-monitoring activities. In recent years, they have increasingly provided direct patient care, in the dearth of more qualified clinical staff that has resulted from emigrations, deaths, and mass resignations from the public health sector.

CHAPTER 2

1. Bauer and Taylor (2005) make a compelling argument for treating the whole south of Africa, bounded to the north by a line from Mozambique to Angola, as a historically and politically cohesive region. For the purposes of analysis here, I focus primarily on literature from Malawi and from three countries in the region with which it has had strong and long-standing trading, migration, and political ties: Zambia, Zimbabwe, and South Africa. Its other neighbors (Tanzania and Mozambique) are less closely linked, although patterns of migration—especially the large influx of Mozambican refugees during the civil war in that country—do forge important connections.

2. This breadth can make the literature on African healing hard to confine as well as nonsensical to constrict under the label "medical anthropology." Readers can find important analyses of healing practices in works primarily concerned with politics (Ashforth 2005; Feierman 1990), witchcraft or sorcery (Evans-Pritchard 1937; West 2005), religion (Pfeiffer 2006; Ranger 1981), or spirit possession (Englund 1998).

3. See Janzen 1982 and 1992 for historical perspectives on healing traditions, and V. Turner 1968 or Spring 1978 for relatively early ethnographic work on cults of affliction and healing of the social body. Kaspin 1996 provides a recent cosmology of body, land, and society from Malawi. Several Africanists who contributed to the edited collection *Modernity and Its Malcontents* (Comaroff and Comaroff 1993) advanced the argument that witchcraft-related healing represented a push for social change rather than social cohesion. See Englund 1996 for an opposing argument grounded in fieldwork in central Malawi.

4. Belief in witchcraft is not inevitably stamped out by conversion to monotheism nor by education, two assumptions common among those—Africans and non-Africans— who see it as a destructive force in African societies. Ashforth (2005) gives a particularly thoughtful analysis of the interplay of witchcraft beliefs, modernity, democratic politics, and rationality in Soweto. In Malawi, as in Soweto, official denials of witchcraft's existence sometimes seem to give witches the upper hand. Malawi's legal system, like most in the region, makes witch killings and accusations subject to prosecution, while being a witch is not. Religious interdictions may have a similar effect. Several educated Malawians I have spoken with over the years lamented that, as Christians, they were left

particularly vulnerable to injury by witches: their religion forbade the use of protective amulets as a form of false idolatry while providing no effective substitute.

5. See also Ashforth 2005, Davis 2000, and Prins 1992. Geschiere (1997) addresses a similar duality of occult power in West Africa.

6. For the use of colonial medicine to control movements and practices of African subjects, see, for example, Comaroff 1993 and Lyons 1992. (An extensive transregional literature explores colonial medicine's roles in imperial projects. The volumes edited by MacLeod and Lewis [1988] and Arnold [1988] were two early and classic collections on the topic.) For the argument that colonial medicine in southeast Africa was not particularly relevant to the lives of Africans, see Ranger 1992 and Vaughan 1991; Feierman (1985) makes the same argument for *all* colonial-era healing systems in southeast Africa. Vaughan (1991), drawing extensively on Nyasaland material, usefully complicates both traditional histories of progressive triumph over tropical disease and Foucault-inspired analyses that depict medicine as relentless producer of colonial subjects and subjectivities. For examples of the linkage between biomedicine and Christian mission, see Hunt 1999, Ranger 1981, and Langwick 2006. Van Dijk (1992), Pfeiffer (2002, 2006), and Ranger (1992) explore Christian nonbiomedical—or even antibiomedical—healing in southeast Africa. For the view of biomedicine as an essentially white European endeavor, and for the complication of this view when Africans increasingly began to train and practice as clinicians, see De Craemer and Fox 1968, Flint 2001b, Hunt 1999, Iliffe 1998, and Marks 1994.

7. Livingstone is often credited, both within and outside Malawi, with being the first non-African to explore the region. In fact, he was long preceded by Portuguese explorers and slave traders, who traversed the area by the early seventeenth century (Pachai 1973).

8. Maravi is variously referred to as a state, an empire, and a community. Some authors have suggested that the legend of the great Maravi state was magnified as part of an overtly romanticized precolonial past to facilitate postindependence nationalism (Forster 1994). In any case, by the 1860s, it was a functional trading unit, well integrated into coastal-central networks. Trade in ivory had been going on since the eighteenth century, trade in slaves at least since 1840 and probably considerably earlier.

9. *Medical dresser* is a nonspecific term indicating a doctor's assistant with relatively minimal and usually nonformalized training. Some simply dressed wounds or sores with bandages. Others gave out medicines or assisted in surgery.

10. Some evidence suggests that medical missionaries to Nyasaland were considerably less hostile to African healing traditions than is often assumed (Hokkanen 2004).

11. For a time, politicians in Britain's foreign office had leaned toward allowing the Portuguese, who also held established trading interests in the area, to claim control over the area that is now Malawi. British and Scottish missionaries, opposed to the slave trade, successfully urged British control instead (Ross 1997). Slavery was much reduced in Nyasaland after armed British forces under the protectorate's first commissioner, Harry Johnston, defeated the slave trader Mlozi in 1895. It was not outlawed until 1906, however.

12. At the onset of formal rule, the country's official name was the British Central Africa Protectorate, and it was run by the British South Africa Corporation. The region was reorganized in 1907, claimed by Britain itself rather than a corporate proxy, and

renamed the British Protectorate of Nyasaland in 1907. I refer to it consistently if anach-
ronistically as Nyasaland to avoid unnecessary confusion. The discussion of the colonial
period that follows draws primarily upon Bauer and Taylor 2005, Johnston 1898, Rafael
1980, and T. Williams 1978. Additional sources are noted in the text.

13. A copy of the "quarterly mortality report for Blantyre" produced by the city hospital in 1897 (reproduced in Lamport-Stokes 1989) reports only deaths among whites.

14. Christian mission medicine changed over the latter half of the nineteenth
century. Narrowly targeted to expatriates at first, it was later strategically expanded to
Africans and ultimately widely regarded as a basic service. (Colonial medicine under-
went a parallel shift to some extent in the decades just before independence.) Doctors
were first sent on missions to protect the health of the missionaries, whose mortality
rates—especially in Africa—were extremely high. Mission medicine then came to be used
tactically, as an enticement for people resistant to evangelism but susceptible to disease,
although such an approach was controversial. (The success of this strategy, of course,
depended on clinicians' ability to have an effect on disease—or at least to appear to have
such an effect. Thus, the dramatic although temporary effect of treatment for yaws initially seemed to be a great success for the missions [Vaughan 1992]. And the utter failure
of medicine to save victims of the 1918 influenza pandemic not only led many Africans
away from medical missions, it also sparked Christian antimedicine movements that
rejected any form of healing other than that of the Holy Spirit [see Ranger 1992].) A still
later philosophy was to see care of the sick simply as part of God's work on earth.

15. The southern missions left a rather different legacy. In central and southern
Malawi, the Dutch Reformed Church was more active than the various Scots churches
of the north. The Dutch Reformed Church leadership, although perhaps less malignant
in Malawi than in South Africa, did not view Africans as capable of real intellectual
achievement. Education was a much less significant emphasis of the southern missions,
and mission schools tended to be set up much more on vocational-technical lines than
those in the north (Chimwenje 1990). By the end of the nineteenth century, Islam also
was spreading, especially among Yao-speaking people of the south. Unlike the Islam of
northern Africa, it was not associated with a strong educational tradition. These regional
differences in educational background meant that northerners were significantly overrepresented in the late colonial and early postcolonial civil service. They continue to be
important in Malawian politics, medicine, and higher education. In several interviews,
Malawians connected regional differences to mission history. Edward Batumbo, a College
of Medicine consultant, told me in an interview that northerners valued education more.
When I asked why he thought that might be, his answer was succinct: "Livingstone.
He came, he started a school right away up in the north, and he showed the people they
could learn anything."

16. Hut taxes for Africans had been introduced in the Nyasaland Protectorate by
the 1880s. To pay the taxes, Africans had to enter into the cash economy, sometimes by
selling goods or cash crops but usually by undertaking wage labor for European planters.
In 1901, these taxes were doubled to pay for the increasingly large colonial bureaucratic
apparatus (Shepperson and Price 1987) and to mobilize more African labor. Africans who
worked for a European for at least a month were exempted from half the tax. This system
of forced labor, called *thangata*, ensured that many Nyasaland farmers were away from

their land during the crucial planting and harvest seasons each year, causing diminished yields and increases in malnourishment (T. Williams 1978). *Thangata*, unsurprisingly, was a huge focus of anticolonial unrest from the turn of the twentieth century to the collapse of British rule. Grievances were exacerbated by the essential absence of formal channels through which Africans could protest such injustice. By the time of the Chilembwe rebellion, African taxes provided 70 percent of the protectorate's income, but it was taxation without representation. Although the government included executive and legislative councils for Europeans, African interests were represented solely by a Scottish missionary appointed by the governor. Nyasaland's African population did not find this representation adequate. Indigenous chiefs and other authorities, together with the new elite of mission-educated medical assistants, clerks, and teachers, formed regional "native associations" to inform the state of African opinions on taxes, labor, and other rulings. The protectorate's district commissioners responded by attempting unsuccessfully to abolish these associations in the 1930s. A decade later, the regional associations banded together to form the Nyasaland African Congress Party, a nationalist movement with the goal of native representation, racial equality, and development.

17. One Malawi medical history states that Malekebu never practiced medicine in Nyasaland again (Mulwafu and Muula 2001). In an interview in the 1950s, however, the doctor himself reported that he *did* practice at the mission, if rather unsuccessfully. His clinic was so poorly stocked that he rarely had drugs or even bandages, and so those seeking assistance were more likely to go to nonbiomedical healers in the area (Macdonald 1975). Macdonald's history also confirms that Malekebu, far from remaining apolitical, was in fact the organizer and "leading spirit" of the Chiradzulu Native Association.

18. After the early 1900s, government no longer sponsored such training, probably because of protests by whites in Nigeria. Nigerians trained as doctors in Britain served in the West African military at the turn of the twentieth century, but the prospect that they might give commands to white officers or sit with them in mess halls raised so much outrage that the colonial government stopped sponsoring medical training for Africans (Adeloye 1977; Patton 1982).

19. Returning migrants in the 1930s also brought the Pentecostal movement to Nyasaland. This movement was to grow in strength and numbers of adherents over the subsequent decades, and prophet leaders who claim to heal through the power of the Holy Spirit are major figures on Malawi's medical scene today. In recent years, the articulation of healing rituals and inequality has come under scholarly scrutiny. (See van Dijk 2006 and Pfeiffer 2002 for conflicting arguments on the role of Pentecostal healing; the impact of witchcraft cleansing on perceptions of inequality has also been controversial.)

20. A particularly contentious law in Nyasaland was a 1929 amendment to the penal code that punished sexual relations between black men and white women while ignoring relations between white men and black women.

21. Marsh (2008; see also Ngalande Banda and Simukonda 1994) details the effects of federation on health systems in Central Africa. The push toward federation of small and less economically productive colonies was empirewide. British leaders saw increased productivity of the colonies as essential to pay for the postwar reconstruction of their own country and to help pay for the huge trade deficit incurred with the United States during the war. Settlers in the two Rhodesias, their population augmented by demobilized

soldiers seeking opportunities abroad, were also vocal proponents of federation, which they believed would facilitate migration of laborers from Nyasaland to their own farms, mines, and factories. Nyasaland itself never had enough industry or plantation agriculture to absorb the labor force that taxation and other new requirements for cash mobilized. It therefore served—and to some degree continues to serve—as a labor reserve for other nations. Some scholars have argued that this long history of migration in fact helps create more sense of national unity than is found in some neighboring states. A man might have been a Ngoni or a Tonga at home, but underground in the Kabwe copper mines or assisting surgeons at a Tanganyikan hospital, he was just a Nyasalander.

22. The discussion of Banda's reign that follows is indebted to Sindima (2002), T. Williams (1978), Pachai (1973), Posner (1995), and Bauer and Taylor (2005: chapter 3). Other references are cited in the text and in footnotes. No material even tangentially critical of the president was available within Malawi during Banda's reign. The students I interviewed would have been more likely to learn their Malawian history as schoolchildren from a book by Rafael (1980), a short, largely pro-European, very pro-missionary, and exclusively pro-Banda text approved by the autocratic leader himself. Doctors David Livingstone, Robert Laws, and of course Hastings Banda were major figures in that text.

23. Banda paid his way at the University of Chicago in part by acting as a Chichewa language and culture consultant for ethnographers and ethnomusicologists at the university. The complexities and ambiguities of his story are fascinating, although beyond the purview of this book. For a brief and accessible introduction to his twelve-year sojourn in the United States—during which he connected with wealthy patrons, represented the Chewa people for scholars and Africa for wealthy white audiences to whom he spoke for pay, saw a lynching, attended an African Methodist Episcopal church, and learned from radical African-Americans in the antiracist movement—see Henderson 1996. Exploration of the strong ties between African anticolonial movements and African-American missionaries on the continent would also take this book too far afield, but they illustrate well the importance of transnational movements of people and ideas. Interested readers are referred to Killingray 2003.

24. Estimated life expectancy for 1960 Nyasaland is from Alubo 1990, based on UNICEF data. Like many other details of his biography, Banda's age was a matter of dispute. He was probably actually sixty-six by the time he became leader of the newly independent Malawi. Although his official birth date was 1906, there were no birth records. His biographer Philip Short and others, including those officials who wrote his death certificate in 1997, concluded that his most likely birth date was 1898.

25. Henderson (1996) believes that Banda honed these skills during his American sojourn, when ethnographers applauded (and paid) him for his mastery of African linguistic and musical traditions, while church audiences were more inclined to support him the more he looked and acted like them—out of respect for all he had "overcome."

26. Likely confirming the fears of the MCP, in the mid-1980s a new figure appeared among the costumed dancers: "Kamuzu," a powerful and rapacious beast who threatened the village and demanded money.

27. Auslander (1993; cf. Friedson 1996) supplies a fascinating postscript. Chikanga escaped his virtual house arrest in Blantyre by fleeing to Southern Rhodesia and later to South Africa. In the late 1980s, however, he returned to northern Malawi—apparently

under the aegis of the same regime that had exiled him. Some Malawians believed that the orchestration of Chikanga's return was part of a belated and unsuccessful bid to augment Banda's popularity in the increasingly hostile northern regions. Whatever the means of his return, more than two decades after his exile, Chikanga once again established a thriving practice in Malawi.

28. The structural adjustment programs and their successors ("expanded structural adjustment facilities" and "poverty reduction strategy papers") mandated by the international financial institutions are ironic—or perhaps tragic—when viewed in light of the history of those institutions. In 1944, when the defeat of Germany and Japan was imminent, representatives from forty-four nations met at Bretton Woods to discuss ways to prevent another global calamity on the scale of World War II. Germany's National Socialism, those attending agreed, filled a vacuum created by the disastrous interwar poverty and consequent destabilization of German society. The Bretton Woods conference led to the formation of the World Bank and the International Monetary Fund. The IMF was to provide short-term loans to prevent disruption of state services in countries where currencies became devalued on international markets. The World Bank was to provide poor nations with long-term loans to aid in development projects. Over time, however, contributor countries pushed both lending agencies to a shift of mission. Rather than aiding development to reduce poverty, the new goal was to encourage nations to participate in the international marketplace, on the grounds that this participation would both encourage democracy and create openings for international capital. (I use the term *contributor* rather than *donor* because of the structure of these institutions. All member countries contribute an annual fee proportionate to the size of their economies, and all are eligible for loans from this revolving fund. Because of the size of the US economy, the United States is the largest contributor to both institutions, and American neoliberal economic theory has set their philosophical agenda for three decades [Scher and Baxandall 2000]. In practice, however, no wealthy country has taken an IMF or World Bank loan since the late 1970s. Other lenders, offering comparable terms without any accompanying policy requirements, are readily available to the large economies felt to be good risks.) For poor countries, which, like Malawi, may depend on donor aid for over half the national budget and over three-quarters of development funding, the policies and ideologies of international lending agencies can be profound influences upon social services, including health planning and health care delivery.

29. Laissez-faire economics was roundly rejected by John Maynard Keynes, the influential British economist and architect of the Bretton Woods conference. Keynes blamed this form of liberal economics for the worldwide depression of the 1930s and indirectly for bringing into being the fascist states of Europe.

30. It is important to note that deterioration of health indicators is *not* simply due to poverty, either at the state or at the household level. The Indian state of Kerala provides the classic example of high human development despite extensive poverty and demonstrates the impact of government decision making on health. In the 1980s, India in general refused most loans that required structural adjustment agreements (Kolko 1999). Kerala took matters further. Rejecting free-market arguments, the state government's socialist agenda pushed women's literacy and provision of basic (but free) professional care as most likely to have a beneficial impact on overpopulation, morbidity, and mortality.

By the turn of the millennium, the gap between male and female literacy rates in Kerala was minimal, and literacy rates among women were three or more times higher than in the rest of the country. Despite a GDP below India's average, Kerala's births per woman were half and infant mortality one-fifth that of India as a whole, while life expectancies were more than a decade greater. In fact, by 2000, Keralans survived longer on average than did African-Americans (Evans 1995; Sen 2001).

31. For more detail on SAPs in Malawi, see Chinsinga 2002. Schoepf, Schoepf, and Millen (2000) give a detailed, extensively documented historical analysis of structural adjustment programs and their effects on sub-Saharan Africa more generally. In a series of heartbreaking case studies, the authors link structural adjustment to increasing social and political violence, worsened nutrition, the spread of HIV/AIDS, decreased access to biomedical care, and decreased quality of care for all but the elite (as supplies run out in local clinics and staff leave due to frustration). In every category, poor women are dispro-portionately affected (Schoepf, Schoepf, and Millen 2000; Turshen 1999; Wall 1998). In part, the lower status of women means that when limited funds are available, resources are likely to go to the males of the household. In part, women have less access to the cash economy in much of the world, so that the imposition of user fees for hospitals is not offset by the possible use of fee-for-service care. And in part, when families cannot afford professional health care of any variety, the burden of caring for the ill falls on women.

32. In 1990, I spent several months in Malawi. Even to a naïve American medical student, the atmosphere felt explosive. The government's displays of glory had increased to the point that many parents who lived in Blantyre and Lilongwe tried to arrange for their school-age children to stay with relatives in more rural areas: urban children missed too much time at school because they were expected to line the streets to sing and cheer whenever the president's motorcade drove through the cities. Discussions of this and other negative impacts of the regime only took place out of doors, in whispers, after a careful look around to check for eavesdroppers—and even then without using proper names. (The president was "H.E."—an abbreviation of his very long title, His Excellency the Life President of the Republic of Malawi Ngwazi Dr. Hastings Kamuzu Banda.) For-eign magazines arrived with articles about the deteriorating situation in Malawi neatly cut out of them, while domestic newspapers featured such blandly positive headlines as "Ngwazi: Youth Should Respect Elders," presented as if newsworthy in an inch-high banner. A fellow student was deported for jotting a note on a five-kwacha bill, as it was a treasonous crime to deface the image of the president on it. Everyone knew the conse-quences would have been much worse had she not been protected by a white skin and a European passport. At the hospital, certain surgical procedures could not be offered be-cause the only surgeon trained in them was languishing in prison on no charge, suspected of treason. Yet the gaps in Banda's reign of terror were also becoming visible, and some of them were technological. Shortwave radios that got BBC Africa news, fax machines that could send and receive material unscreened by government censors: these were two of the technologies that some have since argued played vital roles in the demise of the dictator-ship (see, e.g., Posner 1995).

33. For a summary of the events that led to this largely peaceful transition, see van Donge 1995 or Posner 1995. Steve and Moira Chimombo (1996) give an account of the remarkable flowering of the arts that took place just before the Banda regime ended, and

the ways that the visual arts, dance, music, and journalism both reflected the country's turmoil and contributed to public political debate. The heady excitement and sense of infinite possibility in this era are hard to overestimate; the gap between hope and subsequent reality may explain some of the bitterness Malawians often expressed toward their government during my fieldwork in 2001–3.

34. UNAIDS-sponsored studies in central Africa report that when the mother dies, two-thirds of households dissolve within a year.

35. The 2002 GNP is from UNDP 2003; when adjusted for purchasing power parity, a calculation designed to compensate for the transnational economic differences that make tomatoes cheaper and cars more expensive in Malawi than in the United States, per-capita GNP was US$570. Debt data are from World Bank 2003: in 2000, loan repayments made up 3.1 percent of Malawi's exports, but new disbursements still exceeded repayments. Repayments would have exceeded disbursements beginning in 2002, but some of this debt was forgiven as part of the Highly Indebted Poor Countries Initiative (HIPC), partially in 2001 and fully in 2006. The budget improvement following HIPC loan forgiveness allowed the reopening of the nursing and clinical officer training schools in fall 2001 after a nine-month suspension for lack of electricity, water, and staff salaries (field notes, August 2001). To meet conditions for loan forgiveness, however, Malawi's government had to agree to cut health and education spending by 15 percent from 1998 levels.

36. Several of my informants reported that by 2003 this figure was up to six out of seven dollars. I can find no published information to support their statement, but it would not be surprising, given that by some calculations, overseas development assistance accounted for 89 percent of *all* government expenditures by 1999 (Bräutigam and Knack 2004). Official Malawi government plans for public health sector management acknowledged that the country-based or "bilateral" donors (such as DFID, USAID, and others) provided over half the state's health budget. The total additional amount provided by multilateral organizations, hundreds of nongovernmental organizations, and church-based charities was probably greater than either Malawi government or bilateral aid contributions (Malawi Ministry of Information 2001). A precise number would probably not be particularly useful in any case. Some NGOs (such as MACRO, a Malawi-based AIDS-counseling program) provided services directly, while others (such as JHPIEGO, a Johns Hopkins women's health outreach project) funded research projects that provided limited services as part of their research mission. A few donor countries, like the United States, spent the great majority of "donated" funds on the salaries of expatriate experts on short-term loan to Malawi. Others, like the United Kingdom, channeled funds directly to Malawi's government. Some NGOs (such as United States–based Direct Relief International) provided goods in kind without any cash transaction, while other groups (such as the United Kingdom's Voluntary Service Overseas or the United States' Peace Corps) provided personnel but not goods or cash. The patchwork nature of health services funding was very visible on the ground—not in the proliferation of paperwork seen in the United States but in the inconsistent availability and provenance of various drugs, levels of services, and equipment. Anything was better than nothing, and clinicians consistently expressed gratitude for donor support, but its piecemeal nature had serious drawbacks. For instance, I once helped my midwife partner try to stop a pregnant patient's seizure by drawing up the relatively toxic drug magnesium sulfate from three different vials, in three

different strengths, with instructions written in three different languages. A fatal error in dose calculations under such circumstances is only a matter of time.

37. Given the scope of this book, I can do no more than hint at the richness and diversity of healing practices used in contemporary Malawi. I hope to treat this issue more adequately in future work.

38. For forty years after Malawi's independence, hospitals around the country were supervised mostly by expatriate physicians or Malawians trained as clinical officers. (Smaller clinics and health posts were run entirely by nurses or medical assistants.) Clinical officers were clinicians who after an intensely practical three-year training course could perform many of the duties of physicians, including common surgical procedures such as Cesarean sections and hernia repairs. They are still in many ways the clinical and administrative backbone of Malawi's health care system, even since the opening of the medical school. The clinical officer was also an important foil against whom medical students constructed their doctor identities, as later discussion will show.

39. I found no reliable data on the number of Malawian doctors that ever existed; different sources report that there were either four or five at the time of independence in 1964. One of these was the head of state, who no longer practiced, and two others were exiled that same year after disagreements with Banda (Lwanda 2005:83). Another was the first Malawian doctor to work in a district hospital; political threats soon led this man to flee to the United Kingdom, but he eventually returned to Malawi in the 1990s. One common estimate is that about three-quarters of those who were trained abroad never came back (Mulwafu and Muula 2001). This estimate may be high. An unpublished Ministry of Health document reports that of seventy-six Malawians trained as general practitioners abroad from 1960 to 1980, forty-five returned at some point and thirty-one did not. Especially high rates of nonreturn were reported for students trained in the United Kingdom (62 percent) compared with students learning at medical schools in other developing countries (17 percent). These figures exclude those trained as specialists, for whom no reliable data could be found (Planning Unit 1984). Rates of nonreturn were likely to have become higher as the political situation deteriorated after 1980.

40. Several planners involved in the early stages of the College of Medicine believed that the school took so long to establish in part because Banda quietly opposed the idea. Some suggested to me that this opposition was rooted in a sincere belief that physician training was an inappropriate drain on Malawi's scarce resources; others saw it as yet another attempt to avoid grooming potential rivals.

41. Historical continuities with colonial medical education, donor priorities and systems of evaluation, and transnational movement of medical faculty, researchers, and graduates are among the important factors sustaining these widely if tacitly accepted markers of medical educational "excellence." All of these factors have been studied more thoroughly, and their consequences explored at greater length, in the medical systems of Southern and Southeast Asia than in Africa (see, e.g., Goldstein and Donaldson 1979; Tan 1990; cf. van Niekerk 1999). That such international standards for medical education are neither published nor agreed to be important by medical educators does not mean—as Blizard (1991) has concluded—that they do not exist.

42. Gusau (1994) argues that the demise of the alternative medical school program in Ife, Nigeria, was also related to another important factor: the establishment of monetary

prizes in highly specialized research areas, sponsored by pharmaceutical companies. Such prizes pushed early and inappropriate specialization, and again held up basic science research as the sine qua non of a medical school. Both effects undercut the leadership's determination to focus on primary care and community health.

43. Suspicions about second-rate expatriates in Malawi are not confined to medicine, as an incident recorded in my field notes suggests. On the southern end of Victoria Avenue in Blantyre stood several of the city's large banks: imposing buildings with colonnades, porticos, polished brass-and-glass doors, and public hours from ten until two. Security guards kept the street urchins and tomato sellers away from the shade offered by the trees in planters on the front sidewalk. I walked by the National Bank one day and heard two Malawian bank employees in suits and ties sitting on one of the planters talking vehemently about their new boss. "He's a failure. A failure!" one of the men said, throwing his hands in the air as I walked past. "I tell you, no proper white man would come to Malawi unless he's a failure!"

CHAPTER 3

1. The College of Medicine actively recruited foreign nationals at regional preparatory schools, and the enrollment of non-Malawians (although still fairly small) trended upward in recent years. Most foreign students came from countries without medical schools, such as Lesotho, or countries that were politically unstable, such as Zimbabwe. The requirements for entry were the same, the fees different: in 2003, foreign students (or those few Malawian medical students from whom the government withheld sponsorship) paid US$8,000 per year, while in-country students paid US$263 (MK25,000).

2. None identified openly as gay or lesbian. It is not clear that these are meaningful categories for most Malawians who have not spent time in the West, although sexual orientation has begun to be a topic of more conversation—and condemnation—since South Africa legalized same-sex marriages.

3. Tuition fees in 2003 were typically MK2,000 (US$21) per term for government and MK5,000 (US$53) per term for mission schools, not including book and uniform fees or other expenses. While these fees may seem small, they represent a substantial portion of the typical family's total expenditures.

4. Only a few older students had taken this route to secondary certification, which was at the time of my initial research temporarily defunct. Students learned partially by correspondence and partially in classrooms; poorly qualified teachers earned a little extra pay by teaching mostly adult learners in the primary school buildings after hours, nearly always without any lab facilities and often without lights or books.

5. Bruce Fuller (1991) and others have characterized school systems in much of Africa as caricatures of Western education, designed to demonstrate to lenders and donors a state's commitment to meritocracy and opportunity but in fact serving a primarily symbolic function. Many Malawians would agree with Fuller's harsh assessment. The blame for this situation cannot be wholly laid upon the government of Malawi. Dire shortages of cash and staff have left educational systems in the poorest countries particularly vulnerable to the whims of donors, whose activities may be intermittent and uncoordinated (Hango 2004). At the time of my initial fieldwork, UNICEF was building toilets in

some schools of Malawi's central region, Icelandic aid was funding school construction near Lake Malawi, and the Canadian development agency CIDA had supplied books and pencils to a number of Malawian primary schools. (Three years later, a survey showed that these supplies were gone; schools had no secure places to store books, pencils, or any supplies.) These were only a few of the agencies at work in Malawi's school system at the time. Teachers' pay, like that of health workers, was subject to similar constraints and confusions; Adamolekun, Kulemeka, and Laleye (1997:218) point out that by the late 1990s, seven different donors were working, without coordination, in the area of civil service payroll restructuring. Policy was also constrained by donor priorities: a UNESCO requirement for aid was that funding to the educational system reach 27 percent of the total budget by a given date, while DFID and WHO required that a certain proportion be targeted to primary education, and other donors specified the amount that was to go directly toward recruitment of girls into primary schools. These requirements raise interesting questions about the meaning of sovereignty in very poor states: does the concept of sovereignty also serve a primarily symbolic function? Problematic and patchworked as they are, however, schools are still seen as the primary route by which students without wealth or powerful family connections have a shot (if a long shot) at escaping poverty.

6. Students from wealthier families are likely to be younger than their peers at each grade level, because it is not uncommon to pull primary and secondary students out of class for a term or two to allow time for families to accumulate the necessary fees. I did not have family income data for the students, nor did the college. Occupation was a less useful status marker than it might have been elsewhere, in part because Malawi's formal-sector employment rate is very low: "businessman" covered everyone from the president, who owned a string of gas stations and several large houses, to the homeless teenager selling stolen goods at the roadside. Parents of students—especially female students—did seem to be overrepresented in the professions, especially teaching and nursing.

Another clue to the relative privilege of these students was their parents' high educational levels. Postsecondary education is rare among Malawians, especially Malawian women (see table 3.1). Among older cohorts, it is rarer yet. Among the medical students, a fifth of fathers and a third of mothers had a primary education or less, but just under half of mothers and over half of fathers had at least some postsecondary education. (Parents with secondary or postsecondary education were more common among women students than among men.) Compared to parental education levels for American or European students, these are low. Compared to Malawians as a whole, they are extraordinarily high. In fact, medical students' mothers must represent about one of every eight Malawian women of their generation with postsecondary education (calculated by comparing questionnaire results with population data from National Statistical Office [Malawi] and ORC Macro [2001], tables 2.1 and 2.4).

7. It was not just the curriculum that was British. Students played cricket and rugby, and wore uniforms featuring blazers and straw boaters.

8. Students with actual baccalaureate degrees in the sciences, whether from Chancellor or elsewhere, were also eligible for admissions interviews. A baccalaureate was never required, however. Unlike most North American medical schools, but like medical schools in the United Kingdom, the College of Medicine was a postsecondary institu-

tion. It was not uncommon to begin medical school at seventeen or eighteen, and a few students were even younger.

9. A faculty member's report corroborates their accounts (Phiri 2000) and suggests the depth of the problem: when Phiri gave a radio interview discussing her findings about harassment of women on and off campus, the repercussions included serious vandalism to her home and office and threats to her family by enraged male students.

10. The rumors were not confined to the grounds of the college. The headmaster of one exclusive private school was blunt:

> That premed program has got to be crap. They took nine of our young ladies last year. Three of them were good students—excellent students. Two? Well, maybe. Maybe it's possible they could make it. The other four, there's no way they were capable of making it through. Scholastically. Intellectually. No way. But all nine of them passed—they're in the first year now. (field notes June 2003)

This man proclaimed that the college had been training far below capacity (measured in terms of hostel blocks and faculty) for many years and was, in terms of cost to the government and donors per student trained, the most expensive medical school in Africa. (I am unable to substantiate or refute his claim, although I think it unlikely. See below for further discussion of per-student costs and the difficulties in calculating them.) Pressure was very high to show better returns or lose funding, he argued, and in a do-or-die burst of effort to increase output, the school had let standards slip below an acceptable level.

11. My data do not support the belief that socioeconomic diversity was increasing. Typical educational levels were higher for the parents of students in the earlier years of training, but the degree of variance found was not different among classes. In years past, however, students from humbler socioeconomic backgrounds usually arrived at the medical school through the elite training grounds of Kamuzu Academy. By 2002, poorer students generally arrived at the premedical program straight from work as clinical officers. I believe it likely that *perceived* differences among students were greater as the role of KA in indoctrinating lower-class students into high-class behaviors, dress, and language receded.

12. At the time of this research, tuition for Malawian students was MK25,000 (US$263) at all constituent branches of the University of Malawi, and MK43,000 (US$452) at Mzuzu University.

13. Dreams were taken very seriously as sources of guidance in Malawi, as historical and ethnographic work confirms (see Probst 1999 for an example). They were ubiquitous in popular literature as well. Every weekend, the *Malawi Weekend Nation* newspaper featured short stories submitted by readers; nearly all of them featured guidance by dreams, either ignored by the protagonist with awful consequences or followed just in time to save the day.

14. The limited studies available on this topic suggest that personal experience with illness or injury is a much less common motivating factor for those choosing medical school in the North (see, e.g., Hyppölä et al. 1998). The frequency of this theme among Malawian students—it came up in many conversations and over a third of the formal interviews—echoes the older African traditions of the "wounded healer," in which

becoming a healer is part of the healing process itself (see, e.g., Friedson 1996; Reis 2000; Spring 1978). It may also reflect the commonness of encounters with serious illness.

15. Simonds, Rothman, and Norman's 2007 study of American midwives and Lester's (2005) of Mexican postulants in a Catholic order both provide nuanced analyses of how vocation and volition conflict and coexist.

16. On the questionnaire, 97 percent of students indicated that they were Christians. The rest included one Muslim student; four who checked "other," probably part of the school's small Hindi contingent; two who left the question blank; and none who identified as atheist or agnostic. Several factors may contribute to the apparently disproportionate number of Christians in the college. First, many people believed that the 20 percent figure for Malawi's Muslims was artificially inflated with "temporary Muslims," those who found it expedient to share the faith of then head of state Bakili Muluzi. In a 2004 nationwide survey, 86.5 percent of respondents reported being Christian while only 11.9 percent reported being Muslim (National Statistical Office [Malawi] and ORC Macro [2005], calculated from data in table 3.1). Second, the Muslim strongholds of Malawi, concentrated about the southern shore of Lake Malawi, were among the poorest in the country. School enrollment rates, literacy rates, and measures of school quality (such as student-to-teacher ratios and graduation rates) were even more dismal than they were for the country as a whole (see Benson 2002:43–59). Very few children from this area would be expected to finish secondary school, pass the exams, and find funding for tertiary education. Third, students from Christian schools were probably at an advantage. The history of Christian missions, especially in northern Malawi, was closely linked to the history of education—and specifically, to a vision of education as emancipation. Islam, in contrast, was brought by slave traders and in Malawi (unlike some other Islamic parts of Africa) was not historically associated with a strong educational tradition. For Christian students who could afford them, private religious schools sometimes provided a better alternative to public education and a good springboard to medical school. Malawi's Muslim madrassas did not have this reputation.

17. The MBBS stands for "Bachelor of Medicine, Bachelor of Surgery." It is the basic certification for doctors in Malawi, equivalent to the MD degree or the MBChB degree elsewhere.

18. Location changed to protect Davies's identity.

19. No one I interviewed had doctor parents. In the American studies of the 1950s, both Becker et al. (1961:61) and Rogoff (1957:124) found that about one-fifth of medical students had fathers who were doctors. Neither group seems to have asked about students' mothers. Sinclair (1997:76) noted that among contemporary medical students in the United Kingdom, 20 percent had at least one doctor parent. I have no comparable data for North America or Europe about other types of medical work, such as nursing.

20. The higher a student's parents' level of education, the more likely the student was to report family encouragement to enter medicine. (Women also reported family encouragement as a more significant factor than men did.) American research dating from several decades past showed the opposite: in the United States, students from less privileged families reported greater family encouragement to choose a medical career (Rogoff 1957).

21. A comparable tuition rate, in terms of proportion of average per capita income,

would have been $56,500 in the United States (using per capita income figures for 2001 of US$160 in Malawi and US$34,280 in the United States from World Bank 2003). Including room, board, and transport, one could encounter a yearly total cost this high in certain circumstances—such as that of a student with no financial aid at an expensive private school in an urban setting. It would be at the very top of the range for American medical students overall, however.

22. In 2000, the Ministry of Education instituted a loan system for the first time. Students whose families could not come up with the requisite twenty-five thousand kwacha per year could now borrow it from the government. In theory, this loan was needs-based, but in practice, no student applying had yet been refused, and nearly all students (98 percent by one estimate) did apply. The loan system was new, and poorly understood by both those who administered it and those who borrowed. Neither the students nor the registrar who administered the loans could tell me the interest rate or repayment terms, for instance. One group of students who explained the program was under the impression that their loans would be forgiven if they worked for the government after internship, although the registrar did not believe this to be the case. In the end, that group agreed, it was always possible in Malawi just to evade those looking for loan repayments: "Sometimes you do things through an uncle or an aunt, so you can hide."

The students and their families were not the only ones who paid for their schooling. Examination of the budget for the College of Medicine for 2000–2002 showed a cost of operations averaging US$96,595 per graduate. (The simple calculation I've performed here [total school budget divided by number of graduates] obscures more complicated issues. For instance, should clinical teaching staff wages be wholly attributed to the cost of education when clinical staff are actually providing services to patients as well? Because of considerations of this nature, calculation of the actual cost of educating a medical student—anywhere in the world—is controversial and difficult, which means that useful comparison data are not available. [In 1978, Abel-Smith and Leiserson estimated that the cost of training a doctor in the developing world was about US$60,000. Adjusted for inflation, this figure would now be equivalent to $156,000.]) In 2002, 3.5 percent of this cost was covered by tuition fees and another 2.5 percent defrayed by income the college generated—for instance, by performing autopsies, charging small fees to foreign students who came to Malawi for electives, or hosting conferences. The remaining 94 percent was government subvention and donor aid. Some government officials and representatives from donor countries found the degree of public expenditure on medical education disturbing, as faculty members and expatriate aid workers told me. It was less clear how the taxpayers themselves felt about it, or whether they were aware of the extent to which they subsidized these new doctors.

23. The creative exploitation of connections to gain medical access came up almost constantly for me as a medically qualified field-worker. My field notes from 2002 record several late-night knocks at the door, people looking for help—diagnosis of dysentery, medications for headaches, referrals for an X-ray or an appointment, explanations for why a relative was not yet released from the hospital after having a baby or an operation—from me or from my midwife partner. Our landlady, a nurse well established in the community, was even busier.

24. Little comparative data are available on this point. In an informal study of

student aspirations in a new medical school in the United Arab Emirates, Gallagher (1993) found the desire to help ill family members to be a key goal for many students. The intent of increasing ethnic and socioeconomic diversity in medical-school classes in wealthier countries has in some ways been based on a similar assumption: that someone who was "your family" would want—and feel obliged—to care for you. (Thanks to Stephanie Koczela for this insight.)

25. Location changed to protect Joe's identity.

26. Statistics for physicians per 100,000 population are taken from UNDP 2007, although all three numbers given originate from surveys done in 2000–2004.

27. In the studies of which I am aware, even when African policymakers strongly supported such midlevel categories, African medical personnel almost universally believed they should be eliminated. Most saw them both as relics of colonialism and as socially problematic, beset with frustrations and role ambiguities (primarily related to authority and mobility, and often manifested in unfair salary structures) that drastically limited their efficacy. De Craemer and Fox's 1968 study of medical assistants and ex–medical assistant doctors in newly independent Congo is especially clear on those frustrations, which are beyond the scope of this book. Iliffe (1998), Marks and Andersson (1992), and Frankenberg and Leeson (1974) provide historical perspectives on similar intermediate medical cadres in eastern, southern, and central Africa.

28. Conversations over the years with Jennifer Whitman Foster have helped me think through this concept of identity-within-stories more clearly. See also Somers 1994, Mattingly 1998, and Bruner 1991 on narratives as mechanisms by which humans express desire and through which we construct both identity and reality itself.

29. Arrival narratives, those stories that tell of the ethnographer's arduous journey to the field, are a time-honored yet contested form in the anthropological literature (see, for instance, the useful discussions in Geertz 1988 and Pratt 1986). Characteristically, arrival narratives are full of visual imagery and present a "transparent" view of the site of work, as if the author were showing slides and allowing readers to draw their own conclusions. This very transparency, as Geertz has pointed out, in fact establishes the authority of the ethnographer by implying, "If you had been there, you would have seen the same." Some readers regard such narratives contemptuously as part of the wind-rustling-in-the-palm-trees school of ethnography (to paraphrase a famous dismissal of Margaret Mead's work), hastening past them to get to the theoretical meat. Others wish that the theoretical bits could be half as interesting as the vivid descriptions of arrival were.

I have played with the conventions in this book, inserting several different arrival narratives at various points. The ones that begin and end the book are mine. Two others—including this one—position the reader as a medical student arriving at the college and, later, at the hospital. The use of the second person in these two is a grammatical acknowledgment of the artifice (or hubris) involved. As you, the reader, are well aware, these narratives are also mine. This is a little piece of Malawi through *my* eyes, *my* senses, and it is inevitably and deliberately a partial depiction—I chose to write here the things that struck *me*, in this case on a walk to the College of Medicine on the day before classes began in January 2003 and a minibus ride from Zomba to Blantyre much later. The second person, awkward as it is, invites readers to beware: if you had actually been there, you might very well have noticed something quite different. It also attempts to honor, in the most literal way, the specific request of Malawian medical students who asked that people I spoke with, or wrote for, try to imagine themselves in the students' place.

30. I have not changed these names, as the signs were public. Dr. Mkango's sign was in Chichewa (except for the words *Dr.* and *AIDS*), Apostle Zalimba's in English.

31. The rest of the clearing was grass. By 2007, most of this terrain and some of the surrounding farmland would be torn up by construction, in a sprawling project designed to accommodate the teaching and housing of dramatically expanded medical-school classes.

32. The rains started too late and ended too early, and harvests were disappointing for the second year in a row. The two bad harvests contributed to making this particular time in Malawi exceptionally difficult for many people. I did not fully recognize just how difficult it was until I returned in 2007, when two years of bumper harvests, a new government that was performing better than many people had expected, and the advent of antiretrovirals were among the factors contributing to a much more hopeful feeling among many of the Malawians I knew.

CHAPTER 4

1. Junior faculty members told me that fiercely guarded notions of departmental autonomy undermined curricular coordination and student learning, as they do in many medical schools. "Every department has its own head, and if we elect a coordinator from one department, the other departments will say, 'I don't have to follow what that one is saying.' So it's a bit difficult," commented one basic-science lecturer. The result: workloads were relatively light in one term and crushing in the next, and organ systems that should have been taught together were taught separately.

2. The 5,000-kwacha-per-year book stipend for which students were eligible, at least until budget restructuring eliminated it in 2003, did not go far. One essential textbook, Robbins's *Pathologic Basis of Disease*, cost about 9,000 kwacha ($100), and many of the books could not be bought in Malawi at all.

3. Prentice (forthcoming) explores several fascinating effects of the increasing reliance on virtual or simulated bodies for anatomical and surgical training in the North. Cadavers never look like the atlas, but presumably simulated bodies always will: how will doctors' embodied knowledge change when the body they train on *is* the atlas, when there *is* a truly universal—and also profoundly incorporeal—body?

4. This belief is not unique to Malawian medical students. Studies of medical students in the United Kingdom and the United States also show widespread acceptance of some (not all) ethically questionable behaviors when they are deemed necessary to academic success (Feudtner, Christakis, and Christakis 1994; Rennie and Crosby 2001). I revisit the issue of flexible ethics in the context of resource scarcity in chapter 6.

5. Foucault's 1975 history charted the emergence of an objectifying medical "gaze." The gaze enabled physicians to see cases, illnesses, conditions, rather than humans, and justified a system in which, in return for healing, a patient was expected to make his or her mind or body available to general inspection by others. In this work as elsewhere, Foucault contended that to look in order to know was a form of tacit violence.

6. The habitus, as understood by Bourdieu, has been one widely influential approach to a long-standing social theory dilemma: how can people act (and perceive themselves) as individual agents while at the same time reproducing social structures like those of class or institution or in this case a profession? Bourdieu's answer is in part that individuals do have an infinite number of possible actions and perceptions—but that this infinity is contained within a range defined by the social order and internalized through various bodily disciplines.

> Only in imaginary experience (in the folk tale, for example), which neutralizes the sense of social realities, does the social world take the form of a universe of possibles equally possible for any possible subject. Agents shape their aspirations according to concrete indices of the accessible and the inaccessible, of what is and is not "for us," a division as fundamental and as fundamentally recognized as that between the sacred and profane. (Bourdieu 1990:64)

Infinite possibilities are not the same as all possibilities.

7. Sinclair analyzes his data explicitly in terms of habitus; his major contention is that medical students' acquired dispositions predispose them to mental illness and substance abuse as practicing doctors. Beagan does not use Bourdieu's ideas to frame her work, but her findings can usefully be considered in this light. She shows convincingly that medical socialization works by encouraging—or sometimes forcing—trainee doctors to relinquish markers of previous identities in order to become "neutral" professionals. See also Luke 2003 on the medical habitus of Australian interns and house officers. Physicians also use the word *habitus,* but in a somewhat different sense (and—at least for English speakers—without the French pronunciation social scientists apply to this word): a patient's habitus is a body morphology indicative of an underlying disease. A round face, hump at the back of the neck, and truncal obesity, for instance, is a "cushingoid" habitus because it suggests an excess of corticosteroids such as that resulting from Cushing's disease.

8. Such habits are common among clinicians in the United States as well, at least when they talk with colleagues. Watch obstetricians or midwives discuss the progress of a patient's labor, and one will likely see them mark out the stages of cervical dilation with their fingers (the tools with which dilation is measured). Watch surgeons recount a recent laparoscopic procedure, and one may note them reenacting the motions and postures they used to insert instruments. Rachel Prentice (2007) has argued that embodied practices like these become ways of enacting social roles, important in the process of socialization among surgeons.

9. See Weiss 2009 on the uses of hip-hop style among urban Tanzanian barbers to mark both their global inclusion and their marginality. In the Malawian case, it is likely that some of this stylistic variation reflected differential exposure to Western influences, related both to opportunities for travel and to access to media. Westerners had come and gone from Malawi for centuries, but the flow of images and media had been tightly restricted under Banda, and "globalized" images—while spreading rapidly—were still available only to a few. One student mused on the differences between the Americans she had actually met and the American videos she had recently seen: "I don't believe people

in America really dress like that. All the ones who come here dress like missionaries."
Malawi had no television at all until 1996, and the number of households with regular
access to a television or to films remained small. (In 2000, fewer than one in five men and
one in ten women in a large national survey reported watching television at least once a
week [National Statistical Office (Malawi) and ORC Macro 2001, table 3.4]. Four years
later, both figures had doubled [National Statistical Office (Malawi) and ORC Macro
2005, tables 3.4.1 and 3.4.2].) In 2007, there were still no movie theaters in Blantyre,
although one could find illegal showings of pirated videos—mostly action films or
pornography—by asking around in the slums.

10. Until 1995, women were required by law to wear skirts or dresses that fully
covered the knees. Trousers were forbidden. Eight years later, during the initial period
of this fieldwork, trousers were still considered risqué in most areas. Mainstream styles
for women continued to change very rapidly and to reflect overlapping social class and
urban-rural distinctions; by 2007, it was extremely rare to see national wear on a medical
professional in the city.

11. Like Beagan's (2001:279) Canadian students, the Malawians commented that
dressing in this style both conveyed "respect for the profession" and helped patients to
see them as doctors.

12. Among the clinically experienced students I interviewed, modal maternal education was primary school (compared to secondary school for all others). Modal paternal
education was junior secondary school (compared to college for all others).

13. No male student I asked believed he was treated differently from the females.

14. Anne Akeroyd (2004) has argued that the sexualization of work and school
environments in Africa is an understudied occupational hazard for women; women may
expect or be expected to have workplace relationships with male supervisors or teachers.
The students and interns rarely discussed this topic, and then only obliquely. My field
notes record an exchange that suggests it may happen.

> I was in the computer lab when Frank Kabwe came up to an instructor. "Sir, one of my
> classmates was looking for you earlier, Flora Chikani. She needs your assistance." "Is
> that the short one from Zomba?" asks the instructor, and Frank nods. "Ah—academic as-
> sistance or social assistance?" "Ah, uh, I think perhaps it may be a bit of both," stammers
> Frank, not meeting his eyes. "Here—give her my number, and be sure you pass it on to her
> right away." (field notes 2002, names and places changed)

15. Gallagher (1993) reported a similar expectation in the United Arab Emirates:
women medical students there saw their becoming doctors as a step toward gender equality for all women. It is also reminiscent of the push toward medical education for women
during the first wave of feminism in America.

16. Students eagerly depicted themselves as mature and very consistently linked that
self-described maturation to their medical training. Many said they had "grown up" at
the College of Medicine after entering as "childish." Intern Duncan Kasinja, after remark-
ing that he had completely transformed his clothing, his language, his drinking habits,
and his haircut—all from carefree to constrained—summed the changes up by saying, "I
grew up at College of Medicine. I became a man." I did not often challenge students on

this topic in interviews, but every time I did, they were emphatic about attributing the changes they saw in themselves to medicine rather than simply to time.

17. In fact, it was in their later years, when they worked directly with patients, that students most often reflected on and articulated this early experience of being doctors-as-Malawi-citizens. The timing of this reflection on what it meant to feel oneself a "true Malawian" may indicate that it was one part of a more general questioning of the meaning of nationalism that seemed to take place in the clinical years (and which will be discussed below). The process was similar to the way clinical students retold other aspects of their preclinical time, seeming to sift their experience for underlying meanings and narratives in a way that I encountered much less often among preclinical students.

18. City dwellers, even urban slum residents, were much more likely to access higher education than village dwellers; an urban woman was four times likelier than a rural woman, and an urban man three times likelier than a rural man, to have had at least some secondary education (National Statistical Office [Malawi] and ORC Macro 2005, tables 3.2.1 and 3.2.2). The disparity is likely related to four factors: closer access to schools in urban settings; less need for children's labor in the fields (although in the poorest city families, children are often kept at home to help with other kinds of work); greater perceived benefit of education for urban job opportunities; and disproportionate rural poverty.

19. I owe thanks to the anonymous reader who reminded me of this important work. Compare, for instance, Stacy Pigg's (1997) work on international development projects in Nepal, which also suggests that only social distance makes this embrace of the local desirable. Even as overseas NGO personnel stressed the need for local cultural knowledge and tried to depict themselves as "culturally sensitive," Nepalese intermediaries were distancing themselves from village "backwardness," the better to construct themselves as new and modern people, the educated among the uneducated. See also Ferguson 1999 for a very different take on the meanings of cosmopolitan and localist styles of dress, language, and demeanor in a Zambian context of failed modernity, when rural connections could be a lifeline for urbanites and style a matter of life and death.

20. In the North American literature, medical students rarely report feeling like doctors before their clinical years. Most are first called "doctor" by patients or by teachers, not by family or community members, and most express a discomfort with the title that I found only rarely among Malawian students (see Beagan 1998:113–15; Huntington 1957).

21. The help preclinical students gave those who sought them out was improvisational, sometimes perhaps even dangerous. Students freely admitted they did not really know what to do in many situations but in the absence of any other available clinical resources did it anyway. (I heard several hair-raising tales of bandaging bleeding head wounds at road accidents or improvising homemade splints for fractures on the basis of a year's training in the anatomy lab.) Muula (2005) has suggested that students also often provide erroneous medical advice in community settings without being aware that they are doing so. Medical authority, like *muti*, appears to have the power to hurt as well as the power to help.

22. Notably, the preclinical students who reported *not* feeling like real doctors were those who had previously worked in hospital settings: of those who answered "no" when I asked them whether they ever felt that they were real doctors, most were experienced

clinicians. It is possible that this difference is one facet of the social marginalization members of this group often described: perhaps they were constantly (if subtly) reminded by others that they did not match the "doctor" identity. Becoming a doctor involves submerging identifications inconsistent with that role. Among the Canadians she studied, Beagan noted that those with "deviant" outside identities (most notably those who were older, poor, or working-class) were the most resistant to the process she called "subsuming the former self" (Beagan 2001:285). For all the stigma they encountered, experienced Malawian clinicians often expressed pride in their work histories; perhaps it was harder for them to let go of their identities as clinical officers or nurses than it was for others to let go of the identity of secondary school students.

23. Emily Martin (1987; 1990), Donna Haraway (1992), and others have shown that this mechanical and warlike language is only one of many possible types of imagery that could be used to describe the structures and functions of the body. Indeed, many healing traditions center on ideas of balance and harmony rather than antagonism.

24. Readers whose mothers swore to them that going outside without a hat in January would lead to one's prompt death will understand this risk.

25. Faculty members who used this terminology, expatriates and Malawians alike, anticipated that students would then be emissaries of science back home to their families and communities. But the boundaries between "science" and "superstition" are sometimes unclear and can be crossed in both directions by the educated and uneducated alike. In 2003, a marauding creature killed three people and injured sixteen in a series of rampages outside the Malawian town of Dowa. Survivors of the attacks said it looked like nothing they had seen before and suspected a beast created by witchcraft. While the Dowa MP postulated an aggrieved ancestor spirit and Parks and Wildlife staff suggested a rabid hyena, journalists drew on science and sorcery to call the thing a "genetically modified beast." I recorded in field notes another example of this kind of epistemological boundary crossing. Every few years, rumors about "bloodsuckers" spread through Malawi, as they did in January 2003. (See Blumenthal 2002 for a description of events in Malawi; White 1997 analyzes similar stories in central Africa as a response to technological change.) The bloodsuckers or blood hunters—the *New York Times* called them vampires, but Malawians did not—were believed to roam the countryside, snatching victims and draining them dry. In the 2003 incarnation of the rumors, bloodsuckers then sold the blood to foreign governments in exchange for maize donations (Munthali 2002). It is a startlingly apt metaphor for economic globalization, but many people believed it to be literally true: during one period of my fieldwork, several people were seriously injured from beatings sustained when they were accused of being bloodsuckers. I first heard about these rumors in a faculty interview, when the principal of the college used them as an example of rural superstitions that scientifically educated medical folk had a responsibility to stamp out. Ironically, the next week when the topic came up again, it was in the operating theater, where the urban scientifically educated nurses were all earnestly trying to convince a dubious anesthetist that the rumors were true. By the end of the conversation, the anesthetist seemed half persuaded, wondering aloud whether the bloodsuckers might have been trained to use an internal jugular catheter to drain blood quickly. Both the bloodsuckers using internal jugular lines and the sorcerers genetically modifying beasts support the argument put forth by Adam Ashforth, who holds that education does

not destroy "superstition" but instead "creates new possibilities for shaping structures of plausibility within which the dangers contributing to spiritual insecurity are interpreted" (Ashforth 2005:19).

This creation of new possibilities is by no means exclusive to Africans. In the context of inexplicable increases in autism spectrum disorders, in a part of the world where educated people may see science used as often to cover up the truth as to reveal it, the proliferation of plausible structures of explanation involving vaccines might be considered a parallel (if deliberately provocative) example.

26. Many feminist critics have shown that scientific knowledge construction performs cultural work by locating socially important gender roles in the body (Martin 1987; Schiebinger 2000a) or in other features of the natural world (Haraway 1989), and by naturalizing sexual or racial differences (Fausto-Sterling 1993; Somerville 1997). This kind of cultural work gets done in Malawi, too, where endless research projects and publications document gender or racial-group differences in various anatomical measurements. Though very few of these differences have any appreciable clinical significance, they all subtly confirm that the groupings studied are biologically real and have far-reaching bodily implications. (After all, they show up on X-rays.) It would be difficult to publish a paper showing differences in radiographic measurements between short people and tall people—even though systematic differences almost certainly exist—or between red-haired people and blond people, but those categories are less socially meaningful than gender and race.

27. Krieger and Smith (2004) offer an excellent review of the mechanisms by which social processes are embodied. Sapolsky (1991) points out that anatomical knowledge in Europe and North America has also depended disproportionately on the bodies of the poor and that this dependence has introduced distortions into scientific concepts of the normal. In the early twentieth century, autopsies of wealthy persons showed small, apparently shrunken adrenal glands, and the bodies were posthumously diagnosed with "idiopathic [unexplained] adrenal atrophy." Only later did anatomists realize that poor people's adrenals were abnormally large from the constant excess manufacture of the corticosteroid hormones produced in times of stress. What had been understood as "normal" from dissection of the cadavers of the poor was actually pronounced adrenal hypertrophy.

28. Queens was a referral center, but it was also one of the twenty-three Ministry of Health district hospitals in the country, so both routine and specialty cases were seen there. It was originally built as part of a series of infrastructure projects meant to sweeten the bitter pill of inclusion in the Federation of Northern and Southern Rhodesia and Nyasaland in 1953 (see chapter 2). The new hospital replaced several smaller area clinics and the old Blantyre Mission Hospital, which had been staggering under a large patient load as the Shire Highlands area became more and more heavily populated. The history of the hospital presented here is drawn from my field notes, Dr. Michael King's memoirs (in King and King 2000), McCracken 1998, and Ngalande Banda and Simukonda 1994.

29. White skin also served as an effective entry badge. People the guards knew, or who had made special arrangements, could get in anyway. Vending was not officially allowed in Queens, but the nurses' long shifts, and the danger of wandering the city after

dark to shop, made the hospital staff an irresistible captive market. Over the years, I saw—among other things—shoes, wigs, plastic flowers, live chickens, and hunks of raw meat sold on the wards.

CHAPTER 5

1. They were also extremely uneven in level of faculty oversight and in project quality. I have cited several outstanding fourth-year papers in this book. When I dug recent projects out of the archives in 2007, however, I also found some that were essentially incoherent and one in which substantial portions were plagiarized from my own research.

2. Immunosuppressed people are greatly overrepresented on medical and surgical wards because they are more vulnerable both to various medical complications, like pneumonia or tuberculosis or malaria, and to certain infections (and cancers) requiring surgical attention—abscesses, infections of bones and joints, typhoid-related gut perforations. For similar reasons, although to a lesser extent, pediatric patients are also disproportionately HIV-positive. HIV/AIDS alters the demographics of the wards as well. Where in the United States the average age of hospitalized patients is currently in the midfifties and rising, in Malawi the average patient is in his or her early twenties.

3. This question was usually followed by a list of tools or capabilities I had previously thought essential to a real hospital: a medical records office with numbered patient files in cabinets, a functional telephone system, pregnancy tests. I often thought of Queens as a hospital simulacrum. In some ways, perhaps it was. Yet for all its limits, within that brick-walled compound, some people did get healed and go home, sometimes after illnesses or surgical emergencies that would have been fatal outside the hospital, and other people did provide care, sometimes with impressive dedication and resourcefulness.

4. The issues in education were similar. Parents who had some money could gamble that the expense of sending children to a private school would be repaid when those children were able to get better jobs, or send their children to the public schools and hope for the best. Like the private biomedical *zipatala* (clinics or hospitals), the private schools had proliferated under the neoliberal governance regime of donors and lenders. Also like the *zipatala*, they were extremely uneven in quality.

5. Fansidar is an antimalarial drug (sulfadoxine and pyrimethamine). It is often given presumptively to ill children in Malawi, as many of them will have malaria.

6. About 4.7 percent of surgical procedures involve at least one sharps injury, most of these injuries to the surgeon (average of five prospective studies, calculated from Beltrami et al. 2000: table 1).

7. Obviously, this propensity of a needle to move was even more dangerous for the patient than for the surgeon. In addition to needle-sticks, the dancing needles contributed to tissue injury, lacerations of blood vessels causing excess blood loss or hematoma—especially dangerous in a place where anemia was prevalent and banked blood rarely available—and injury to adjacent organs.

8. A simple calculation suggests that, *contra* the official view, occupational exposure may be quite serious. The risk of seroconversion from sharps injuries in a year should be calculable from the number of surgical cases done, likelihood of sharps injury per case, likelihood of seroconversion in the event of a sharps injury, and HIV seroprevalence in the

surgical (not general) population. Published American prospective series give the likelihood of sharps injury per surgical case as 4.7 percent, of which about two-thirds are to the surgeon, reducing the number to 3.1 percent for purposes of this calculation. (Given the equipment issues discussed above, it is probably higher in Malawian reality.) The risk of seroconversion per injury, in the absence of postexposure prophylaxis, is about 0.46 percent (Beltrami et al. 2000; Consten et al. 1995). For a surgeon doing a typical caseload of three hundred surgical cases per year in a hospital like Queens, where surgical patients are 80 percent HIV-seropositive (using the lower end of the estimated range), that works out to a 3.4 percent annual risk of seroconversion due to occupational exposure. In ten years' full-time practice, using these conservative estimates, one would expect 29 percent of surgeons in this setting to acquire HIV at work. Operating-theater nurses, who attend more cases but have a lower stick-per-case likelihood, should have a fairly similar rate.

9. This is an actual report, except that I have changed the patient's name. "Gravida one para zero" means this was her first pregnancy, and she had never given birth. Septic (infected) abortions could result from spontaneous miscarriage but were more often a result of illegal self-induced abortions, often accomplished with the aid of cassava sticks inserted into the cervix in extremely unsterile conditions.

10. If the Malawians were troubled by this self-protective move, they did not mention it to me. I find it deeply problematic—in fact, unethical—and believe it should not be an option for international students. It reduces the hospital to a sort of zoo: foreign students can watch African patients and clinicians interact, enjoying the spectacle of medicine in a very poor and culturally exotic place while keeping themselves safely on the other side of the bars.

11. It would be fascinating to compare these images with those in a neighboring country like Zambia, more traditionally aligned with the former Soviet states, where most short-term expatriate doctors have been Cuban, Russian, or Chinese. I am unaware of any research of this sort.

12. I do not wish to romanticize this improvisation as some sort of postmodern bricolage. None of these makeshift solutions was ideal (although all of them were better than nothing). The repurposed IV fluid containers used as catheter bags often leaked, leaving patients and staff standing in puddles of urine and increasing risks of bladder and kidney infections for patients. Cardboard sharps boxes were not needleproof and posed particular hazards for the hospital cleaners who had to discard them. Resterilized suture broke easily. Devolving clinical tasks to personnel with less (or even no) formal training, a stopgap solution to human resources problems used widely in African countries, is often advocated in a more systematic form by international experts, under the name "task shifting" (see, e.g., World Health Organization 2006). At Queens, it was a crucially important strategy to get patients necessary services. It also led to lowered standards of care and occasionally to dangerous errors or oversights.

13. Studies in the West and elsewhere show high rates of substance abuse among medical students and practicing physicians, particularly among men (see, for example, Newbury-Birch, Walshaw, and Kamali 2001; Stern, Sloan, and Komm 1993). Alcohol and drug abuse is one of the few aspects of medical-student socialization that researchers have investigated around the world. A 2008 PubMed search showed studies on substance abuse among medical students from twenty-one countries on five continents.

14. Talk of spiritual leadership and pastoral care may strike readers as grandiose coming from eighteen- or nineteen-year-old students. These students' rhetoric fits in well, however, with Malawi's long tradition of fiery adolescent (mostly but not exclusively male) evangelical preachers who promise to restore purity to individuals and to the nation (see, e.g., van Dijk 1992, 1995).

15. Social pressures were not confined to the medical school. Churchgoing (or at least mosque-going) was presumed, to the extent that a denial of religious faith was so rare as to seem perverse. The customary getting-to-know-you questions asked of me repeatedly were: "Where is your husband?" "How many children do you have?" and "What church do you attend?" My answers were not satisfactory.

I probably made a serious misstep on this count in the early days of fieldwork. In the operating theater one morning, as I was helping a woman onto the theater table in preparation for her tubal ligation, a gaggle of students came into the room to observe the procedure. The patient was clearly chronically and severely ill, laboring to breathe; we had been treating her for pulmonary tuberculosis and chronic diarrhea. Her hair was thin and brittle, her skin mottled with the rash common to HIV-positive Africans. She was so wasted and weak, it was surprising she had been able to conceive and carry a pregnancy at all. Although she had only one living child (despite five births, including a stillborn delivered the day before), she was adamant that she wanted no more pregnancies. When the anesthetist gently told us he felt she was too sick to withstand the surgery, she began to weep. I helped the woman back up to return to the ward, and the students—likely realizing they would be unable to check off "tubal sterilization" in their logbooks that day—began gathering up their belongings to leave the room, without a word to the patient. One lingered to ask if I would speak to the Christian Medical and Dental Association meeting that evening. Sad and annoyed, I snapped, "I'm an agnostic." "A *what?*" he asked, and the whole group of students turned back to hear what an agnostic was, frowning and wide-eyed at the answer. I am left to wonder whether the response rate I got from this particular cohort, far lower than from any other medical-student class, was related to that encounter.

16. All of the observations in this section hold true for clinical students. One intern, however, was fully as vocal about his religious beliefs as any of the preclinical students and felt Christian faith was an important attribute of a good doctor. Still, he did not speak about spiritual healing, spiritual counseling of patients, God as consultant, or prayer as the key to clinical efficacy. The difference between his response and those of the inexperienced preclinical students might speak to how thoroughly the biomedical model of healing supplants other models during the course of training, even for the fervent. Given the very small sample, however, this interpretation is speculative.

17. Half of the clinical trainees raised this issue, but only two preclinical trainees (both experienced clinicians) did.

18. This MP did go to jail in 2007 on an unrelated corruption conviction. By that time, most Malawians, including most clinicians I spoke with, expressed a cautious hope in their government. A new president appeared to be seriously cracking down on corruption and also resisting certain aspects of the international neoliberal economic regime that had hurt Malawians badly.

19. Senior doctors, Malawian and expatriate, tended to have a much more ambiva-

lent take on donors and lenders, and many were highly critical. This difference may have reflected their greater experience. It may also have been an artifact of the field situation. If students saw me as both a senior doctor and a representative of the United States, they may have felt uncomfortable expressing criticism. Clinicians who knew me as a peer would likely have felt much less uncomfortable.

20. Health and education expenditures increased as percentages of all government expenditure between 1990 and 2000 because the total government budget dropped, but both decreased as fractions of GNP (see UNDP 2003, 2000). Restrictions on the education budget imposed by various funding agencies probably protected it to a limited extent. Participation in a UNESCO project required that a certain percentage of the total government budget be spent on education, for instance; the World Bank required further shifts of the budget in favor of primary education as a qualification for loans. These restrictions made budget cuts come down all the harder on the health sector.

21. Three-fifths of the clinically experienced students mentioned availability as a characteristic of a good doctor, compared with one-fifth of the students without clinical experience. Conversely, when discussing bad doctors, half of the clinically experienced and only two of the inexperienced students talked about clinicians who were not there when needed. It may be that it had not occurred to preclinical students that consultant absence was a real possibility.

22. DIC is disseminated intravascular coagulopathy, a condition in which the blood does not clot normally and that can be both cause and consequence of catastrophic hemorrhage. A feared and sometimes fatal obstetrical complication, it is typically treated with prompt surgical intervention and blood products.

23. This story and the next are those of people I knew who got ill and were hospitalized. I did no formal interviews with patients, but I knew plenty of people—friends or acquaintances—who had dealings with hospitals, and was often called on informally to help. (Mobilizing medical connections, as discussed above, can be essential to getting care. A 2006 letter to the editor in a national newspaper, pinned to a bulletin board at Queens, expressed the writer's shock and gratitude at obtaining timely medical care for his gravely ill child *without* having to track down a staff member he knew.) These two stories are neither the best nor the worst I knew. I chose them because they are fairly typical illustrations of the social and economic conditions that both limit treatment possibilities and make treatment possible at all.

24. See Hansen (2000) for an analysis of the history, economy, and cultural and social impact of the used-clothing trade in southern Africa. This trade can produce incongruous visual effects. Intern Duncan Kasinja dressed immaculately, wearing a suit to work every day. His tie must have belonged at one time to a small boy; it stopped about eight inches down his chest. On a walk once, I passed a small Malawian girl dressed only in a black T-shirt that hung to her ankles, made into a dress by the simple expedient of belting with a piece of string. The T-shirt logo announced "Lordy Lordy Look Who's Forty."

CHAPTER 6

1. Discussions of work-life balance, already apparent in the earliest studies of medical education, have become more prominent and contentious in recent years (see, for in-

stance, studies by Beagan [1998]; Good and Good [1993]; and Sinclair [1997]). Many older (often male) physicians lament the inadequate work ethic of younger (and often female) doctors. See Jovic, Wallace, and Lemaire 2006 for an accessible discussion exploring gender and generational differences.

2. At the time, Kamuzu Central Hospital (part of it since rebuilt) was generally considered to be in worse shape than Queens. I vividly recall a gynecologist colleague, coming from KCH for his first visit to Queens, who walked into our dilapidated labor ward and blurted in a tone of envious admiration, "Nice!"

3. Staffing was far thinner than in the typical American or European hospital, and no supervisory cadre of residents or registrars was present. (Registrars, where they existed at all, were typically part of the consultants' call rosters.) For much of the year, interns would also have two or three students working with them on night duty. Thanks to increased enrollment, by 2007 interns were usually paired on call, easing the stress and workload slightly.

4. Reasons doctors gave for turning down postings included inadequate housing at the site, no transportation, antagonism from the district's people who wanted a doctor from their own region or ethnic group, or threats from locals to work witchcraft on the new DHO. Sometimes these were serious concerns; at other times, it was hard not to suspect the doctors of coming up with any excuse to turn down an undesirable post. One DHO told me about the search for his successor. The College of Medicine graduate rejected the house he was assigned because it had no electric stove. "Everyone knows he'll never make enough money as a DHO to be able to run the electricity anyway," this man scoffed. "It was just a reason to turn it down."

5. My investigations could not definitively answer the question of graduate disposition. The college kept no database of contact information for graduates (apparently not engaging in the relentless alumni fund-raising found elsewhere). When I tried to find recent COM graduates to interview, I went from office to office asking faculty and staff to look over a list of graduates and tell me if they knew where any of them were. Most responses were vague: "Mmm, that one, I think he was in Embangweni for a while. I don't know if he is still there or if he has gone." More than one college administrator asked for copies of my results once I finally had the list put together. Persistent in-person inquiries at the Malawi Medical Council in Lilongwe enabled me to track down a few more graduates, although many of the addresses the council had were out of date. Given the lack of formal graduate tracking, one wonders about the quality of data sources for the article that claimed eighty-eight graduates were working in Malawi and not one unaccounted for. On my own 2003 list of thirty-three postinternship graduates since 1999, only one was known to have emigrated. This very small pool of graduates otherwise broke down as follows: five were district health officers; seven worked in central hospitals (most as registrars); seven were in mission hospitals; two in NGOs; one was chronically ill and too sick to work; the remaining eight were unknown. These proportions were roughly similar to those reported by Muula and Broadhead (2001) except for the high number of unknowns and the absence of anyone known to be in formal postgraduate training abroad. In 2007, tracking down the graduates I had interviewed four years earlier as students or interns yielded similar results (although there is no way to know whether this sample is representative). One had emigrated permanently; one other was in post-

graduate training abroad. Most were working in district, mission, or central hospitals in Malawi.

6. All foreign students I spoke with did plan to emigrate after internship was complete, most back to their countries of origin. Interns were also very likely to want to emigrate. The interview sample was too small to make correlations reliable, but in the much larger questionnaire sample, desire to emigrate was not predicted by age, gender, parental education, or year in training.

7. The comments students wrote on their questionnaires demonstrated this agreement especially well. Overall, nearly half of all comments were about the inadequate salaries students anticipated, followed in descending order by comments on the inadequacy of drugs or equipment, issues relating to government incapacity or unresponsiveness, and the overload of patients to be seen.

8. Five years later, when I talked with him again, he was still in Malawi. The path to America had not worked out, but he was hopeful about a new recruitment scheme in Dubai.

9. Over time, I came to recognize soap, peanuts, and cars as indicators students used to discuss poverty and wealth. To be too poor to buy soap was a marker of abjection. Students often spoke of traveling to villages where people had to save for months "even to buy soap," and after their return from the Learning by Living week, some discussed girls prostituting themselves to purchase soap. (See Burke 1996 for a fascinating discussion of how soap went from irrelevant to essential among Africans in neighboring Zimbabwe.) A decent professional standard of living, by contrast, would allow one to have a car. Students and interns complained that politicians, accountants, engineers, and others had cars while their own salaries would not allow such an expense. They consistently described medical salaries—enough to buy soap but not enough to buy a car—as "peanuts."

10. Interns' housing allowance was about $80 per month after tax. At the time, an unplumbed, unheated, unfurnished house in good condition in one of the nearby urban townships (or "locations," as they were often called in Malawi) typically rented for about $95 monthly. That cost did not include any utilities or security, the latter an essential in any city neighborhood. Flats, very few in number and located mostly in expatriate neighborhoods, were much more expensive. In or near the city limits, a small apartment or a small house with working plumbing would start at about $300 monthly.

11. This erratic pay was a serious problem for doctors but even more so for nurses. A typical public-sector nurse earned $3–$4 for a twelve-hour shift (typically about $625 yearly) and did not usually get a housing allowance. From this amount, nurses had to subtract about fifty cents a day, on average, for transport to and from the hospital. Continuing to work when salaries were on hold quickly became a serious financial drain. Malawi was already in the throes of a nursing crisis, in part due to active recruitment of trained nurses by research projects, NGOs, and other countries (particularly the United Kingdom), but even more due to trained nurses leaving the profession entirely. Many nurses attributed the attrition to terrible working conditions, especially chronic and severe understaffing. As more nurses left, the few remaining shouldered heavier and heavier loads. In 2007, this crisis showed no signs of abating, and in significance for the public health sector and for Malawi's patients, it easily overshadows the issue of physician brain drain.

12. The salary difference also held for other University of Malawi employees, such

as professors at Chancellor College. It was often explained to me as a historical artifact that had lingered from colonial days and that the current administration felt powerless to rectify. The Ministry of Education could not afford to pay everyone what the expatriates earned, one faculty member explained, but the ministers knew that if they reduced expatriate pay to Malawian levels, they would not be able to retain enough professors to keep the university functioning. Burawoy (1972) described a similar dilemma in newly independent Zambia, as the state tried to keep the mining industry going by offering a dual wage structure, even while trying to "Zambianize" the mines.

13. By 2007, multiparty democracy was often referred to as "so-called democracy," and I heard various people link it with a host of social ills: corruption, teen pregnancy, promiscuity, lack of proper respect for traditional authority, insubordinate wives, and a single shocking call for gay rights. Multiparty democracy co-occurred with other changes (most significantly civil service "reform" that froze many workers' salaries and cost others their jobs). Anders (2002) has argued that these changes increasingly meant that civil servants needed to run outside businesses, sometimes engaging in corrupt practices. In short, scholarship and conventional wisdom both see a correlation between multiparty democracy, laissez-faire capitalism, and social breakdown.

14. The term *social capital* has been defined and used in many ways. Here I follow Bourdieu (1990:35), who considers it to be the "effective possession of a network of kinship (or other) relations capable of being mobilized" to desirable material or symbolic ends.

15. By law, any clinician with full-time employment in the public sector was restricted to one half day per week for private practice. This restriction was flagrantly violated without disciplinary action for the doctors involved. While there was no consequence for consultant physicians, serious consequences sometimes befell the patients, as well as the interns and medical students whose clinical instructors were effectively absent from their teaching positions. Some specialists failed to show up for scheduled clinics, scheduled ward rounds, scheduled surgical cases, and unscheduled emergencies when they were on call because they were busy with private work. Faculty members and administrators explained that the rule was not enforced because it was so difficult to support a family on an MOH salary that if their more lucrative private work were restricted, fewer physicians would work in the public sector at all. Thus, work in the private sector funded the *appearance* of work in the public sector.

16. One large US-based research NGO, for instance, had a reputation for facilitating approval of building plans and project proposals by offering cash and other favors to people who could make the wheels of Malawi's bureaucracy turn a little faster. This group also routinely recruited top-quality nurses from the government hospitals by offering over four times the public-sector salary. There is no question this latter practice hurt Ministry of Health staffing badly, and officials resented the "poaching" of nurses. The ethics of it were contested, however. Quadrupling a local salary still came to only about $14.00 per twelve-hour shift for a nurse, easy to justify given the difficulties of nursing work in Malawi. (In fact, offering the public-sector salary of $3.50 for a twelve-hour shift would be difficult for American researchers to get past their institutional review boards, or in many cases their consciences.) Even though contracts were of variable length and a research nurse could be out of a job quickly, these posts were highly coveted; both my

partner and I were often approached by nurses asking us to use any contacts we had to find them work in NGOs. Jobs for doctors were less readily available but just as desirable. Emigration attracts more research attention, but the role of NGOs in facilitating a sort of internal brain drain merits more analysis.

17. In fact, part of the attraction of administration may be that it presented a way to do one's job while avoiding frightening or overwhelming work with patients. Around the time most of this fieldwork was done, members of the Malawi Medical Council interviewed COM graduates who were working as DHOs in response to district-level complaints about their excessive focus on administrative rather than clinical work. The consensus from graduates was that they felt well prepared for administrative work but inadequately prepared to do surgical cases, and that they would prefer to leave the latter for the clinical officers to do.

18. James Pfeiffer has provided a damning indictment of the mechanisms by which international NGOs in neighboring Mozambique undermine primary care, the per diem system and the use of government staff in NGO research among them. By 1998, he notes, "there were week-long periods in which no community health program heads were conducting routine health system work; all were either conducting NGO-sponsored surveys, or attending training seminars put on by NGOs to prepare for NGO projects"—which the NGOs could then sell to their donors as capacity building (Pfeiffer 2003:733).

19. John Iliffe, in a history of East African doctors, has argued that the conditions of work there produced similarly polarized responses among doctors and nurses. In Uganda's Mulago Hospital in the 1990s, he reported, one could find side by side selfless heroes and corrupt and insensitive clinicians (Iliffe 1998).

20. By 2007, some of this clinical impunity was beginning to erode. One specialist was known to have lost his Malawi license despite good political connections after repeated complaints of negligence were brought by other doctors (including interns who had much to lose by challenging him). A handful of obstetrical malpractice cases against Queens Hospital, although prosecuted unsuccessfully, had brought talk of lawyers into our department's monthly "morbidity and mortality" meetings, albeit rarely. It is too early to say whether these changes will have a substantial impact on how physicians practice.

21. Or just to get away. An American who wrote a memoir about his stint as the only psychiatrist at Harare Central Hospital (Linde 2002) described how one could become so overwhelmed by the magnitude of need and the impossibility of meeting it that taking a long break for tea at eleven and leaving for the day at one came to seem only right.

22. The prevalence of military metaphors for clinical training and clinical work in America is actually quite striking. Many commentators have analyzed and criticized the use of military metaphors to depict the doctor—or the drug or the patient or the patient's immune system—battling the enemy onslaught (see, e.g., Martin 1990). Military terms go beyond combat with disease, however, to refer to the antagonistic relationships doctors have with trainers and with patients. Medical school, internship, and residency are often called "boot camp." The emergency room or the trauma center becomes a battlefield when those working there are referred to as being "in the trenches" or "on the front lines." People who require hospital admission are referred to by the on-call team as "hits" (as in "How many hits did you take last night?"). The tales of horrible patients or medical

care gone wrong, the sharing of which is both force for socialization and resource of collective knowledge, are "war stories."

23. Medical trainees typically categorize derogatory slang as "humor," although much of it does not sound especially funny to nonclinicians. Wear and colleagues (2006; see also Parsons et al. 2001; Sinclair 1997) provide a helpful analysis of this humor:

> Students enter the clinical world full of enthusiasm and optimism for what medicine can achieve and are met with obstacles of all sorts, including cynical faculty, uncooperative or unappreciative patients, and their own unanticipated emotional responses to the experience of hospital-based medicine. Every day they encounter something that should be otherwise, and humor may be one way of managing these incongruencies. (Wear et al. 2006:460)

Most of the medical literature on the topic argues that cynical humor has corrosive effects on junior doctors and their patients and that it should be changed through better education in "professionalism." This approach seems to me to put the cart before the horse. If derogatory talk is an attempt to cope with the enormous gap between medical ideals and medical reality by blaming patients for that gap, then rather than having corrosive effects, it may itself be seen as an effect of a corrosive problem: the touting of medicine as having extraordinary curative powers. Treating cynicism about patients as a simple failure of professional etiquette perpetuates the gap between ideal and reality by ignoring students' lived experiences of medicine's failures and leaving unchallenged medicine's unrealistic promises. It also risks forcing students' vulnerability and horror and disgust and grief even further underground to an untouchable and unallowable place.

24. This response, of course, could also leave an idealized picture of curative medicine—always accomplished somewhere else, where there were resources—unchallenged.

25. Controversy attends this "appropriate technologies" movement in the international health arena. Some analysts regard "appropriate technology" (usually meaning locally produced and sustainable low-cost health interventions) as perpetuating and naturalizing unjustifiable inequities between rich countries and poor ones. One Malawian faculty member I interviewed strongly agreed with this view and believed "the best thing we could do is to be bringing First World medicine into Queens." Others, including all students who discussed it, took for granted that the development of locally appropriate technologies was a worthy goal. There are solid arguments on both sides.

26. An ectopic pregnancy is one that has implanted outside the uterus (most commonly in a Fallopian tube), where it may rupture and bleed. Bridget's case was a complicated one. The pregnancy was large, and it was attached not just to one but to both tubes, which were heavily scarred. She made the difficult choice to remove both tubes, leaving her young patient without fertility and with no living children, but saving her life after a substantial blood loss. A more experienced surgeon might have been able to spare the patient's fertility. Bridget knew as much and was angry: "There is something really wrong with this system. I don't know how, but this system must be changed." She spoke to me on her way to lodge a formal complaint. (Even as a student some years earlier, Bridget had raised concerns about "the system," although at that time, her concerns were more related to lack of tools than to lack of supervisory doctors. She was the student I have

quoted as asking whether people from "advanced" countries who advised Malawi to train doctors would be willing to become doctors there themselves, given the conditions of work.)

27. An old medical joke (told to me by a faculty member when I was an intern) illustrates the position of the intern in an American hospital. Q: What's the difference between dog shit and an intern? A: Nobody goes out of his way to step on dog shit.

28. That said, my impression from watching them at work was that female students were more, not less, likely than males to listen to nurses' or clinical officers' opinions on clinical questions.

29. The concept of heart or love is not one I have come across in Northern medical education. (In anthropology, Behar's [1996] call for "anthropology that breaks your heart" does seem to ask for similar acts of imaginative empathy.) Love has been suggested—if not generally accepted—as one principle of medical ethics, however. Rothman (1991:210), in a discussion of situational ethicist Joseph Fletcher's contention that love should be the guiding principle of decisions, has cautioned that "so amorphous a concept as 'love' suited the exercise of a very traditional kind of paternalism." His warning is worth considering in the Malawian context as well.

In most of the Northern research, medical students begin to acquire detachment in the cadaver lab and at their first autopsies (see, e.g., Hafferty 1991). The process accelerates in the hospital, where the need for objectivity, the expectations of their supervisors, and the intensity of contact with patients produce for most trainees a sharp decline in empathy (see, e.g., Hojat et al. 2004; Newton et al. 2008). One study of medical residents has linked emotional numbness and loss of empathy with the perception of having made a major medical error (West et al. 2006). If this link is a generalizable one, then perhaps among the Malawians, love and clinical impunity are not unrelated.

30. Lwanda (2005:68) gives the five essential conditions of humanness as "form (thupi), spirit (mzimu), community (mudzi), integrity (chilungamo) and productivity (nchito)"; note that thupi also means "body" and mudzi also means "village." He attributes conflict between indigenous Africans and colonial medics in part to the difference between uMunthu (in his spelling, umuntu) and European individualism, which made colonial medical care unsatisfactory. In recent years, Dr. Bandawe has begun to incorporate uMunthu philosophy and Chewa culture teaching into the first-year social and behavioral science curriculum (Bandawe 2005).

31. Some students argued that the College of Medicine itself should take the lead in holding the state to account, even if that put college leaders in an uncomfortable position. One noted that in America, "If George Bush makes a statement, you find people somewhere, somebody from the university, will comment on that." Malawi's frequent epidemics and outbreaks, he thought, were opportunities for members of the college to speak publicly, both to educate the populace and to hold the government accountable for a response. In this way, it would become "a college for the people." Students and faculty have in the years since begun a popular radio program on health. In 2007, it was still a new program, however, and had been far more educational than confrontational.

32. Hospital work stoppages are illegal in Malawi, and at the time, little public sympathy for the strikers was apparent. In Queens, however, there was enormous indignation

over the punishment of the so-called strike leaders. Nurses on one of the wards gave some background on the issue in this field-note excerpt (from March 2003).

"Everyone was sitting down right there, on the outside of the hospital," said [one of the nurses], gesturing toward the little obscure side door that serves as the main entrance to Chatinkha maternity ward, since the formal main entrance is always kept locked. "The people from the Ministry of Health came, and they said, 'Where are your spokespeople, because we want to negotiate?' And everyone said, 'We have no spokespeople—you have to negotiate with all of us. Every time we have certain people be our representatives, you make scapegoats out of them.' But the ministry people promised that this time they would not fire representatives, they just wanted to be able to negotiate with a smaller group. So this is what happens—we have lost twelve workers, we still have no raises." I'm shaking my head at this perfidy and asking what happens now—will there be more industrial action? "No, they have made their point. No more union activity here. But, instead, people just wait for their chance, they find some other work, they slip away one by one, and we hire no new people, because everybody knows what the conditions are like."

Four years later, when a group of interns struck because their salaries had gone unpaid for months, public opinion seemed more on their side. Two major newspapers printed editorials sympathetic to the interns, and the issue was quickly resolved without any arrests.

33. Zaithwa was probably referring to Peter Davies (2002), who had recently described physicians' work as dealing with "end stage social pathology." Davies's opinion piece includes a memorable summing-up of medicine from a fellow doctor: "Our patients spend most of their lives drowning in excrement. Our job is to direct them to the shallow end."

CHAPTER 7

1. Margaret Lock's discussion of moral economy (Lock 2002) brought Daston's use of this term to my attention. The web of values Daston describes is a collective one into which novice scientists are collectively schooled. It is made relatively stable and coherent by the ties between values and activities (like quantification and measurement) that "anchor and entrench but do not determine" them (Daston 1995:4). In her analysis, the moral economy necessary for scientific objectivity routinely draws upon and reworks the values of society at large but is specifically scientific: it does not then reach back out into, and change, the larger society.

2. This sense of *moral economy* is similar to one often used in science and technology studies (see, e.g., Kohler 1999). In that literature, moral economies are assumed to be local, flexible if durable, changing. Such uses sometimes downplay the impact of broader cultural norms on communities of scientists, however, and often lack the more anthropological emphasis on relations of power.

3. It is no longer accepted by most anthropologists or historians (see Chakrabarty 2000; Escobar 1992; Gupta 1998).

4. This distinction between the art and science of medicine is widely used to frame both problems in medical education (loss of empathy among trainees, for instance, is

read to reflect ascendancy of science over art) and laments over a lost—and perhaps imaginary—golden age of caring physicians. It also has a number of practical effects. First, it positions humanities education (the arts) as the solution to the deficiencies of contemporary (scientific) medicine (although when the "arts" *are* made part of a medical curriculum, they tend to be a part no one ever fails, confirming for students that the *real* guts of medicine are in the "sciences"). Second, like the related dichotomy between caring and competence (Good and Good 1993), or the "two cultures" distinction between humanities and sciences made famous by C. P. Snow (1964), it confirms and entrenches a divide that is not always nearly so clear in practice. It glosses over the evidentiary base for much of medicine's "art" as it does the intuitive and subjective elements in biomedical "science." And third, in the appealingly Manichean way it divides all of medicine in two, it leaves no room for the urgent questions of justice and health inequities that cannot easily be categorized as either art or science. (In this respect, the fate of the second half of Snow's famous lecture is revealing. After discussing the "two cultures," Snow turned to the huge gap between wealthy countries and poor ones, which he saw as a great social evil and for which he proposed several remedies. This entire part of his analysis, so important that Snow considered renaming the whole lecture "The Rich and the Poor," is almost always omitted in discussion of his work.)

5. This transition could instead be theorized using Pierre Bourdieu's analysis of *orthodoxy* and *heterodoxy*. When heterodox knowledge struggles against orthodox knowledge for scientific legitimacy, Bourdieu argues, the very field of struggle is itself determined by a shared "doxa": "the aggregate of the presuppositions which the antagonists regard as self-evident and outside the area of argument" (Bourdieu 1999:41). This analysis has the advantage of stressing what remains unquestioned as the Malawian students reconfigure the role of the doctor: the universal truth of biological knowledge. Where Gramsci's contradictory consciousness seems more apt to me, however, is in its stress on knowledge as means to a political end. Although Malawians did sometimes characterize their own version of medicine as "better," it did not usually seem to me that they were taking sides against a mainstream in a battle for scientific legitimacy. It seemed more a matter of finding a pathway by which they could work toward something else: the improvement of conditions among Malawi's poor, inside and outside of Malawi's hospitals and health centers.

6. T. M. Luhrmann, comparing psychopharmacology and analytic psychiatry in America, comes to a provocatively similar conclusion: "If the moral authority of the scientist derives from the knowledge he acquires, the moral authority of the analyst derives from the love he gives" (Luhrmann 2001:202).

7. Vincanne Adams (1998:224) notes a related ambivalence in the model of "science in the service of the poor" espoused by doctors in Nepal.

8. Julie Livingston (2005), in a fascinating analysis of changing ideas about debility in colonial and contemporary Botswana, uses the term *moral imagination* to describe the way people imagine better or worse possible worlds—whether past or future. The term is very useful, but it does not capture how these imaginings also inevitably craft moral *trajectories* of improvement or decline when they are compared with "the way things are now." Did the students who depicted their own version of medicine as "better"—because they could see the larger causes of illness and disease, because they were flexible in the absence of technology—see it as an end point or as a necessary stopping place on the way

to somewhere else? I read them as seeing their own flexible, resourceful, loving version of medicine as simply *better*, but I cannot be sure that they did not see it as a point on a moral trajectory to modernity, better *only for this place and at this time.*

9. These were stories people told; written and filmed stories were also different. No medical dramas had yet made it to Malawian television, and the books available without a trip to South Africa were quite limited. The few medical biographies I located in libraries and bookstores were triumphalist narratives of tropical medicine's conquest of disease, hagiographies of Christian martyrs or politically prominent heroes, or some combination of the two.

10. At first glance, the fact that I can do the same surgical procedure on a Navajo-speaking woman in New Mexico and a Chichewa-speaking woman in Blantyre, and expect to be able to find basically the same anatomy and use basically the same techniques, may seem to confirm that this science really is universal. The catch is in that word *basically*, of course. It must be acknowledged that the tools I use will be different and have different names, the consequences of missteps will be different, the expected course of healing and the potential recourses if healing goes poorly will be different, the personal and familial impacts of surgery—say, perhaps a tubal sterilization procedure or a Cesarean section—will be different, the amount of bleeding I consider acceptable will be different, and the type of anesthesia used will be different. I believe in the science of biomedicine, but the closer I look at what can safely be considered "universal," the narrower I must draw its bounds. In this regard, perhaps medical knowledge is less like the laws of thermodynamics and more like the technology of the Zimbabwean water pump described by Marianne de Laet and Annemarie Mol (2000): recognizable everywhere as a "Zimbabwe bush pump" but constantly revised, jury-rigged, reworked by individuals and collectives, a technology so entangled in its circumstances that even the question of whether it worked or not had to be answered, "That depends."

11. When I speak to American undergraduates and medical students, the news that nearly all the doctors and nurses working in Africa are Africans often comes to them as a surprise; it is not at all uncommon for students never to have considered the possibility of an African doctor or medical school at all. We could interpret this as evidence of American education's remarkable parochialism, and perhaps it is. I believe it more likely reflects a worldview in which "African knowledge" and "medical science" are conceptualized as inherently separate spheres.

12. Ivan Illich's *Medical Nemesis* (1976) is the classic statement of the latter position. See Lewis 2007 for a contemporary version of the argument with specific reference to the twenty-first-century push for "global health."

13. GNP growth *does* correlate positively with health, at least using the crude measure of longevity, but the effect of income is strongly mitigated by social and community arrangements, and especially by structural inequality. Sudhir Anand and Martin Raval-lion (1993) have shown that the positive effect of GNP growth functions primarily—in fact, almost exclusively—through two mediators: (1) increased income for the poor and (2) increased public expenditure, especially although not solely expenditure on health care. Where these two mediators are lacking (e.g., in pre-Lula Brazil or in South Africa), one finds high economic growth without improvements in the length or quality of life. Where public expenditure on health care and improved incomes for the poorest are found,

longevity and health can improve even in the absence of rapid economic growth (e.g.,
in Kerala, Costa Rica, or Sri Lanka). A lecture by Amartya Sen (2001) is an accessible
introduction to this analysis, and Gustav Ranis, Frances Stewart, and Alejandro Ramirez
(2000) provide a more detailed examination of the relationship between economic inputs
and human development outcomes.

   14. A related debate over technology and responsibility on the international scale
questions what constitutes sustainability in health care. Until the late 1990s, many
influential voices in international health policy took the position that high-technology
medicine was tragically misguided in poor countries, an inappropriate technology for the
resource-strapped. The devastating effects of the HIV epidemic in Africa, and the with-
holding of antiretroviral therapies on what looked more and more like racist grounds,
were among the most important factors that prompted a partial reversal of this position
by the turn of the millennium. With the recent resurgence of interest in "global health,"
some influential leaders have argued very strongly for provision of high-technology
biomedical care around the world as a human right. Essential to the reversal was a
shift in the concept of sustainability. Conventional ideas of sustainability meant that
recipient countries would need to gradually take over any internationally funded health
intervention. Because the cost of vaccines and AIDS drugs is so high, programs involving treatment of AIDS or prevention of childhood infections were clearly not going to be
sustainable by this definition anytime soon. An innovation of the new funders was to
consider programs "sustainable" if they could be paid for indefinitely at the *international*
level. If wealthy countries made long-term pledges to buy drugs and vaccines, the poorest
recipients would only have to be sustainably responsible for provision of basic health-
system needs like transport, nutritional support, infrastructure, and health care staffing.
This shift essentially relied on the idea that *technologies* (not people) were the sine qua
non of global health, and while it has indeed resulted in reductions in HIV deaths and improvements in vaccination rates in targeted areas, it has for two reasons also exacerbated
some long-standing primary health problems (Ooms, Van Damme, and Temmerman
2007; Piller and Smith 2007). First, the disease-specific or intervention-specific "vertical"
programs funded through these new mechanisms keep their staff lean and their programs
efficient by refusing to integrate other kinds of care. Where transport is difficult, villagers
may walk for hours to bring a sick or starving child in for a mass vaccination campaign
but be unable to speak to anyone about their child's malnutrition, seizure disorder, or
diarrhea—not to mention the mother's new pregnancy. These essential primary health
tasks shift downward to untrained laypeople, or to no one at all, and health systems
become more fragmented. Second, public health sector staffing is hurt. When vertical
programs such as those providing antiretrovirals are part of the public health system,
donors pay for the drugs but not the new staff needed to distribute them and monitor
patients. When these programs are nongovernmental, they hire qualified nurses and
doctors away from the public sector, because they can afford to pay more than the local
salary. In either case, a ministry of health must train, recruit, and pay salaries for new
staff even as existing doctors and nurses are being hired away. But many governments
are required by the international financial institutions from which they borrow to keep
the total civil service wage bill at prespecified caps. Governments are left with two ugly
choices: violate the salary cap to recruit and retain health workers, but lose development

loans; or keep salaries low and risk ongoing hemorrhage of qualified health professionals
into the nongovernmental sector, not to mention the strikes, retirements, and emigration
that take their toll on the well-being of patients in public hospitals and clinics. Malawians in general are very happy to have the internationally funded antiretroviral programs
present—at last—to treat the infected. But health workers understand the costs. As a doctor in Malawi told me flatly, talking about hospital staffing and the impact on maternal
deaths there, "These NGOs are killing us."

15. This framing of the state as locus of both culpability and responsibility for redress
also limits human rights approaches to health, practically if not rhetorically. While, in
theory, health is a universal human right (as are those conditions necessary for it, such
as basic health care, clean water, etcetera), in practice application is up to the state. This
framing requires those least able to do so to make formal claims upon governments
that—whether powerful or powerless, receptive or hostile to such claims—are typically
bureaucratically opaque. It also places the burden of fulfilling those claims squarely upon
national governments while diverting attention from transnational policies that entrench
health inequities (Mackintosh 2001; Wendland 2008; cf. Englund 2006 for similar concerns with human rights and social justice beyond the realm of health).

16. A useful if preliminary exploration of this question can be found in Donald Pollock's (1996) article on American "training tales," or physician autobiographies of medical training. This genre (as opposed to physician autobiographies in general, which have
a much longer history) is a fairly recent invention: the first did not appear until 1965, but
by the mid-1980s, there were many of them. These tales tend to be critical of medical
training, a factor that may account in part for their appearance during an era of consumer
activism over dehumanized medicine. However, as Pollock points out, "their critique is
essentially a conservative one, calling less for a radical change in medicine than a return
to traditional forms of medical practice and power" (Pollock 1996:340). Pollock sees training tales as social acts that legitimate the social positions and values of physicians to the
readers. The tales follow a consistent arc: doctors-in-training are faced with an ever more
enormous burden of knowledge and technical expertise to master; the author manages
to survive this nightmare, learning while doing no serious harm; ultimately, he emerges
a competent physician, albeit one who has learned that technology is both amazing and
dehumanizing and that "the system," variously defined, is corrupt. The physician-author
usually takes herself to be unique, a humble hero who manages to retain her compassion
and individualism against the heartless machinery of medical education, and who is thus
able to comment upon the moral failings of her colleagues or even medicine more generally. Pollock makes the very interesting argument that medical socialization as a "technology of self" may in fact produce exactly this response: that each graduated physician
sees himself as uniquely resisting what the rest succumb to, while never realizing that
everyone else feels the same way (a claim he supports by referring to the many interviews
with medical students he conducted). The stories of training that students consume and
circulate may be part of this very technology of self-making.

17. My suspicion is that a materialist analysis might reveal America's medical
marketplace to be very well served by graduating generation after generation of efficient,
"productive," nine-to-five doctors who stay clear of the complicated, inefficient messi-
ness of their patients' lives and the system-threatening potentials of political question-

ing. The moral economy of American medicine may well be one in which the power and prestige of medicine, and the associated high salaries for doctors, are compensation in a negotiation that specifically *requires* physicians to be detached, authoritative, and reductionistic. Most American physicians are not civil servants—as most of the Malawians are—nor are most, today, entrepreneurs. Rather, they are increasingly the manipulators of technology in a medical-industrial bureaucracy in which standardization, depersonalization, and automation trump authentic relationship (not to mention creative resourcing or political activism) at every point. In this system, "heart" would be no moral good, although the *performance* of empathy might be valued as a means to the moral good of market share.

Does this suggestion sound cynical? Let me quote, from a recent study lamenting the loss of empathy among medical students during training, the sentence in which the authors explain why we should care: "Empathy is one of the most highly desirable professional traits that medical education should promote, because empathic communication skills promote patient satisfaction and adherence to treatment plans while decreasing the likelihood of malpractice suits" (Newton et al. 2008:244). The need to defend empathy by citing measures that administrators can count, tout, and trot out for the shareholders makes it pretty clear that the bottom line here is the bottom line.

18. Although this is a commonly stated mission, anyone who read the previous footnote will know that I am not at all convinced it is really on the agenda of most academic medical centers in North America. Perhaps it would be worth opening this issue up for some kind of public discussion rather than simply assuming it to be a worthy goal. Do patients and policymakers really want humanistic and socially responsible doctors? Do we prefer adequate technicians? (The two are often understood as mutually incompatible or at least in conflict; see Good 1994 on the competing values of competence and care.) There is some ambivalence in the North, both within (R. Smith 2001) and outside biomedicine (Scheper-Hughes 1990), about the idea that doctors should be actively involved in attempts to remedy larger social ills. What *should* the goals of medical education really be, and whose ends *should* be served?

19. Curricular reforms ostensibly intended to make more humanistic doctors typically repeat the failed efforts of other institutions without challenging any of the material reward structures, social hierarchies, or political allegiances of the academic medical center. Perhaps not surprisingly, the result is what Samuel Bloom (1989) once summed up as "reform without change." In this respect, medical-school reforms are oddly similar to "development" projects, depoliticizing real problems while expanding bureaucratic apparatuses, raising the hopes of the powerless while insulating the powerful from criticism, performing important social work even (or perhaps especially?) through failed or inefficient interventions (Ferguson 1990; cf. Justice 1999).

20. Some medical educators and clinicians believe that student-run programs incorporating social activism (Small 2000) or international health experiences (C. Taylor 1994) create more empathetic and socially responsible physicians. These reports are mostly anecdotal. In the rare cases in which evidence supports the idea, like Davenport's 2000 paper, it is restricted by small sample sizes, significant self-selection bias, and limited or no long-term follow-up. These very serious limitations do not mean that the conclusions are wrong, however. If the cynical, detached physician is no longer a foregone conclusion,

medical educators might consider activities like homeless-clinic work, international health experiences in poor communities, or student-run outreach programs to be worthy of serious long-range testing (and perhaps, if results are favorable, wider implementation).

They also might be less likely to treat such experiences as optional niceties; even educators who argue strongly that community health experiences of various kinds will produce better physicians tend to use language that reinforces the construction of these experiences as peripheral. Often they seem to imagine the medical school as separate from the world outside and try to meet the school's obligation to the community (or fulfill the terms of what they see as the school's social contract) by sending students *out* from the school and the teaching hospital *into* "the community" (see, e.g., Wasylenki, Byrne, and McRobb 1997). This language of inside and outside may well reinforce an imagined separation between medicine and society, and play a role in convincing students that such experiences are irrelevant to the real process of becoming doctors.

21. Exchanges of medical goods, ideas, and people have often been formalized in collaborative projects between medical schools in the North and in the South. Such links run the risk of an intellectual neocolonialism uncomfortably reminiscent of other forms of exploitation. Often enough, a medical school in a wealthy country will bring funds and equipment to a medical school in an impoverished country. In return, Southern hospitals and universities become sites for Northern researchers to do research impossible (whether for epidemiological or regulatory reasons) at home, and for Northern medical students to practice procedures they would not be allowed to do on their own educated and entitled patients. The assumption here is that the Northern institution has not just the financial but the *intellectual* capital, while the Southern institution has the raw materials (including exotic patients and pathogens) ready to be extracted. This kind of relationship is by no means inevitable—there are many responsible, egalitarian, and innovative research and teaching partnerships, including some in Malawi—but it is common.

22. Writings by Cole (2003), Errington and Gewertz (2004), Mattingly (1998), and Davis-Floyd (1998) have been extremely helpful to me in thinking through how narratives work to position people in history, to make community, to enlarge possibility.

GLOSSARY

adokotala (sing. *dokotala*)	doctors (Plural is also respectful address.)
asing'anga (sing. *sing'anga*)	traditional healers (Plural is also respectful address.)
azungu (sing. *mzungu*)	white people (Plural is also respectful address.)
chipatala (pl. *zipatala*)	hospital or clinic
chitenji	length of fabric used as a wrap
dzina laMulungu	the name of God
gule wamkulu	great dance of the *Nyau*
mai	madam, mother
mankhwala	medication, curative or protective
mankhwala achikuda	African medicine (literally, "medicine of the blacks")
mankhwala achizungu	European medicine (literally, "medicine of the whites")
matola	informal transport (usually in the back of a truck)
mbumba	roughly, matriline; later, women's political praise groups
mchape	poison ordeal, witch-cleansing movement
mopani (also *mopane*)	a southern African tree, *Colophospermum mopane*
mudzi	village or community
Muthu umodzi susenza denga.	One head cannot carry the roof. (Chewa proverb)
muti	medicine, remedy, poison
Ndilibe.	I have nothing.

ndiwo	sauce that goes with *nsima*—usually translated as "relish"
ngwazi	hero, lion-killer
nsima	ground-maize porridge, a staple food
Nyau	Chewa male secret society
Sindikumva.	I don't understand. (From *kumva*, to hear.)
sing'anga	See *asing'anga*.
Thandizani.	Please help. (From *kuthandiza*, to help.)
thangata	forced plantation labor
thupi	form or body
ufa	maize flour
uMunthu	humanity
Walira mvula walira matope.	To cry for rain is to cry for mud. (Chewa proverb)
zipatala	See *chipatala*.

Approximate pronunciations:

- Vowels are pronounced roughly as follows: *a* = ah, *e* = eh, *i* = ee, *o* = oh, *u* = oo.
- *Ch* and *sh* are pronounced as they are in English (as in *cheek* or *ship*); *kh*, *ph*, and *th* are pronounced like the *k*, *p*, and *t* in *kin*, *person*, and *top*.
- When an *n* or *m* precedes another consonant, it is barely voiced; speakers new to Chichewa who cannot manage the combinations can usually be understood even if they omit the *m* or *n* (so Zaithwa Mthindi's name should be pronounced "Zah-eet-wa Mtin-dee" but will still be comprehensible without the M sound that begins his surname).

REFERENCES

Abel-Smith, Brian, with Alcira Leiserson. 1978. *Poverty, development, and health policy.* Geneva: World Health Organization.

Abu-Lughod, Lila. 1991. Writing against culture. In *Recapturing anthropology*, ed. Richard G. Fox, 137–62. Santa Fe: School of American Research Press.

Adamolekun, Lapido, Noel Kulemeka, and Mouftaou Laleye. 1997. Political transition, economic liberalization and civil service reform in Malawi. *Public Administration and Development* 17 (2): 209–22.

Adams, Vincanne. 1998. *Doctors for democracy: Health professionals in the Nepal revolution.* Cambridge, UK: Cambridge University Press.

Adeloye, Adelola. 1977. *Nigerian pioneers of modern medicine: Selected writings.* Ibadan, Nigeria: Ibadan University Press.

Akeroyd, Anne V. 2004. Coercion, constraints, and "cultural entrapments": A further look at gendered and occupational factors pertinent to the transmission of HIV in Africa. In *HIV and AIDS in Africa: Beyond epidemiology*, ed. Ezekiel Kalipeni, Susan Craddock, Joseph R. Oppong, and Jayati Ghosh, 89–103. Malden, MA: Blackwell Publishing.

Alubo, S. Ogoh. 1987. Drugging the people: Pills, profits, and underdevelopment in Nigeria. In *The impact of development and modern technologies in Third World health*, ed. Barbara E. Jackson and Antonio Ugalde, 89–113. Williamsburg, VA: Department of Anthropology, College of William and Mary.

———. 1990. Debt crisis, health and health services in Africa. *Social Science and Medicine* 31 (6): 639–48.

———. 1994. The medical profession and health policy in Nigeria. In *Physicians and health care in the Third World*, ed. Antonio Ugalde and S. Ogoh Alubo, 3–17. Williamsburg, VA: Department of Anthropology, College of William and Mary.

Anand, Sudhir, and Martin Ravallion. 1993. Human development in poor countries: On the role of private incomes and public services. *Journal of Economic Perspectives* 7 (1): 133–50.

Anders, Gerhard. 2002. Freedom and insecurity: Civil servants between support networks, the free market and the civil service reform. In *A democracy of chameleons:*

Politics and culture in the new Malawi, ed. Harri Englund, 43–61. Uppsala, Sweden: Nordiska Afrikainstitutet (The Nordic Africa Institute).

Anderson, Benedict. 1983. *Imagined communities: Reflections on the origin and spread of nationalism.* London: Verso.

Anderson, Warwick. 2000. The Third-World body. In *Medicine in the twentieth century,* ed. Roger Cooter and John Pickstone, 235–45. Amsterdam: Harwood Academic Publishers.

———. 2002. Introduction: Postcolonial technoscience. *Social Studies of Science* 32 (5–6): 643–58.

———. 2003. How's the empire? An essay review. *Journal of the History of Medicine and Allied Health Sciences* 58:459–65.

Anspach, Renee R. 1988. Notes on the sociology of medical discourse: The language of case presentation. *Journal of Health and Social Behavior* 29:357–75.

Apker, Julie, and Susan Eggly. 2004. Communicating professional identity in medical socialization: Considering the ideological discourse of morning report. *Qualitative Health Research* 14 (3): 411–29.

Archampong, E. Q. 1990. *Medical education and national development in Africa.* Accra: Ghana Academy of Arts and Sciences.

Arnold, David, ed. 1988. *Imperial medicine and indigenous societies.* Manchester, UK: Manchester University Press.

———. 1993. *Colonizing the body: State medicine and epidemic disease in nineteenth-century India.* Berkeley and Los Angeles: University of California Press.

Ashforth, Adam. 2005. *Witchcraft, violence, and democracy in South Africa.* Chicago: University of Chicago Press.

Auslander, Mark. 1993. "Open the wombs!": The symbolic politics of modern Ngoni witchfinding. In *Modernity and its malcontents: Ritual and power in postcolonial Africa,* ed. Jean Comaroff and John L. Comaroff, 167–92. Chicago: University of Chicago Press.

Baer, Hans A. 1989. The American dominative medical system as a reflection of social relations in the larger society. *Social Science and Medicine* 28 (11): 1103–12.

Baer, Hans A., Merrill Singer, and Ida Susser. 1997. *Medical anthropology and the world system: A critical perspective.* Westport, CT: Bergin & Garvey.

Bandawe, Chiwoza R. 2005. Psychology brewed in an African pot: Indigenous philosophies and the quest for relevance. *Higher Education Policy* 18 (3): 289–300.

Bauer, Gretchen, and Scott D. Taylor. 2005. *Politics in southern Africa: State and society in transition.* Boulder, CO: Lynne Rienner Publishers.

Beagan, Brenda L. 1998. Personal, public, and professional identities: Conflicts and congruences in medical school. PhD diss. in sociology, University of British Columbia.

———. 2000. Neutralizing differences: Producing neutral doctors for (almost) neutral patients. *Social Science and Medicine* 51:1253–65.

———. 2001. "Even if I don't know what I'm doing I can make it look like I know what I'm doing": Becoming a doctor in the 1990s. *Canadian Review of Sociology & Anthropology* 38 (3): 275–92.

Beck, Ann. 1970. *A history of the British medical administration of East Africa, 1900–1950.* Cambridge, MA: Harvard University Press.

Becker, Howard S., Blanche Geer, Everett C. Hughes, and Anselm L. Strauss. 1961. *Boys in white: Student culture in medical school*. Chicago: University of Chicago Press.

Behar, Ruth. 1996. *The vulnerable observer: Anthropology that breaks your heart*. Boston: Beacon Press.

Beltrami, Elise M., Ian T. Williams, Craig N. Shapiro, and Mary E. Chamberland. 2000. Risk and management of blood-borne infections in health care workers. *Clinical Microbiology Reviews* 13 (3): 385–407.

Benson, Todd, with James Kaphuka, Shelton Kanyanda, and Richmond Chinula. 2002. *Malawi: An atlas of social statistics*. Zomba, Malawi: National Statistical Office and Washington, DC: International Food Policy Research Institute.

Bernard, H. Russell. 1995. *Research methods in anthropology: Qualitative and quantitative approaches*. 2nd ed. Walnut Creek, CA: Alta Mira Press.

Biagioli, Mario, ed. 1999. *The science studies reader*. New York: Routledge.

Bickel, Janet, and Ann J. Brown. 2005. Generation X: Implications for faculty recruitment and development in academic health centers. *Academic Medicine* 80 (3): 205–10.

Blizard, Peter J. 1991. International standards in medical education or national standards / primary health care—Which direction? *Social Science and Medicine* 33 (10): 1163–70.

Bloom, Samuel W. 1989. The medical school as a social organization: The sources of resistance to change. *Medical Education* 23 (3): 228–41.

———. 1973. *Power and dissent in the medical school*. New York: Free Press.

Blumenthal, Ralph. 2002. A fear of vampires can mask a fear of something much worse. *New York Times*, December 29, WK2.

Bosk, Charles L. 1979. *Forgive and remember: Managing medical failure*. Chicago: University of Chicago Press.

Bourdieu, Pierre. 1974. The school as a conservative force: Scholastic and cultural inequalities. In *Contemporary research in the sociology of education*, ed. John Eggleston, trans. J. C. Whitehouse, 32–46. London: Methuen.

———. 1977. *Outline of a theory of practice*. Trans. Richard Nice. Cambridge, UK: Cambridge University Press.

———. 1990. *The logic of practice*. Trans. Richard Nice. Stanford, CA: Stanford University Press.

———. 1999. The specificity of the scientific field and the social conditions of the progress of reason. In *The science studies reader*, ed. Mario Biagioli, 31–50. New York: Routledge.

Boyes, Kit. 2007. Medicine's heretic bible nearly 30 years onward. *New Zealand Medical Student Journal* 1:39–41.

Bräutigam, Deborah A., and Stephen Knack. 2004. Foreign aid, institutions, and governance in sub-Saharan Africa. *Economic Development and Cultural Change* 52:255–85.

Broadhead, R. L. 1998. Community-based paediatric curriculum: The Malawi experience. *Annals of Tropical Paediatrics* 18 (supplement): S27–S32.

Bruner, Jerome. 1991. The narrative construction of reality. *Critical Inquiry* 18 (1): 1–21.

Burawoy, Michael. 1972. *The colour of class on the copper mines, from African advancement to Zambianization*. Manchester, UK: Manchester University Press for the University of Zambia Institute for African Studies.

Burke, Timothy. 1996. *Lifebuoy men, Lux women: Commodification, consumption, & cleanliness in modern Zimbabwe*. Durham, NC: Duke University Press.

———. 2003. Eyes wide shut: Africanists and the moral problematics of postcolonial societies. *African Studies Quarterly* 7 (2 & 3). http://web.africa.ufl.edu/asq/v7/ v7i2a12.htm.

Bynum, J., and G. Sheets. 1985. Medical school socialization and the new physician: Role, status, adjustments, personal problems, and social identity. *Psychological Reports* 57 (1): 182.

Campos-Outcalt, Douglas, Janet Senf, Arleen J. Watkins, and Stan Bastacky. 1995. The effects of medical school curricula, faculty role models, and biomedical research support on choice of generalist physician careers: A review and quality assessment of the literature. *Academic Medicine* 70 (7): 611–19.

Carroll, Rory. 2002. The Eton of Africa reinvents itself. *Guardian Weekly*, December 19–25, 15.

Casper, Monica J. 1998. Working on and around human fetuses: The contested domain of fetal surgery. In *Differences in medicine: Unraveling practices, techniques, and bodies*, ed. Marc Berg and Annemarie Mol, 28–52. Durham, NC: Duke University Press.

Castel, Robert. 1991. From dangerousness to risk. In *The Foucault effect: Studies in governmentality*, ed. Graham Burchell, Colin Gordon, and Peter Miller, 281–98. Chicago: University of Chicago Press.

Chakrabarty, Dipesh. 2000. *Provincializing Europe: Postcolonial thought and historical difference*. Princeton, NJ: Princeton University Press.

Chambliss, J. E. 1881. *The lives and travels of Livingstone and Stanley, covering their entire career in southern and central Africa*. Boston: DeWolfe, Fiske & Company, Publishers.

Chanock, M. L. 1975. Ambiguities in the Malawian political tradition. *African Affairs* 74 (296): 326–46.

Chimombo, Steve, and Moira Chimombo. 1996. *The culture of democracy: Language, literature, the arts and politics in Malawi, 1992–94*. Zomba, Malawi: WASI Publications.

Chimwenje, Dennis. 1990. Curriculum planning and decision-making process in secondary schools in Malawi. EdD thesis, University of Massachusetts at Amherst.

Chinsinga, Blessings. 2002. The politics of poverty alleviation in Malawi: A critical review. In *A democracy of chameleons: Politics and culture in the new Malawi*, ed. Harri Englund, 25–42. Uppsala, Sweden: Nordiska Afrikainstitutet (The Nordic Africa Institute).

Chipolombwe, John. 2004. Medical personnel knowledge, attitude and beliefs towards traditional medicine in Lilongwe. MBBS Year IV Project, on file with the Department of Community Health, College of Medicine, University of Malawi.

Chirwa, Wiseman Chijere. 1997. "No TEBA . . . Forget TEBA": The plight of Malawian ex-migrant workers to South Africa, 1988–1994. *International Migration Review* 31 (3): 628–54.

Chokani, Angela C. V. 1998. Local medicines audit: Reasons for going to the *sing'anga* first. MBBS Year IV Project, on file with the Department of Community Health, College of Medicine, University of Malawi.

Cole, Jennifer. 2003. Narratives and moral projects: Generational memories of the Malagasy 1947 rebellion. *Ethos* 31 (1): 95–126.

Comaroff, Jean. 1982. Medicine: Symbol and ideology. In *The problem of medical knowledge: Examining the social construction of medicine*, ed. Peter Wright and Andrew Treacher, 49–68. Edinburgh: Edinburgh University Press.

———. 1993. The diseased heart of Africa: Medicine, colonialism, and the black body. In *Knowledge, power and practice: The anthropology of medicine and everyday life*, ed. Shirley Lindenbaum and Margaret Lock, 305–29. Berkeley and Los Angeles: University of California Press.

Comaroff, Jean, and John Comaroff. 1991. *Of revelation and revolution: Christianity, colonialism, and consciousness in South Africa*. Chicago: University of Chicago Press.

———, eds. 1993. *Modernity and its malcontents: Ritual and power in postcolonial Africa*. Chicago: University of Chicago Press.

Conrad, Peter. 1988. Learning to doctor: Reflections on recent accounts of the medical school years. *Journal of Health and Social Behavior* 29 (12): 323–32.

Consten, E. C., J. J. van Lanschot, P. C. Henny, J. G. Tinnemans, and J. T. van der Meer. 1995. A prospective study on the risk of exposure to HIV during surgery in Zambia. *AIDS* 9 (6): 585–88.

Cunningham, Andrew, and Bridie Andrews. 1997. Introduction: Western medicine as contested knowledge. In *Western medicine as contested knowledge*, ed. Andrew Cunningham and Bridie Andrews, 1–23. Manchester: Manchester University Press.

Dahlenburg, Geoffrey W. 1993. Letter from . . . Malawi: The first year of the College of Medicine of the University of Malawi. *Tropical Doctor* 23:4–6.

Daston, Lorraine. 1995. The moral economy of science. *Osiris* 10:3–26.

Davenport, Beverly Ann. 2000. Witnessing and the medical gaze: How medical students learn to see at a clinic for the homeless. *Medical Anthropology Quarterly* 14 (3): 310–27.

Davies, Peter. 2002. The big picture of health. *Caduceus* 55 (Spring): 38–39.

Davis, Christopher O. 2000. *Death in abeyance: Illness and therapy among the Tabwa of central Africa*. Edinburgh: Edinburgh University Press.

———. *See also* Davis-Roberts, Christopher.

Davis-Floyd, Robbie E. 1992. *Birth as an American rite of passage*. Berkeley and Los Angeles: University of California Press.

———. 1998. Storying corporate futures: The Shell scenarios. In *Corporate futures: The diffusion of the culturally sensitive corporate form*, ed. George E. Marcus, 141–76. Chicago: University of Chicago Press.

Davis-Roberts, Christopher. 1992. *Kutambuwa ugonjuwa*: Concepts of illness and transformation among the Tabwa of Zaire. In *The social basis of health and healing in Africa*, ed. Steven Feierman and John Janzen, 376–92. Berkeley and Los Angeles: University of California Press.

Davison, Jean. 1993. School attainment and gender: Attitudes of Kenyan and Malawian parents toward educating girls. *International Journal of Educational Development* 13 (4): 331–38.

De Craemer, Willy, and Renée C. Fox. 1968. *The emerging physician*. Stanford, CA: The Hoover Institution on War, Revolution and Peace.

de Laet, Marianne, and Annemarie Mol. 2000. The Zimbabwe bush pump: Mechanics of a fluid technology. *Social Studies of Science* 30 (2): 225–63.

Dillman, Don A. 1983. Mail and other self-administered questionnaires. In *Handbook of survey research*, ed. Peter H. Rossi, James D. Wright, and Andy B. Anderson, 359–78. New York: Academic Press.

Doran, Marissa C. M. 2007. Reconstructing *Mchape '95*: AIDS, Billy Chisupe, and the politics of persuasion. *Journal of Eastern African Studies* 1 (3): 397–416.

Dufort, Francine, and Brigitte Maheux. 1995. When female medical students are the majority: Do numbers really make a difference? *Journal of the American Medical Women's Association* 50 (1): 4–6.

Dyrbye, Liselotte N., Matthew R. Thomas, and Tait D. Shanafelt. 2006. Systematic review of depression, anxiety, and other indicators of psychological distress among U.S. and Canadian medical students. *Academic Medicine* 81 (4): 354–73.

Englund, Harri. 1996. Witchcraft, modernity and the person: The morality of accumulation in central Malawi. *Critique of Anthropology* 16 (3): 257–79.

———. 1998. Death, trauma and ritual: Mozambican refugees in Malawi. *Social Science and Medicine* 46 (9): 1165–74.

———. 2006. *Prisoners of freedom: Human rights and the African poor.* Berkeley and Los Angeles: University of California Press.

Enstad, Nan. 2009. On grief and complicity: Notes toward a visionary cultural history. In *The cultural turn in U.S. history: Past, present, and future*, ed. James W. Cook, Lawrence B. Glickman, and Michael O'Malley, 319–42. Chicago: University of Chicago Press.

Errington, Frederick, and Deborah Gewertz. 2004. *Yali's question: Sugar, culture, and history.* Chicago: University of Chicago Press.

Escobar, Arturo. 1992. Imagining a post-development era? Critical thought, development and social movements. *Social Text* 31–32:20–56.

Evans, Imogen. 1995. SAPping maternal health. *Lancet* 346 (8982): 1046.

Evans-Pritchard, E. E. 1937. *Witchcraft, oracles and magic among the Azande.* Oxford, UK: Clarendon Press.

Farmer, Paul. 1999. *Infections and inequalities: The modern plagues.* Berkeley and Los Angeles: University of California Press.

———. 2004. An anthropology of structural violence: Sidney W. Mintz lecture for 2001. *Current Anthropology* 45 (3): 305–25.

Fausto-Sterling, Anne. 1993. The five sexes: Why male and female are not enough. *The Sciences*, March–April, 20–24.

Feierman, Steven. 1985. Struggles for control: The social roots of health and healing in modern Africa. *African Studies Review* 28 (2–3): 73–147.

———. 1990. *Peasant intellectuals: Anthropology and history in Tanzania.* Madison: University of Wisconsin Press.

———. 1995. Healing as social criticism in the time of colonial conquest. *African Studies* 54 (1): 73–88.

———. 2006. Afterword: Ethnographic regions—healing, power, and history. In *Borders and healers: Brokering therapeutic resources in southeast Africa*, ed. Tracy J. Luedke and Harry G. West, 185–94. Bloomington: Indiana University Press.

Feldman, Kenneth A., and Theodore M. Newcomb. 1969. *The impact of college on students*. San Francisco: Jossey-Bass.

Ferguson, James. 1990. *The anti-politics machine: "Development," depoliticization, and bureaucratic power in Lesotho*. Cambridge, UK: Cambridge University Press.

———. 1999. *Expectations of modernity: Myths and meanings of urban life on the Zambian copperbelt*. Berkeley and Los Angeles: University of California Press.

Feudtner, Chris, and Dimitri A. Christakis. 1994. Making the rounds: The ethical development of medical students in the context of clinical rotations. *Hastings Center Report* 24 (1): 6–12.

Feudtner, Chris, Dimitri A. Christakis, and Nicholas A. Christakis. 1994. Do clinical clerks suffer ethical erosion? Students' perceptions of their ethical environment and personal development. *Academic Medicine* 69:670–79.

Finkler, Kaja. 1991. *Physicians at work, patients in pain: Biomedical practice and patient response in Mexico*. Boulder, CO: Westview Press.

Flint, Karen. 2001a. Competition, race, and professionalization: African healers and white medical practitioners in Natal, South Africa, in the early twentieth century. *Social History of Medicine* 14 (2): 199–221.

———. 2001b. Negotiating a hybrid medical culture: African healers in southeastern Africa from the 1820s to the 1940s. PhD diss. in history, University of California at Los Angeles.

Forster, Peter G. 1994. Culture, nationalism, and the invention of tradition in Malawi. *Journal of Modern African Studies* 32 (3): 477–97.

———. 1997. Religion and the state in Tanzania and Malawi. *Journal of Asian and African Studies* 32 (3–4): 163–84.

Fortin, Alfred J. 1991. Ethics, culture, and medical power: AIDS research in the Third World. *AIDS and Public Policy Journal* 6 (1): 15–24.

Foucault, Michel. 1975. *The birth of the clinic: An archaeology of medical perception*. New York: Vintage Books.

Fox, Renée C. 1957. Training for uncertainty. In *The student-physician: Introductory studies in the sociology of medical education*, ed. Robert K. Merton, George G. Reader, and Patricia L. Kendall, 207–41. Cambridge, MA: Harvard University Press.

———. 1979. *Essays in medical sociology: Journeys into the field*. New York: John Wiley.

———. 1989. *The sociology of medicine: A participant observer's view*. Englewood Cliffs, NJ: Prentice-Hall.

Fox, Renée C., and J. P. Swazey. 1984. Medical morality is not bioethics—medical ethics in China and the United States. *Perspectives in Biology and Medicine* 27 (3): 336–60.

Frankenberg, Ronald. 1988. Rejoinder. *Medical Anthropology Quarterly* 2 (4): 454–59.

Frankenberg, Ronald, and Joyce Leeson. 1974. The sociology of health dilemmas in the post-colonial world: Intermediate technology and medical care in Zambia, Zaire, and China. In *Sociology and development*, ed. Emanuel de Kadt and Gavin Williams, 255–78. London: Tavistock.

Friedman, Jonathan. 1999. Indigenous struggles and the discreet charm of the bourgeoisie. *Journal of World-Systems Research* 5 (2): 391–411.

Friedson, Steven M. 1996. *Dancing prophets: Musical experience in Tumbuka healing*. Chicago: University of Chicago Press.

Fujimura, Joan H. 2006. Sex genes: A critical sociomaterial approach to the politics and
    molecular genetics of sex determination. *Signs: Journal of Women in Culture and
    Society* 32 (1): 49–82.
Fuller, Bruce. 1991. *Growing up modern: The Western state builds Third-World schools.*
    London: Routledge.
Gallagher, Eugene B. 1988. Convergence or divergence in Third World medical education?
    An Arab study. *Journal of Health and Social Behavior* 29:385–400.
———. 1993. Curricular goals and student aspirations in a new Arab medical college. In
    Health and health care in developing countries: Sociological perspectives, ed. Peter
    Conrad and Eugene B. Gallagher, 135–53. Philadelphia: Temple University Press.
Gawande, Atul. 2002. *Complications: A surgeon's notes on an imperfect science.* New
    York: Henry Holt and Company.
Geertz, Clifford. 1988. *Works and lives: The anthropologist as author.* Stanford, CA:
    Stanford University Press.
———. 2000. *Available light: Anthropological reflections on philosophical topics.* Prince-
    ton, NJ: Princeton University Press.
Geissler, P. Wenzel. 2005. "*Kachinja* are coming!": Encounters around medical research
    work in a Kenyan village. *Africa* 75 (2): 173–202.
Geschiere, Peter. 1997. *The modernity of witchcraft: Politics and the occult in postcolo-
    nial Africa.* Charlottesville: University of Virginia Press.
Gibson-Graham, J. K. 1996. *The end of capitalism (as we knew it): A feminist critique of
    political economy.* Oxford, UK: Blackwell.
Gilman, Sander L. 1999. *Making the body beautiful: A cultural history of aesthetic sur-
    gery.* Princeton, NJ: Princeton University Press.
Gisselquist, David, Richard Rothenberg, John Potterat, and Ernest Drucker. 2002. HIV
    infections in sub-Saharan Africa not explained by sexual or vertical transmission.
    International Journal of STD and AIDS 13 (10): 657–66.
Glaser, Barney G., and Anselm L. Strauss. 1967. *The discovery of grounded theory: Strat-
    egies for qualitative research.* Chicago: Aldine.
Goffman, Erving. 1961. *Asylums: Essays on the social situation of mental patients and
    other inmates.* Garden City, NY: Doubleday.
Goldstein, Michael S., and Peter J. Donaldson. 1979. Exporting professionalism: A case
    study of medical education. *Journal of Health and Social Behavior* 20 (4): 322–37.
Good, Byron J. 1994. *Medicine, rationality and experience: An anthropological perspec-
    tive.* Cambridge, UK: Cambridge University Press.
Good, Byron J., and Mary-Jo DelVecchio Good. 1993. "Learning medicine": The con-
    structing of medical knowledge at Harvard Medical School. In *Knowledge, power and
    practice: The anthropology of medicine and everyday life,* ed. Shirley Lindenbaum
    and Margaret Lock, 81–107. Berkeley and Los Angeles: University of California Press.
Gordon, Deborah R. 1988. Tenacious assumptions in Western medicine. In *Biomedicine
    examined,* ed. Margaret Lock and Deborah Gordon, 19–56. Dordrecht, Netherlands:
    Kluwer Academic Publishers.
Gould, Stephen Jay. 1996. *The mismeasure of man.* Rev. and exp. ed. New York:
    W. W. Norton.

Gramsci, Antonio. 1971. *Selections from the prison notebooks*. Ed. Quintin Hoare and Geoffrey Newell-Smith. London: Lawrence and Wishart.

———. 1988. *The Antonio Gramsci reader: Selected writings, 1916–1935*. Ed. David Forgacs. New York: New York University Press.

Groopman, Jerome. 2007. *How doctors think*. New York: Houghton Mifflin.

Gupta, Akhil. 1998. *Postcolonial developments: Agriculture in the making of modern India*. Durham, NC: Duke University Press.

Gusau, G. A. 1994. Physician training and health care in post-colonial Nigeria. In *Physicians and health care in the Third World*, ed. Antonio Ugalde and S. Ogoh Alubo, 19–38. Williamsburg, VA: Department of Anthropology, College of William and Mary.

Haas, Jack, and William Shaffir. 1977. The professionalization of medical students: Developing competence and a cloak of competence. *Symbolic Interaction* 1 (1): 71–88.

Hafferty, Frederic W. 1988. Cadaver stories and the emotional socialization of medical students. *Journal of Health and Social Behavior* 29:344–56.

———. 1991. *Into the valley: Death and the socialization of medical students*. New Haven, CT: Yale University Press.

Hafferty, Frederic W., and Ronald Franks. 1994. The hidden curriculum, ethics teaching, and the structure of medical education. *Academic Medicine* 69 (11): 861–71.

Hahn, Robert A. 1987. Divisions of labor: Obstetrician, woman, and society in *Williams Obstetrics*, 1903–1985. *Medical Anthropology Quarterly* 1 (3): 256–82.

Haiken, Elizabeth. 1997. *Venus envy: A history of cosmetic surgery*. Baltimore and London: Johns Hopkins University Press.

Hango, Ruben Dyson. 2004. Changes and challenges facing the education system in Malawi, 1994–2003. *Malawi Update Newsletter*, January 13. http://www.malawi-update.org/docs/EducationSystem.doc.

Hansen, Karen Tranberg. 2000. *Salaula: The world of secondhand clothing and Zambia*. Chicago: University of Chicago Press.

Haraway, Donna J. 1988. Situated knowledges: The science question in feminism and the privilege of partial perspective. *Feminist Studies* 14 (3): 575–600.

———. 1989. *Primate visions: Gender, race, and nature in the world of modern science*. New York: Routledge.

———. 1992. The promises of monsters: A regenerative politics for inappropriate/d others. In *Cultural studies*, ed. Lawrence Grossberg, Cary Nelson, and Paula A. Treichler, 295–337. New York: Routledge.

Harries, A. D. 2002. High death rates in health care workers and teachers in Malawi. *Transactions of the Royal Society of Tropical Medicine and Hygiene* 96:34–37.

Hawkins, Anne Hunsaker. 2002. The idea of character. In *Stories matter: The role of narrative in medical ethics*, ed. Rita Charon and Martha Montello, 69–76. New York: Routledge.

Heath, Deborah, Rayna Rapp, and Karen-Sue Taussig. 2004. Genetic citizenship. In *A companion to the anthropology of politics*, ed. David Nugent and Joan Vincent, 152–67. London: Blackwell.

Helkama, Klaus, Antti Uutela, Esa Pohjanheimo, Simo Salminen, Anne Koponen, and Leena Rantánen-Väntsi. 2003. Moral reasoning and values in medical school:

A longitudinal study in Finland. *Scandinavian Journal of Educational Research* 47 (4): 399–411.

Henderson, Clara. 1996. A contribution to the discourse on "colonial situations": Hastings Kamuzu Banda's interaction with ethnographers and laypersons in America during the 1930s. *Resound: A Quarterly of the Archives of Traditional Music* 15 (1–2): 1–10.

Hill, Amelia. 2001. Blantyre, where the living is easy, named the world's best city. *Guardian Weekly*, April 19–25, 11.

Hochschild, Adam. 1998. *King Leopold's ghost: A story of greed, terror, and heroism in colonial Africa.* New York: Houghton Mifflin.

Hojat, Mohammedreza, Salvatore Mangione, Thomas J. Nasca, Susan Rattner, James B. Erdmann, Joseph S. Gonella, and Mike Magee. 2004. An empirical study of decline in empathy in medical school. *Medical Education* 38 (9): 934–41.

Hokkanen, Markku. 2004. Scottish missionaries and African healers: Perceptions and relations in the Livingstonia mission, 1875–1930. *Journal of Religion in Africa* 34 (3): 320–47.

Horn, David G. 1995. This norm which is not one: Reading the female body in Lombroso's anthropology. In *Deviant bodies: Critical perspectives on difference in science and popular culture*, ed. Jennifer Terry and Jacqueline Urla, 109–28. Bloomington and Indianapolis: Indiana University Press.

Hunt, Nancy Rose. 1999. *A colonial lexicon of birth ritual, medicalization, and mobility in the Congo.* Durham, NC: Duke University Press.

Hunter, Robert E., C. Ross Anthony, and Nicole Lurie. 2002. Make world health the new Marshall Plan. *RAND Review* (Summer). http://www.rand.org/publications/randreview/issues/rr.08.02/worldhealth.html.

Huntington, Mary Jean. 1957. The development of a professional self-image. In *The student-physician: Introductory studies in the sociology of medical education*, ed. Robert K. Merton, George G. Reader, and Patricia L. Kendall, 179–87. Cambridge, MA: Harvard University Press.

Hutchinson, Sharon E. 1996. *Nuer dilemmas: Coping with money, war, and the state.* Berkeley and Los Angeles: University of California Press.

Hyppölä, Harri, Esko Kumpusalo, Liisa Neittaanmäki, Kari Mattila, Irma Virjo, Santero Kujala, Riitta Luhtala, Hannu Halila, and Mauri Isokoski. 1998. Becoming a doctor—Was it the wrong career choice? *Social Science and Medicine* 47 (9): 1383–87.

Iliffe, John. 1998. *East African doctors: A history of the modern profession.* Cambridge, UK: Cambridge University Press.

Illich, Ivan. 1976. *Medical nemesis: The expropriation of health.* New York: Pantheon Books.

Imber, Jonathan B. 1998. Medical publicity before bioethics: Nineteenth-century illustrations of twentieth-century dilemmas. In *Bioethics and society: Constructing the ethical enterprise*, ed. Raymond DeVries and Janardan Subedi, 16–37. Upper Saddle River, NJ: Prentice Hall.

The Institute of Medicine. 2000. *To err is human: Building a safer health system.* Washington, DC: National Academy Press.

Jackson, Barbara, and Antonio Ugalde. 1987. Health development and technologies: An appraisal. In *The impact of development and modern technologies in Third World health*, ed. Barbara E. Jackson and Antonio Ugalde, ix–xviii. Williamsburg, VA: Department of Anthropology, College of William and Mary.

Janzen, John M. 1978. *The quest for therapy: Medical pluralism in lower Zaire*. Berkeley and Los Angeles: University of California Press.

———. 1982. *Lemba, 1650–1930: A drum of affliction in Africa and the New World*. New York: Garland Publishing.

———. 1992. *Ngoma: Discourses of healing in central and southern Africa*. Berkeley and Los Angeles: University of California Press.

Jeal, Tim. 1973. *Livingstone*. London: Heinemann.

Jefferys, Margot, and Mary Ann Elston. 1989. The medical school as a social organization. *Medical Education* 23 (3): 242–51.

Johnston, Sir Harry H. 1898. *British Central Africa: An attempt to give some account of a portion of the territories under British influence north of the Zambesi*. London: Methuen & Co.

Jordan, Brigitte. 1993. *Birth in four cultures: A crosscultural investigation of childbirth in Yucatan, Holland, Sweden and the United States*. Prospect Heights, IL: Waveland Press.

Jovic, Emily, Jean E. Wallace, and Jane Lemaire. 2006. The generation and gender shifts in medicine: An exploratory survey of internal medicine physicians. *BMC Health Services Research* 6:e55.

Justice, Judith. 1999. Neglect of cultural knowledge in health planning: Nepal's assistant nurse-midwife program. In *Anthropology in public health: Bridging differences in culture and society*, ed. Robert A. Hahn, 327–44. New York: Oxford University Press.

Kaspin, Deborah. 1993. Chewa visions and revisions of power: Transformations of the Nyau dance in central Malawi. In *Modernity and its malcontents: Ritual and power in postcolonial Africa*, ed. Jean Comaroff and John Comaroff, 34–57. Chicago: University of Chicago Press.

———. 1996. A Chewa cosmology of the body. *American Ethnologist* 23 (3): 561–78.

Kaufman, Sharon R. 1993. *The healer's tale: Transforming medicine and culture*. Madison: University of Wisconsin Press.

Keller, Richard C. 2006. Geographies of power, legacies of mistrust: Colonial medicine in the global present. *Historical Geography* 34:26–48.

Killingray, David. 2003. The Black Atlantic missionary movement and Africa, 1780s–1920s. *Journal of Religion in Africa* 33 (1): 3–31.

Kim, Jim Yong, Joyce V. Millen, Alec Irwin, and John Gershman, eds. 2000. *Dying for growth: Global inequality and the health of the poor*. Monroe, ME: Common Courage Press.

King, Michael, and Elspeth King. 1992. *The story of medicine and disease in Malawi: The 150 years since Livingstone*. Blantyre, Malawi: Montfort Press.

———. 2000. *The great rift*. Cambridge, UK: Arco Publishing.

Kitching, Gavin. 2000. Why I gave up African studies. *African Studies Review and Newsletter* 22 (1): 21–26.

Klass, Perri. 1987. *A not entirely benign procedure: Four years as a medical student*. New York: Putnam.

Kleinman, Arthur. 1993. What is specific to Western medicine? In *Companion encyclo-pedia of the history of medicine*, ed. W. F. Bynum and Roy Porter, 15–23. London: Routledge.

———. 1999. Moral experience and ethical reflection: Can ethnography reconcile them? A quandary for "the new bioethics." *Daedalus* 128 (4): 69–97.

———. 2009. Care-giving and the moral impoverishment of medicine. Project Syndicate. http://www.project-syndicate.org/commentary/kleinman1.

Kohler, Robert E. 1999. Moral economy, material culture, and community in *Drosophila* genetics. In *The science studies reader*, ed. Mario Biagioli, 243–57. New York: Routledge.

Kolko, Gabriel. 1999. Ravaging the poor: The International Monetary Fund indicted by its own data. *International Journal of Health Services* 29 (1): 51–57.

Konner, Melvin. 1987. *Becoming a doctor: A journey of initiation in medical school.* New York: Viking.

Kressin, Nancy R. 1996. The effect of medical socialization on medical students' need for power. *Personality and Social Psychology Bulletin* 22 (1): 91–98.

Krieger, Nancy, and George Davey Smith. 2004. "Bodies count," and body counts: Social epidemiology and embodying inequality. *Epidemiologic Reviews* 26:92–103.

Lamport-Stokes, Barbara. 1989. *Blantyre: Glimpses of the early days*. Blantyre, Malawi: Society of Malawi, Historical and Scientific.

Langwick, Stacey. 2006. Geographies of medicine: Interrogating the boundary between "traditional" and "modern" medicine in colonial Tanganyika. In *Borders and healers: Brokering therapeutic resources in southeast Africa*, ed. Tracy J. Luedke and Harry G. West, 143–65. Bloomington: Indiana University Press.

Leape, Lucian L., and Donald M. Berwick. 2005. Five years after *To err is human*: What have we learned? *JAMA: Journal of the American Medical Association* 293 (19): 2384–90.

LeBaron, Charles. 1981. *Gentle vengeance: An account of the first year at Harvard Medical School*. New York: Penguin.

Leserman, Jane. 1981. *Men and women in medical school: How they change and how they compare*. New York: Praeger.

Lester, Rebecca J. 2005. *Jesus in our wombs: Embodying modernity in a Mexican convent*. Berkeley and Los Angeles: University of California Press.

Lewis, Bradley. 2007. The new global health movement: Rx for the world? *New Literary History* 38 (3): 459–77.

Light, Donald. 1980. *Becoming psychiatrists: The professional transformation of self*. New York: Norton.

Likert, R. 1932. A technique for the measurement of attitudes. *Archives of Psychology* 140:5–53.

Linde, Paul R. 2002. *Of spirits and madness: An American psychiatrist in Africa*. New York: McGraw-Hill.

Lindenbaum, Shirley, and Margaret Lock, eds. 1993. *Knowledge, power and practice: The anthropology of medicine and everyday life*. Berkeley and Los Angeles: University of California Press.

Livingston, Julie. 2005. *Debility and the moral imagination in Botswana*. Bloomington: Indiana University Press.

Lo, Ming-Cheng M. 2002. *Doctors within borders: Profession, ethnicity, and modernity in colonial Taiwan*. Berkeley and Los Angeles: University of California Press.

Lock, Margaret. 2002. *Twice dead: Organ transplants and the reinvention of death*. Berkeley and Los Angeles: University of California Press.

Lock, Margaret, and Deborah Gordon. 1988. *Biomedicine examined*. Dordrecht, Netherlands: Kluwer Academic Publishers.

Lock, Margaret, and Nancy Scheper-Hughes. 1996. A critical-interpretive approach in medical anthropology: Rituals and routines of discipline and dissent. In *Medical anthropology: Contemporary theory and method*, rev. ed., ed. Carolyn F. Sargent and Thomas M. Johnson, 41–70. Westport, CT: Praeger.

Ludmerer, Kenneth M. 1999. *Time to heal: American medical education from the turn of the century to the era of managed care*. Oxford, UK: Oxford University Press.

Luedke, Tracy J. 2006. Presidents, bishops, and mothers: The construction of authority in Mozambican healing. In *Borders and healers: Brokering therapeutic resources in southeast Africa*, ed. Tracy J. Luedke and Harry G. West, 43–64. Bloomington: Indiana University Press.

Luhrmann, T. M. 2001. *Of two minds: An anthropologist looks at American psychiatry*. New York: Vintage Books.

Luke, Haida. 2003. *Medical education and sociology of medical habitus: "It's not about the stethoscope!"* Dordrecht, Netherlands: Kluwer Academic Publishers.

Lupton, Deborah. 2003. *Medicine as culture: Illness, disease and the body in Western societies*. 2nd ed. London: Sage Publications.

Lutz, Catherine. 1992. Motivated models. In *Human motives and cultural models*, ed. Roy D'Andrade and Claudia Strauss, 181–90. Cambridge, UK: Cambridge University Press.

Lwanda, John. 2005. *Politics, culture and medicine in Malawi: Historical continuities and ruptures with special reference to HIV/AIDS*. Zomba, Malawi: Kachere.

Lyons, Maryinez. 1992. *The colonial disease: A social history of sleeping sickness in northern Zaire, 1900–1940*. Cambridge, UK: Cambridge University Press.

Macdonald, Roderick J. 1975. Rev. Dr. Daniel Sharpe Malekebu and the re-opening of the Providence Industrial Mission, 1926–39: An appreciation. In *From Nyasaland to Malawi: Studies in colonial history*, ed. Roderick J. Macdonald, 215–33. Nairobi: East African Publishing House.

Mackintosh, Maureen. 2001. Do health care systems contribute to inequalities? In *Poverty, inequality, and health: An international perspective*, ed. David Leon and Gill Walt, 175–93. Oxford, UK: Oxford University Press.

MacLeod, Roy, and Milton Lewis, eds. 1988. *Disease, medicine, and empire: Perspectives on Western medicine and the experience of European expansion*. London and New York: Routledge.

Maheux, B., and F. Beland. 1987. Changes in students' sociopolitical attitudes during medical school: Socialization or maturation effect? *Social Science and Medicine* 24 (7): 619–24.

Maier, Birga. 1988. Gesundheit für Alle und Kolonisierung für Wenige—das Dilemma der traditionellen Medizin? *Curare* 11 (4): 196–206.

Malawi Ministry of Information. 2001. Home page. http://www.maform.malawinet.com.

Marks, Shula. 1994. *Divided sisterhood: Race, class and gender in the South African nursing profession.* New York: St. Martin's Press.

Marks, Shula, and Neil Andersson. 1992. Industrialization, rural health, and the 1944 National Health Services Commission in South Africa. In *The social basis of health and healing in Africa,* ed. Steven Feierman and John M. Janzen, 131–61. Berkeley and Los Angeles: University of California Press.

Marsh, B. D. 2008. "Multiracial partnership" and African health care in the Central African Federation, 1953–1963. In *Health knowledge and belief systems in Africa,* ed. Toyin Falola and Matthew M. Heaton, 261–76. Durham, NC: Carolina Academic Press.

Martin, Emily. 1987. *The woman in the body: A cultural analysis of reproduction.* Boston: Beacon Press.

———. 1990. Toward an anthropology of immunology: The body as nation state. *Medical Anthropology Quarterly* 4 (4): 410–26.

———. 2006. The pharmaceutical person. *BioSocieties* 1:273–87.

Marwick, M. G. 1952. The social context of Cewa witch beliefs. *Africa* 22 (2): 120–35.

Marx, Karl, and Friedrich Engels. 1970. *The German ideology: Part one: With selections from parts two and three, together with Marx's "Introduction to a critique of political economy."* Ed. and with an intro. by C. J. Arthur. New York: International Publishers. (Orig. written 1845; first pub. 1932.)

Masambo, L., Y. Chimalizeni, P. Kayange, and A. Nyaka. 2004. The cost of congenital heart disease (letter). *Malawi Medical Journal* 13 (3): 53.

Matos, Narciso. 2000. The nature of learning, teaching and research in higher education in Africa. In *African voices in education,* ed. P. Higgs, N.C.G. Vakalisa, T. V. Mda, and N. T. Assie-Lumumba, 12–38. Lansdowne, Cape Town: Juta & Co.

Mattingly, Cheryl. 1998. *Healing dramas and clinical plots: The narrative structure of experience.* Cambridge, UK: Cambridge University Press.

Mauss, Marcel. 1973. Techniques of the body. Trans. Ben Brewster. *Economy and Society* 2 (1): 70–88.

McCracken, John. 1998. Blantyre transformed: Class, conflict and nationalism in urban Malawi. *Journal of African History* 39:247–69.

Merton, Robert K., George G. Reader, and Patricia L. Kendall, eds. 1957. *The student-physician: Introductory studies in the sociology of medical education.* Cambridge, MA: Harvard University Press.

Mizrahi, Terry. 1986. *Getting rid of patients: Contradictions in the socialization of physicians.* New Brunswick, NJ: Rutgers University Press.

Morgan, Lynn M. 1998. Latin American social medicine and the politics of theory. In *Building a new biocultural synthesis: Political-economic perspectives on human biology,* ed. Alan H. Goodman and Thomas L. Leatherman, 407–24. Ann Arbor: University of Michigan Press.

Morsy, Soheir A. 1988. Islamic clinics in Egypt: The cultural elaboration of biomedical hegemony. *Medical Anthropology Quarterly* 2 (4): 355–69.

————. 1996. Political economy in medical anthropology. In *Medical anthropology: Contemporary theory and method*, rev. ed., ed. Carolyn F. Sargent and Thomas M. Johnson, 21–40. Westport, CT: Praeger.

Mulwafu, Wakisa, and Adamson Muula. 2001. *The first medical school in Malawi.* Lilongwe, Malawi: Sunrise Publications.

Munthali, Gedion. 2002. No blood hunters around—Muluzi. *Nation* (Malawi), December 23, 1.

Mutha, Sunita, and John I. Takayama, with Edward H. O'Neil. 1997. Insights into medical students' career choices based on third- and fourth-year students' focus-group discussions. *Academic Medicine* 72 (7): 635–40.

Muula, Adamson S. 2005. Five-year experience of Malawi College of Medicine with "Learning by Living" program. *Croatian Medical Journal* 46 (6): 1010–14.

Muula, Adamson S., and Robert L. Broadhead. 2001. The first decade of the Malawi College of Medicine: A critical appraisal. *Tropical Medicine and International Health* 6 (2): 155–59.

Mwanza, Gollie Mkhutchwa. 1982. Traditional and Western medicine in a changing society: The Jandalala case studies. In University of Malawi final year sociology research papers, 1981–1982. Available at Malawiana archives, Chancellor College, University of Malawi, Zomba.

Nagel, Thomas. 1986. *The view from nowhere.* New York: Oxford University Press.

Nandy, Ashis. 1988. Introduction: Science as a reason of state. In *Science, hegemony and violence: A requiem for modernity*, ed. Ashis Nandy, 1–23. Delhi: Oxford University Press.

National Statistical Office [Malawi] and ORC Macro. 2001. *Malawi Demographic and Health Survey 2000.* Zomba, Malawi, and Calverton, MD: National Statistical Office and ORC Macro.

————. 2005. *Malawi Demographic and Health Survey 2004.* Calverton, MD: NSO and ORC Macro.

Newbury-Birch, Dorothy, David Walshaw, and Farhad Kamali. 2001. Drink and drugs: From medical students to doctors. *Drug and Alcohol Dependence* 64 (3): 265–70.

Newton, Bruce W., Laurie Barber, James Clardy, Elton Cleveland, and Patricia O'Sullivan. 2008. Is there hardening of the heart during medical school? *Academic Medicine* 83 (3): 244–49.

Ngalande Banda, Elias E., and Henry P. M. Simukonda. 1994. The public-private mix in the health care system in Malawi. *Health Policy and Planning* 9 (1): 63–71.

Nguyen, Vinh-Kim. 2005. Antiretroviral globalism, biopolitics, and therapeutic citizenship. In *Global assemblages: Technology, politics, and ethics as anthropological problems*, ed. Aihwa Ong and Stephen J. Collier, 124–44. Malden, MA: Blackwell.

Nussbaum, Martha C. 2001. *Upheavals of thought: The intelligence of emotions.* Cambridge, UK: Cambridge University Press.

Ooms, Gorik, Wim Van Damme, and Marleen Temmerman. 2007. Medicines without doctors: Why the Global Fund must fund salaries of health workers to expand AIDS treatment. *PLoS Medicine* 4 (4): e128.

The overseas elective: Purpose or picnic? 1993. *Lancet* 342 (8874): 753–54.

Pachai, Bridglal. 1973. *Malawi: The history of the nation.* London: Longman.

Pakenham, Thomas. 1991. *The scramble for Africa: White man's conquest of the dark continent from 1876 to 1912.* London: Weidenfield and Nicolson.

Paley, Julia. 2001. *Marketing democracy: Power and social movements in post-dictatorship Chile.* Berkeley and Los Angeles: University of California Press.

Parsons, Genevieve Noone, Sara B. Kinsman, Charles L. Bosk, Pamela Sankar, and Peter A. Ubel. 2001. Between two worlds: Medical student perceptions of humor and slang in the hospital setting. *Journal of General Internal Medicine* 16 (8): 544–49.

Patton, Adell, Jr. 1982. Howard University and Meharry medical schools in the training of African physicians, 1868–1978. In *Global dimensions of the African diaspora,* ed. Joseph E. Harris, 142–62. Washington, DC: Howard University Press.

Peard, Julyan G. 1997. Tropical disorders and the forging of a Brazilian medical identity, 1860–1890. *Hispanic American Historical Review* 77 (1): 1–44.

Perry, William G., Jr. 1968. *Forms of intellectual and ethical development in the college years: A scheme.* New York: Holt, Rinehart and Winston.

Petersen, Alan, and Deborah Lupton. 1996. *The new public health: Health and self in the age of risk.* London: SAGE Publications.

Petryna, Adriana. 2002. *Life exposed: Biological citizens after Chernobyl.* Princeton, NJ: Princeton University Press.

———. 2009. *When experiments travel: Clinical trials and the global search for human subjects.* Princeton, NJ: Princeton University Press.

Pfeiffer, James. 2002. African independent churches in Mozambique: Healing the afflictions of inequality. *Medical Anthropology Quarterly* 16 (2): 176–99.

———. 2003. International NGOs and primary health care in Mozambique: The need for a new model of collaboration. *Social Science and Medicine* 56:725–38.

———. 2006. Money, modernity, and morality: Traditional healing and the expansion of the Holy Spirit in Mozambique. In *Borders and healers: Brokering therapeutic resources in southeast Africa,* ed. Tracy J. Luedke and Harry G. West, 81–100. Bloomington: Indiana University Press.

Phiri, Isabel Apawo. 2000. Gender and academic freedom in Malawi. In *Women in academia: Gender and academic freedom in Africa,* ed. Ebrima Sall, 47–63. Dakar: CODESRIA.

Pickering, Andrew, ed. 1992. *Science as practice and culture.* Chicago: University of Chicago Press.

Pigg, Stacy Leigh. 1997. "Found in most traditional societies": Traditional medical practitioners between culture and development. In *International development and the social sciences: Essays on the history and politics of knowledge,* ed. Frederick Cooper and Randall Packard, 259–90. Berkeley and Los Angeles: University of California Press.

Piller, Charles, and Doug Smith. 2007. Unintended victims of Gates Foundation generosity. *Los Angeles Times,* December 16. http://www.latimes.com/news/nationworld/nation/la-na-gates16dec16,0,3743924.story.

Planning Unit, Ministry of Health and Management Sciences for Health. 1984. Medical school feasibility study and alternative solutions. Technical document A-2. Available at Malawiana archives, Chancellor College, University of Malawi, Zomba.

Pollock, Donald. 1996. Training tales: U.S. medical autobiography. *Cultural Anthropology* 11 (3): 339–61.

Posner, Daniel N. 1995. Malawi's new dawn. *Journal of Democracy* 6 (1): 131–45.

Pratt, Mary Louise. 1986. Fieldwork in common places. In *Writing culture: The poetics and politics of ethnography*, ed. James Clifford and George E. Marcus, 27–50. Berkeley and Los Angeles: University of California Press.

Prentice, Rachel. 2007. Drilling surgeons: The social lessons of embodied surgical learning. *Science, Technology, and Human Values* 32:534–53.

———. Forthcoming. *Bodies in formation: An ethnography of anatomy and surgery training and practice*. Durham, NC: Duke University Press.

Prins, Gwyn. 1992. A modern history of Lozi therapeutics. In *The social basis of health and healing in Africa*, ed. Steven Feierman and John M. Janzen, 339–65. Berkeley and Los Angeles: University of California Press.

Probst, Peter. 1999. *Mchape '95*, or, the sudden fame of Billy Goodson Chisupe: Healing, social memory and the enigma of the public sphere in post-Banda Malawi. *Africa* 69 (1): 108–38.

Qualitative Solutions and Research International. 2002. QSR N6 Student. Doncaster, Victoria, Australia.

Rafael, B. R. 1980. *A short history of Malawi*. Limbe, Malawi: Popular Publications.

Ranger, Terence O. 1981. Godly medicine: The ambiguities of medical mission in southeast Tanzania, 1900–1945. *Social Science and Medicine* 15B:261–77.

———. 1992. Plagues of beasts and men: Prophetic responses to epidemic in eastern and southern Africa. In *Epidemics and ideas: Essays on the historical perception of pestilence*, ed. Terence Ranger and Paul Slack, 241–68. Cambridge, UK: Cambridge University Press.

Ranis, Gustav, Frances Stewart, and Alejandro Ramirez. 2000. Economic growth and human development. *World Development* 28 (2): 197–219.

Rapp, Rayna. 1999. *Testing women, testing the fetus: The social impact of amniocentesis in America*. New York: Routledge.

Redmayne, Alison. 1970. Chikanga: An African diviner with an international reputation. In *Witchcraft confessions and accusations*, ed. Mary Douglas, 103–28. London: Tavistock.

Reis, Ria. 2000. The "wounded healer" as ideology: The work of Ngoma in Swaziland. In *The quest for fruition through Ngoma: The political aspects of healing in southern Africa*, ed. Rijk van Dijk, Ria Reis, and Marja Spierenburg, 61–75. Athens: Ohio University Press.

Reiser, Stanley Joel. 1978. *Medicine and the reign of technology*. Cambridge, UK: Cambridge University Press.

———. 1993. Science, pedagogy, and the transformation of empathy in medicine. In *Empathy and the practice of medicine: Beyond pills and the scalpel*, ed. Howard M. Spiro, Mary G. McCrea Curnen, Enid Peschel, and Deborah St. James, 121–32. New Haven, CT: Yale University Press.

Rennie, S. C., and J. R. Crosby. 2001. Are "tomorrow's doctors" honest? Questionnaire study exploring medical students' attitudes and reported behaviour on academic misconduct. *BMJ: British Medical Journal* 322:274–75.

Rhodes, Lorna Amarasingham. 1996. Studying biomedicine as a cultural system. In *Medical anthropology: Contemporary theory and method*, rev. ed., ed. Carolyn F. Sargent and Thomas M. Johnson, 165–80. Westport, CT: Praeger.

Richards, Audrey I. 1935. A modern movement of witch-finders. *Africa* 8 (4): 448–61.

Robichaud, Allyson. 2003. Healing and feeling: The clinical ontology of emotion. *Bioethics* 17 (1): 59–68.

Rogoff, Natalie. 1957. The decision to study medicine. In *The student-physician: Introductory studies in the sociology of medical education*, ed. Robert K. Merton, George G. Reader, and Patricia L. Kendall, 109–29. Cambridge, MA: Harvard University Press.

Rose, Nikolas, and Carlos Novas. 2005. Biological citizenship. In *Global assemblages: Technology, politics, and ethics as anthropological problems*, ed. Aihwa Ong and Stephen J. Collier, 439–63. Malden, MA: Blackwell.

Ross, Kenneth R. 1997. Crisis and identity—Presbyterian ecclesiology in southern Malawi, 1891–1993. *Missionalia* 25 (3): 381–97.

Rothman, David J. 1991. *Strangers at the bedside: A history of how law and bioethics transformed medical decision making*. New York: Basic Books.

Sapolsky, Robert M. 1991. Anecdotal evidence: Poverty's remains. *The Sciences* 31 (September–October): 8–10.

Schafer, Arthur. 2004. Biomedical conflicts of interest: A defence of the sequestration thesis—learning from the cases of Nancy Olivieri and David Healy. *Journal of Medical Ethics* 30:8–24.

Schaffer, Simon. 1994. *From physics to anthropology—and back again*. Prickly Pear pamphlet no. 3. Cambridge, UK: Prickly Pear Press.

Schensul, Jean J., Margaret D. LeCompte, Bonnie K. Nastasi, and Stephen P. Borgatti. 1999. *Enhanced ethnographic methods: Audiovisual techniques, focused group interviews, and elicitation techniques*. Walnut Creek, CA: AltaMira Press.

Scheper-Hughes, Nancy. 1990. Three propositions for a critically applied medical anthropology. *Social Science and Medicine* 30 (2): 189–97.

———. 1992. *Death without weeping: The violence of everyday life in Brazil*. Berkeley and Los Angeles: University of California Press.

Scher, Abby, and Phineas Baxandall. 2000. Excerpts from Joseph Stiglitz's speech to the World Bank, April 1999. *International Journal of Health Services* 30 (2): 253–56.

Schiebinger, Londa, ed. 2000a. *Feminism and the body*. Oxford, UK: Oxford University Press.

———. 2000b. Skeletons in the closet: The first illustrations of the female skeleton in eighteenth-century anatomy. In *Feminism and the body*, ed. Londa Schiebinger, 25–57. Oxford, UK: Oxford University Press.

Schoepf, Brooke G., Claude Schoepf, and Joyce V. Millen. 2000. Theoretical therapies, remote remedies: SAPs and the political ecology of poverty and health in Africa. In *Dying for growth: Global inequality and the health of the poor*, ed. Jim Yong Kim, Joyce V. Millen, Alec Irwin, and John Gershman, 90–125. Monroe, ME: Common Courage Press.

Schroeder, Steven A. 2002. Primary care at a crossroads. *Academic Medicine* 77 (8): 767–73.

Scott, James C. 1976. *The moral economy of the peasant: Rebellion and subsistence in Southeast Asia*. New Haven, CT: Yale University Press.

Self, Donnie J., Dawn E. Schrader, De Witt C. Baldwin Jr., and Fredric D. Wolinsky. 1991. A pilot study of the relationship of medical education and moral development. *Academic Medicine* 66 (10): 629.

Sen, Amartya. 2001. Economic progress and health. In *Poverty, inequality, and health: An international perspective*, ed. David Leon and Gill Walt, 333–45. Oxford, UK: Oxford University Press.

Shah, Sonia. 2006. *The body hunters: Testing new drugs on the world's poorest patients*. New York: New Press.

Shapin, Steven. 1993. Essay review: Personal development and intellectual biography: The case of Robert Boyle. *British Journal for the History of Science* 26:335–45.

Shapin, Steven, and Simon Schaffer. 1985. *Leviathan and the air-pump: Hobbes, Boyle, and the experimental life*. Princeton, NJ: Princeton University Press.

Shapiro, Martin. 1987. *Getting doctored: Critical reflections on becoming a physician*. Santa Cruz, CA: New Society Publishers.

Shaywitz, D. A., and D. A. Ausiello. 2002. Global health: A chance for Western physicians to give—and receive. *American Journal of Medicine* 113 (4): 354–57.

Shem, Samuel. 1978. *The house of God*. New York: Putnam.

Shepperson, George, and Thomas Price. 1987. *Independent African: John Chilembwe and the Nyasaland rising of 1915*. Edinburgh: University Press.

Shiva, Vandana. 1988. Reductionist science as epistemological violence. In *Science, hegemony and violence: A requiem for modernity*, ed. Ashis Nandy, 232–56. Delhi: Oxford University Press.

Simonds, Wendy, Barbara Katz Rothman, and Bari Meltzer Norman. 2007. *Laboring on: Birth in transition in the United States*. New York: Routledge.

Sinclair, Simon. 1997. *Making doctors: An institutional apprenticeship*. Oxford, UK: Berg Publishers.

Sindima, Harvey J. 2002. *Malawi's first republic: An economic and political analysis*. Lanham, MD: University Press of America.

Singer, Merrill, Freddie Valentín, Hans Baer, and Zhongke Jia. 1998. Why does Juan García have a drinking problem? The perspective of critical medical anthropology. *Medical Anthropology* 14 (1): 77–108.

Small, Parker A. 2000. Another view on teaching social responsibility (letter), *Academic Medicine* 75 (10): 957.

Smith, Dorothy E. 1990. *The conceptual practices of power: A feminist sociology of knowledge*. Boston: Northeastern University Press.

Smith, Richard. 2001. Why are doctors so unhappy? There are probably many causes, some of them deep. *BMJ: British Medical Journal* 322:1073–74.

Snow, C. P. 1964. *The two cultures and a second look*. Cambridge, UK: Cambridge University Press.

Somers, Margaret R. 1994. The narrative constitution of identity: A relational and network approach. *Theory and Society* 23 (5): 605–49.

Somerville, Siobhan. 1997. Scientific racism and the invention of the homosexual body.

In *The gender/sexuality reader: Culture, history, political economy*, ed. Roger N. Lancaster and Micaela di Leonardo, 37–52. New York: Routledge.

Spring, Anita. 1978. Epidemiology of spirit possession among the Luvale of Zambia. In *Women in ritual and symbolic roles*, ed. Judith Hoch-Smith and Anita Spring, 165–90. London: Plenum Press.

Stacey, Judith. 1988. Can there be a feminist ethnography? *Women's Studies International Forum* 11 (1): 21–27.

Stark, Evan. 1982. Doctors in spite of themselves: The limits of radical health criticism. *International Journal of Health Services* 12 (3): 419–57.

Starn, Orin. 1992. Missing the revolution: Anthropologists and the war in Peru. In *Rereading cultural anthropology*, ed. George E. Marcus, 152–80. Durham, NC: Duke University Press.

Starr, Paul. 1982. *The social transformation of American medicine*. New York: Basic Books.

Stata Corporation. 2001. STATA 7.0. College Station, TX: Stata Corporation.

Stein, Howard F. 1990. *American medicine as culture*. With ed. assistance of Margaret A. Stein. Boulder: Westview Press.

Stern, Marilyn, Norman Sloan, and Christina Komm. 1993. Medical students' differential use of coping strategies as a function of stressor type, year of training, and gender. *Behavioral Medicine* 18 (4): 173–80.

Strauss, Anselm, and Juliet Corbin. 1998. *Basics of qualitative research: Techniques and procedures for developing grounded theory*. 2nd ed. Thousand Oaks, CA: Sage Publications.

Takakuwa, Kevin M., Nick Rubashkin, and Karen E. Herzig, eds. 2004. *What I learned in medical school: Personal stories of young doctors*. Berkeley and Los Angeles: University of California Press.

Tan, C. M. 1990. Academic standards and changing patterns of medical school admissions in Malaysia: A Malaysian study. *Medical Education* 24 (4): 319–27.

Taussig, Michael T. 1980. Reification and the consciousness of the patient. *Social Science and Medicine* 14B (1): 3–13.

Taylor, Carl E. 1994. International experience and idealism in medical education. *Academic Medicine* 69 (8): 631–34.

Taylor, Janelle S. 2003. Confronting "culture" in medicine's "culture of no culture." *Academic Medicine* 78 (6): 555–59.

Terry, Jennifer. 1999. *An American obsession: Science, medicine, and homosexuality in modern society*. Chicago: University of Chicago Press.

Thompson, E. P. 1971. The moral economy of the English crowd in the 18th century. *Past & Present* 50:76–136.

Traweek, Sharon. 1988. *Beamtimes and lifetimes: The world of high energy physicists*. Cambridge, MA: Harvard University Press.

Turner, Leigh. 2005. From the local to the global: Bioethics and the concept of culture. *Journal of Medicine and Philosophy* 30:305–20.

Turner, Victor Witter. 1968. *The drums of affliction: A study of religious processes among the Ndembu of Zambia*. Oxford, UK: Clarendon Press and The International African Institute.

Turshen, Meredeth. 1999. *Privatizing health services in Africa*. Piscataway, NJ: Rutgers University Press.

Ugalde, Antonio, and S. Ogoh Alubo. 1994. Introduction. In *Physicians and health care in the Third World*, ed. Antonio Ugalde and S. Ogoh Alubo, viii–ix. Williamsburg, VA: Department of Anthropology, College of William and Mary.

UNAIDS (Joint United Nations Programme on HIV/AIDS). 2003. Report on the global HIV/AIDS epidemic 2002. http://data.unaids.org/pub/Report/2002/brglobal_aids _report_en_pdf_red_en.pdf.

UNDP (United Nations Development Program). 2000. *Human development report 2000. Human rights and human development*. New York: Oxford University Press for the United Nations Development Program.

———. 2003. *Human development report 2003. Millennium development goals: A compact among nations to end human poverty*. New York: Oxford University Press for the United Nations Development Program.

———. 2007. *Human development report 2007/2008. Fighting climate change: Human solidarity in a divided world*. New York: Palgrave Macmillan for the United Nations Development Program.

van Binsbergen, Wim. 1991. Becoming a *sangoma*: Religious anthropological field-work in Francistown, Botswana. *Journal of Religion in Africa* 21 (4): 309–44.

van der Geest, Sjaak. 1997. Is there a role for traditional medicine in basic health services in Africa? A plea for a community perspective. *Tropical Medicine and International Health* 2 (9): 903–11.

van Dijk, Rijk. 1992. *Young Malawian puritans: Young born-again preachers in a present-day African urban environment*. Utrecht, Netherlands: ISOR.

———. 1995. Fundamentalism and its moral geography in Malawi: The representation of the diasporic and the diabolical. *Critique of Anthropology* 15 (2): 171–91.

———. 2006. Transnational images of Pentecostal healing: Comparative examples from Malawi and Botswana. In *Borders and healers: Brokering therapeutic resources in southeast Africa*, ed. Tracy J. Luedke and Harry G. West, 101–24. Bloomington: Indiana University Press.

van Donge, Jan Kees. 1995. Kamuzu's legacy: The democratization of Malawi: Or, searching for the rules of the game in African politics. *African Affairs* 94 (375): 227–57.

van Niekerk, J. P. DeV. 1999. Missions of a medical school: An African perspective. *Academic Medicine* 74 (8 supplement): S38–S44.

Vaughan, Megan. 1991. *Curing their ills: Colonial power and African illness*. Oxford, UK: Polity Press.

———. 1992. Syphilis in colonial east and central Africa: The social construction of an epidemic. In *Epidemics and ideas: Essays on the historical perception of pestilence*, ed. Terence Ranger and Paul Slack, 269–302. Cambridge, UK: Cambridge University Press.

———. 1994. Healing and curing: Issues in the social history and anthropology of medicine in Africa. *Social History of Medicine* 7 (2): 283–95.

Visweswaran, Kamala. 1994. *Fictions of feminist ethnography*. Minneapolis: University of Minnesota Press.

Wacquant, Loïc. 2003. Pugilistic incarnation: Skill, pain, and desire in the making of professional boxers. Presentation given at the 102nd Annual Meeting of the American Anthropological Association, Chicago.

Waitzkin, Howard. 1981. The social origins of illness: A neglected history. *International Journal of Health Services* 11 (1): 77–103.

Wall, L. Lewis. 1998. Dead mothers and injured wives: The social context of maternal morbidity and mortality among the Hausa of northern Nigeria. *Studies in Family Planning* 29 (4): 341–59.

Wasylenki, D., N. Byrne, and B. McRobb. 1997. The social contract challenge in medical education. *Medical Education* 31:250–58.

Wear, Delese, Julie M. Aultman, Joseph D. Varley, and Joseph Zarconi. 2006. Making fun of patients: Medical students' perceptions and use of derogatory and cynical humor in clinical settings. *Academic Medicine* 81 (5): 454–62.

Weiss, Brad. 2009. *Street dreams & hip hop barbershops: Global fantasy in urban Tanzania.* Bloomington: Indiana University Press.

Wendland, Claire L. 2004. Making doctors in Malawi: Local exigencies meet global identities in an African medical school. PhD diss. in anthropology, University of Massachusetts–Amherst.

———. 2007. The vanishing mother: Cesarean section and "evidence-based obstetrics." *Medical Anthropology Quarterly* 21 (2): 218–33.

———. 2008. Research, therapy, and bioethical hegemony: The controversy over perinatal AZT trials in Africa. *African Studies Review* 51 (3): 1–23.

West, Colin P., Mashele M. Huschka, Paul J. Novotny, Jeff A. Sloan, Joseph C. Kolars, Thomas M. Habermann, and Tait D. Shanafelt. 2006. Association of perceived medical errors with resident distress and empathy: A prospective longitudinal study. *JAMA: Journal of the American Medical Association* 296 (9): 1071–78.

West, Harry G. 2005. *Kupilikula: Governance and the invisible realm in Mozambique.* Chicago: University of Chicago Press.

West, Harry G., and Tracy J. Luedke. 2006. Introduction: Healing divides: Therapeutic border work in southeast Africa. In *Borders and healers: Brokering therapeutic resources in southeast Africa*, ed. Tracy J. Luedke and Harry G. West, 1–20. Bloomington: Indiana University Press.

White, Luise. 1997. Cars out of place: Vampires, technology, and labor in east and central Africa. In *Tensions of empire: Colonial cultures in a bourgeois world*, ed. Frederick Cooper and Ann Laura Stoler, 436–60. Berkeley and Los Angeles: University of California Press.

Williams, Raymond. 1977. *Marxism and literature.* Oxford, UK: Oxford University Press.

Williams, T. David. 1978. *Malawi: The politics of despair.* Ithaca, NY: Cornell University Press.

Willis, Roy G. 1999. *Some spirits heal, others only dance: A journey into human selfhood in an African village.* Oxford, UK, and New York: Berg.

World Bank. 1982. *Accelerated development in sub-Saharan Africa: An agenda for action.* Washington, DC: World Bank.

———. 1994. *Better health in Africa: Experience and lessons learned.* Washington, DC: World Bank.

―――. 1999. *Confronting AIDS: Public priorities in a global epidemic.* New York: Oxford University Press for the World Bank

―――. 2003. *World development indicators 2003.* http://www.worldbank.org/data.

World Health Organization. 2006. *The world health report 2006: Working together for health.* http://www.who.int/whr/2006/whr06_en.pdf.

Wright, Peter, and Andrew Treacher, eds. 1982. *The problem of medical knowledge: Examining the social construction of medicine.* Edinburgh: Edinburgh University Press.